Terminology of Communication Disorders
Speech-Language-Hearing

FIFTH EDITION

Terminology of Communication Disorders
Speech-Language-Hearing

FIFTH EDITION

Lucille Nicolosi, M.A.
Speech and Language Clinician (ret.)
Rockford, Illinois

Elizabeth Harryman, M.A.
Speech and Language Clinician
Private Practice
Ely, Minnesota

Janet Kresheck, Ph.D.
Professor (ret.)
Department of Communicative Disorders
Northern Illinois University
DeKalb, Illinois

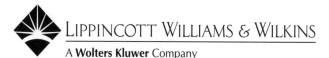
LIPPINCOTT WILLIAMS & WILKINS
A **Wolters Kluwer** Company
Philadelphia · Baltimore · New York · London
Buenos Aires · Hong Kong · Sydney · Tokyo

Senior Acquisitions Editor: Pamela Lappies
Managing Editor: Linda S. Napora
Marketing Manager: Mary Martin
Project Editor: Bill Cady
Designer: Doug Smock
Compositor: Maryland Composition
Printer: R. R. Donnelley

Copyright © 2004 Lippincott Williams & Wilkins

351 West Camden Street
Baltimore, MD 21201-2436 USA

530 Walnut Street
Philadelphia, PA 19106-3621 USA

Printed in China

First Edition, 1978   Third Edition, 1989
Second Edition, 1983   Fourth Edition, 1996

Library of Congress Cataloging-in-Publication Data

Nicolosi, Lucille.
    Terminology of communication disorders : speech-language-hearing / Lucille Nicolosi, Elizabeth Harryman, Janet Kresheck.—5th ed.
       p. ; cm.
      ISBN-13: 978-0-7817-4196-5
      ISBN-10: 0-7817-4196-3

    1. Communicative disorders—Dictionaries. I. Harryman, Elizabeth. II. Kresheck, Janet. III. Title.
    [DNLM: 1. Communication Disorders—Dictionary—English. 2. Speech-Language Pathology—Dictionary—English. WM 13 N651t 2004]
    RC423.N52 2004
    616.85′5′003—dc22

                                                                    2003060782

The publishers have made every effort to trace the copyright holders for borrowed material. If they have inadvertently overlooked any, they will be pleased to make the necessary arrangements at the first opportunity.

To purchase additional copies of this book, call our customer service department at **(800) 638-3030** or fax orders to **(301) 824-7390**. International customers should call **(301) 714-2324**.

Visit Lippincott Williams & Wilkins on the Internet: http://www.LWW.com. Lippincott Williams & Wilkins customer service representatives are available from 8:30 am to 6:00 pm, EST.

4 5 6 7 8 9 10

IN MEMORY

OF

MILDRED FREBURG BERRY, Ph.D.
(1902–1993)

A wife

A mother

A pioneer in Speech/Language Pathology

A scholar

A woman before her time

An advocate for children

A lecturer

An author

A woman who would not settle for mediocrity

Preface

The "Little Blue Book" has come of age. It has been almost 25 years since the first publication of *Terminology of Communication Disorders: Speech-Language-Hearing.* Little did we dream in 1978 that this "Little Blue Book" would be so widely accepted. May we reiterate? It is our sincere wish that we may have contributed, in some small measure, to the understanding of the Speech, Language, and Hearing professions.

The time has come, if we are to continue our original purpose, "to provide a comprehensive Dictionary/Sourcebook containing definitions of the terminology in the fields of Speech, Language, and Hearing" to update terms, add new terms, delete obsolete terms, and add new charts and illustrations. Thus a fifth edition.

Any reference work relies heavily on previous publications. We regret that it is not feasible to cite individually all of the many glossaries, compendia, references, texts, journals, and other sources from which our entries are derived. Our gratitude is extended to the authors, editors, and publishers of the anonymous publications for their indirect contributions.

We remain indebted to many people for encouraging and supporting this work over the past 24 + years. Their suggestions and contributions, especially their encouragement, have been invaluable and enabled us to "carry on." Our sincere thanks to our publishers, editors, consultants, families, and friends.

L. Nicolosi, E. Harryman, and J. Kresheck

Consultants

James R. Andrews, Ph.D.
Professor and Chairman (ret.)
Department of Communicative Disorders
Northern Illinois University
DeKalb, Illinois

Carl W. Asp, Ph.D.
Professor
Director, Verbotonal Research Lab
University of Tennessee
Knoxville, Tennessee

Harold Bauer, M.S.
School Psychologist
Rockford Public Schools
Rockford, Illinois

Richard J. Blank, M.D., FACR
Radiologist
Ely Bloomenson Community Hospital
Ely, Minnesota

Martha Burns, Ph.D.
Associate Professional Staff
Evanston Hospital
Evanston, Illinois
Adjunct Faculty
Department of Communication Sciences and Disorders
Northwestern Illinois University
Evanston, Illinois

Janet De Palma, M.A.
Clinical Audiologist
Northwestern Illinois Association
St. Charles, Illinois

Patricia Handley-Gabrielse, M.S.
Private Practice
Olympia, Washington

Joan Frost
Speech and Language Clinician
Private Practice
Rockford, Illinois

Denise Hove, Au.D.
Clinical Audiologist
Duluth Clinic
Virginia, Minnesota

Edna McManus, M.A.
Supervisor
Speech, Hearing, and Language
Louisiana State Department of Education
Baton Rouge, Louisiana

M. P. Montaleone, D.D.S.
Orthodontist
Rockford, Illinois

Cheryl Orr Nelson, M.A.
Diagnostic Consultant
DeKalb, Illinois

William M. Shearer, Ph.D.
Professor (ret.)
Department of Communicative Disorders
Northern Illinois University
DeKalb, Illinois

Eugene C. Sheeley, Ph.D.
Professor
Department of Communicative Disorders
University of Alabama
Tuscaloosa, Alabama

Betty J. Waters, M.A.
Supervisor, Clinical Practice (ret.)
Department of Communicative Disorders
Northern Illinois University
DeKalb, Illinois

J. David Williams, Ph.D.
Professor (ret.)
Department of Communicative Disorders
Northern Illinois University
DeKalb, Illinois

Roman Zerebny, M.A.
Clinical Audiologist
Northwestern Illinois Association
Rockford, Illinois

List of Figures

List of Tables

Contents

Explanatory Notes

Location of Entries

All of the words, terms, and abbreviations comprising the vocabulary are set in **boldface** and alphabetized in standard dictionary sequence.

Logic suggested that certain words or terms, particularly compounds, related by classification and/or a common term appear as indented alphabetized **boldface** subentries under that **boldface** main entry. Such subentries are cross referenced from their respective alphabetical location in the vocabulary. When the subentry is related to the main entry by a common term, that common term is abbreviated; *e.g.,* **amnesic a.,** under **aphasia.** When the subentry is related to the main entry by classification, it is spelled out; *e.g.,* **contiguity disorder** under **aphasia;** subentries under **audiogram configurations.** Occasionally, certain complex classifications have necessitated use of sub-subentries, which are additionally indented under the subentry with the **boldface** term spelled out and run in to the definition in a paragraph format; *e.g.,* **Cardiac evoked response audiometry (CERA)** under **electrophysiologic a.,** under **audiometry.**

Standardized abbreviations and some common abbreviations of clinical terms are included as **boldface** cross reference entries to the spelled-out terms which they represent and where they are also indicated in **boldface** in parentheses immediately following the **boldface** term.

Appendices containing developmental charts, tests, procedures, measures, etc. follow the vocabulary. Key material in the appendices is cross referenced from the vocabulary.

Cross References

Liberal use of cross references allows the reader to readily locate the desired term and its definition, as well as synonyms and related terms, from whatever approach is made into the vocabulary. When cross references are made to subentries related by a common term, that portion of the subentry which represents the main entry under which it is located is *italicized; e.g.,* "**auditory selective listening** Auditory figure-ground *discrimination.*" / "**adductor paralysis** See under laryngeal motor *paralysis.*" A number in parentheses at the end of a cross reference indicates the numbered definition to which it refers in a multiply defined entry; *e.g.,* "**articulation resonance** Articulation (2)."

(1) A cross reference from a term to its defined synonym consists solely of the name of that synonym; *e.g.,* "**After-glide** Off-glide." / "**acoustic gain control** Volume control." / "**auditory selective listening** Auditory figure ground *discrimination.*" Each synonym of a defined entry is given at the end of the definition and indicated by "Syn:"

(2) A cross reference for location of a defined term is indicated by "see" if it is a main entry or if it is defined as part of a main entry; *e.g.,* "**acute laryngitis** See laryngitis." "See under" is used to indicate that the defined term sought is a subentry; *e.g.,* "**acoustic reflex** See under reflex." / "**adductor paralysis** See under laryngeal motor *paralysis.*"

(3) A cross reference to related information is indicated by "see also" and is located at the end of a definition; *e.g.,* "**abstraction ladder**. . .See also concept(s)."

(4) The use of *cf.* at the end of a definition suggests that the reader compare the two entries; *e.g.,* "**achievement quotient**. . .*Cf.* intelligence quotient."

Defined Entry Format

Defined vocabulary entries are comprised of the defined term in **boldface** and its definition. Where appropriate, pronunciation and derivation have been included.

PRONUNCIATION is in parentheses and follows the **boldface** term after its abbreviation or symbol (if any). A simplified version of the International Phonetic Alphabet has been used for pronunciation of difficult words or words which are not pronounced as they are spelled.

a	hat, cap	k	kind, seek	TH	then, smooth
ā	age, face	l	land, coal	ů	full, put
ã	care, air	m	me, am	u	rule, move
ä	father, far	n	no, in	v	very, save
b	bad, rob	ŋ	ring, bang	w	will, woman
ch	child, much	o	hot, rock	y	young, yet
d	did, red	ō	open, go	z	zero, breeze
e	let, best	ô	order, all	zh	measure, seizure
ē	equal, see	oi	oil, voice	ə	represents:
ėr	term, learn	ou	house, out		a in about
f	fat, if	p	paper, cup		e in taken
g	go, bag	r	run, try		i in pencil
h	he, how	s	say, yes		o in lemon
i	it, pin	sh	she, rush		u in circus
ī	ice, five	t	tell, it		
j	jam, enjoy	th	thin, both		

DERIVATION is in brackets and follows the **boldface** term's pronunciation, if given, and precedes its definition. The bracketed material includes the abbreviation indicating the language from which the word is derived, the word from which the term is derived in *italics,* and the English translation. When the defined entry has the same or a similar spelling and/or meaning as that of the language from which it is derived, the information which would be understood or redundant is omitted from the derivation. Where a combining form, prefix, or suffix has been included in the vocabulary as a defined entry, its definition is not repeated in the derivations of other terms. For terms of Greek and/or Latin origin, that part of speech most closely resembling the English has been used.

ABBREVIATIONS

A.S.	Anglo-Saxon	L.	Latin
c.	L. *circa,* around	obs.	obsolete
cf.	L. *confer,* compare	pl.	plural
dim.	diminutive	priv.	privative
Eng.	English	q.v.	L. *quod vide,* which see
e.g.	L. *exempli gratia,* for example	sing.	singular
Fr.	French	Sp.	Spanish
fr.	from	thr.	through
G.	Greek	*	birth year when death year not given
Ger.	German		
i.e.	L. *id est,* that is	†	death year when birth year not given
It.	Italian		

EPONYMS have been supplied with available biographical data in brackets; *e.g.,* first initial, nationality, specialty, and birth and/or death years.

DEFINITIONS are comprised of the definition *per se* of the term, any synonym(s), and any cross references, and are separated from the **boldface** term and its abbreviation, pronunciation, or derivation if given. Definitions are numbered in **boldface** when there is more than one distinct meaning or use; the most inclusive and/or most commonly used definition usually is presented first, followed by the more restricted and/or less commonly used meaning(s). Definitions restricted to specialized areas are preceded by labels, such as "In stuttering,. . ." Whenever a definition represents that of a particular proponent or school of thought, each is identified in brackets at the end of the respective definition.

SYNONYMS are given after the definition, preceding any cross reference, and are indicated by "Syn:" Each synonym is also listed as a **boldface** cross reference entry in the vocabulary.

CROSS REFERENCES follow the synonym(s) at the end of the definition.

Phonemes of American Speech

Vowels

Front vowels		Back vowels	
Symbol	Key	Symbol	Key
[i]	heed [hid]	[u]	who'd [hud]
[ɪ]	hid [hɪd]	[ʊ]	hood [hʊd]
[e]	hayed [hed]	[o]	hoed [hod]
[ɛ]	head [hɛd]	[ɔ]	hawed [hɔd]
[æ]	had [hæd]	[ɑ]	hod [hɑd]

Central vowels		Diphthongs	
[ɝ–ɜ]*	hurt [hɝt]	[aɪ]	file [faɪl]
[ʌ]	hut [hʌt]	[aʊ]	fowl [faʊl]
[ɚ–ə]*	under [ʌndɚ]	[ɔɪ]	foil [fɔɪl]
[ə]	about [əbaʊt]	[ju]	fuel [fjul]

Consonants

[p]	pen [pɛn]	[f]	few [fju]
[b]	Ben [bɛn]	[v]	view [vju]
[t]	ten [tɛn]	[θ]	thigh [θaɪ]
[d]	den [dɛn]	[ð]	thy [ðaɪ]
[k]	Kay [ke]	[h]	hay [he]
[g]	gay [ge]	[s]	say [se]
[tʃ]	chew [tʃu]	[ʃ]	shay [ʃe]
[dʒ]	Jew [dʒu]	[z]	bays [bez]
		[ʒ]	beige [beʒ]
[m]	some [sʌm]	[w]	way [we]
[n]	sun [sʌn]	[hw]	whey [hwe]
[ŋ]	sung [sʌŋ]	[j]	yea [je]
[l]	lay [le]	[r]	ray [re]

* [ɝ] and [ɚ] are the "r-colored" vowels. [ɜ] and [ə] are the pronunciations typical of r vowels in Eastern, Southern, and English speech.

α First letter of the Greek alphabet, alpha.

A Ampere.

a- Privative prefix denoting without, not; equivalent of Latin *in-* and English *un-*.

AAC Augmentative and Alternative Communication.

AAMD American Association on Mental Deficiency.

ab- [L. *ab*, from] Prefix denoting off, away from.

abdomen (ab′də-mən) [L.] The belly, the part of the trunk located between the thorax and the pelvis.

abdominal (ab-dom′i-nəl) Relating to the abdomen.

abdominal-diaphragmatic respiration See under respiration.

abducens nerve See *Cranial Nerves* table, under cranial nerves.

abducent (ab-du′sent) Abducting, drawing away.

abduction (ab-dək′shən) [L. *abductio*] A drawing away from the midline of the body or a moving away from each other, *e.g.*, the two vocal folds; opposite of adduction.

abductor (ab-dək′tėr) That which performs abduction, said of various muscles.

abductor paralysis See under laryngeal motor *paralysis*.

aberrant (ab-ėr′ənt) [L. *aberrans*] Deviating from the normal, used primarily in terms of behavior.

ABG Air-bone gap.

ABI Acquired brain injury.

ability (ə-bil′i-tē) [L. *habilitas*, aptitude] The actual power to perform a physical or mental act, either before or after training.

ability test A test designed to measure maximum performance that reveals the present level of functioning, *e.g.*, a test of motor ability.

ABLB Alternate Binaural Loudness Balance.

abnormal (ab-nôr′məl) [L. *ab*, from + *norma*, rule] Diverging from a recognized standard, usually referring to a pathologic condition.

abnormal psychology See under psychology.

ABR Auditory brainstem response.

abrupt topic shift See under topic shift.

absolute construction See under construction.

absolute quantity See under objective *quantity*.

absolute threshold See under threshold.

absorption (ab-sôrp′shən) [L. *absorptio*] **1.** Maintenance of a high level of interest in one object or situation, with little or no attention given to other stimuli. **2.** Penetration of sound energy through material of an obstacle when the impedance of the obstacle is not infinite.

abstraction (ab-strak′shən) **1.** The ability to understand relationships and to react, not only to concrete objects but also to concepts and symbols. **2.** The process of selecting or isolating a certain aspect from a concrete whole.

abstraction ladder A theory which maintains that learning stems from sensations (awareness of a stimulus) and progresses through the levels of perception, imagery, symbolism, and conceptualization; *e.g.*, a child hears a noise (sensation), recognizes the noise as from an animal (perception), envisions the noise to represent the animal as a pig based on past experiences (imagery), sees the pig in his mind and associates it as a farm animal (symbolism), and generalizes to sounds of other farm animals (conceptualization). Symbolism and conceptualization are often difficult for individuals

1

with severe hearing or intellectual impairments. See also concept.

abulia (ə-bu′lē-ə) [a- + G. *boulē*, will] Procrastination in performing certain acts or voluntary movements; may be observed in individuals with severe emotional disorders.

abusive vocal behavior Strenuous or excessive use of the vocal folds, such as shouting, screaming, and throat clearing.

abutting consonants See under consonant.

AC Air conduction; alternating current.

acalculia (ə-kal-kyu′lē-ə) [a- + L. *calculo*, to add] Inability to use mathematical symbols, often as a result of brain injury; in a less severe form, often referred to as dyscalculia.

acatamathesia (ə-kat-ə-mə-thē′zē-ə -zhə) [a + G. *katamathēsis*, thorough understanding] Difficulty in comprehending perceived objects or situations; the ability to understand the meaning of speech may be especially affected. See also aphasia.

acataphasia (ə-kat-ə-fā′zē-ə, -zhə) [a- + G. *kataphasis*, affirmation] 1. Disability characterized by difficulties with phrasing and sentence structure of speech. 2. Inability to express ideas logically.

accelerated speech See under speech.

accelerometer (ak′sel-ėr-om′ə-tėr) 1. Instrument designed to measure and record changes in speed. 2. A device that produces a measurement of units of force; the vibrations are then transduced and delivered to a sound level meter for measurement in dB of sound pressure level.

accent (ak′sent) 1. Prominence, stress, or increased sonority assigned to one syllable of a word or group of words over adjoining syllables. 2. Phonetic traits of an individual's native language carried over into a second, foreign language. 3. Diacritical mark indicating stress.

acceptance approach In stuttering, a hypothesis that although stutterers may not have a choice as to whether they stutter, they do have a choice as to how they stutter.

accessory nerve See *Cranial Nerves* table, under cranial nerves.

accommodation (ə-kom′-ə-dā′shŭn) [L. *accomodo*, to adapt] 1. In cognitive development, creation of new ideas and/or the modification of old ideas resulting in a change in the development of cognitive structures. 2. Making facilities and programs accessible to and usable by persons with disabilities through appropriate modifications.

accusative case See under case.

achievement (ə-chēv′mənt) 1. Level of accomplishment attained in general or specific area. 2. Performance on a standardized series of tests. 3. Success in bringing effort to the desired goal.

achievement age Level of accomplishment attained in a general or specific area and described in an age equivalent.

achievement quotient (AQ) Ratio of the achievement to the chronological age of the individual tested. *Cf.* intelligence quotient.

acouesthesia (a-kyu′es-thē′zē-ə, -zhə) [G. *akouein*, to hear + *aisthēsis*, sensation] Acute sense of hearing.

acoupedic method Acoustic method. See under aural rehabilitation.

acoupedics (a-kyu-pē′diks) [G. *akouein*, to hear + *pais (paid-)*, child] Method of auditory training which emphasizes the utilization of residual hearing at an early age in hearing-impaired infants and children. See also aural rehabilitation.

acoustic, acoustical (ə-ku′stik, ə-ku′ sti-kəl) Denoting the perception of sounds, as opposed to their production; *e.g.*, acoustic phonetics.

acoustic admittance The ease with which sound energy flows through a system.

acoustic agnosia See under agnosia.

acoustic-amnestic aphasia See under aphasia.

acoustic analysis Measurement of the quality of phonation in terms of frequency, intensity, and time.

acoustic contralateral reflex See under reflex.

acoustic energy See under energy.

acoustic feedback See under feedback.

acoustic gain See under gain.

acoustic gain control Volume control.

acoustic immittance measurement 1. Evaluation of middle ear function by measuring the flow of sound energy into the ear (admittance) and the resistance to that flow (impedance); used in diagnosis of middle ear pathology, lesions in cranial nerve VII or VIII, and eustachian tube dysfunction; requires little patient cooperation and can be used with young children, or mentally or physically handicapped individuals. **2**. The ease of, or opposition to, sound flow through a system—refers to acoustic impedance or acoustic admittance or both.

acoustic impedance Physical measurement, requiring no participation by the client, in which a test tone is introduced into the external ear canal, and the sound that is reflected by the tympanic membrane is measured; the amount reflected depends on the mass, the stiffness, and the acoustic resistance of the air.

Three measurements utilized are **static acoustic impedance,** the point of maximum compliance, as compared with the point of least compliance; **acoustic reflex,** the relative contraction of the middle ear muscles; and **tympanometry,** which reveals the resistance to the flow of acoustical energy at the tympanic membrane during various pressure changes. See also tympanogram classifications; impedance tests in *Audiometric Tests and Procedures* in appendices.

acoustic ipsilateral reflex See under reflex.

acoustic method See under aural rehabilitation.

acoustic nerve See *Cranial Nerves* table, under cranial nerves.

acoustic neurilemoma See under neurilemoma.

acousticopalpebral reflex See under reflex, auropalpebral.

acoustic phonetics See under phonetics.

acoustic radiation Air-conducted sound leakage from a bone vibrator or other sound stimulus.

acoustic reflex See under reflex. See also under acoustic impedance.

acoustic reflex amplitude See under amplitude.

acoustic reflex decay Decrease in acoustic reflex amplitude with continuous stimulation; clinically significant decay is a decrement of more than 50% of initial amplitude within 10 seconds of stimulus onset.

acoustic reflex latency Time interval between the presentation of an acoustic stimulus and some index of acoustic reflex activity, usually detected as a change in acoustic immittance of the middle ear at the eardrum; criteria for the index of acoustic reflex activity may vary.

acoustic reflex pattern Collection of acoustic findings for crossed (contralateral) and uncrossed (ipsilateral) measurement conditions for the right and left ears. Analysis of patterns, in combination with other audiometric data, differentiates among abnormalities affecting the afferent (cochlea and cranial nerve VIII), brainstem (caudal pons), and efferent (cranial nerve VII and middle ear) portions of the acoustic reflex arc.

acoustic reflex threshold See under threshold.

acoustics (ə-ku′stiks) [G. *akoustikos*, relating to hearing] Study of the science of sound; includes origin, transmission, modification, and effects of vibrations.

acoustic spectrum 1. Sound heard by the human ear, in contrast to sound that might be recorded only by various measuring instruments; it is an analysis of the frequencies that can be heard in a given sound together with the relative sound pressure of each frequency. **2.** A plot of the energy in each of the frequencies present in a complex tone.

acoustic stapedial reflex See under reflex.

acquired (ə-kwī'ėrd) [L. *acquiro*, to obtain] That which appears after birth as a result of injury, disease, or learning; not congenital.

acquired brain injury Traumatic brain injury.

acrolect (ak'rō-lekt) [G. *akros*, extreme + *(dia) lekt (os)*, language] Any dialect that closely resembles the standard usage of a language; *e.g.*, in Black English, "I be going." = "I am going."

acromegaly (ak'rō-meg'ə-lē) [G. *akros*, extreme + *megas*, large] Overdevelopment of bones and connective tissue; specifically of the head, hands, and feet.

acronym (ak'rō-nim) [G. *akros*, extreme + *-onym*, comb. form of *onoma*, name] Word formed from the initial letters or syllables of successive parts of a compound term; *e.g.*, ASHA for American Speech-Language-Hearing Association.

action-locative See under semantic relations.

action-object See under semantic relations.

action potential See under potential.

active bilingualism See under bilingualism.

active filter See under filter.

active voice See under voice.

acuity (ə-kyu'i-tē) [L. *acutus*, sharpen] Sharpness, clearness, or distinctness; ability to respond to sensory data of low intensity, duration, or extent.
> **auditory a. 1.** Sensitivity of the human ear to auditory stimuli. **2.** Sharpness, clearness, or distinctness with which one is able to hear sound.
> **visual a.** Acuteness of vision, the relative ability of the eye to resolve detail.

acute (ə-kyut') [L. *acutus*, sharpen] Intense and of short duration, usually said of a disease. *Cf.* chronic.

acute laryngitis See under laryngitis.

acute phoneme See under phoneme.

ad- [L. *ad*, to] Prefix denoting to, toward.

Adam's apple [Adam, in *Genesis*] Colloquialism for the larynx; specifically, the prominence on the anterior portion of the neck formed by the thyroid cartilage of the larynx.

adaptation (ə-dap'shən) [L. *adaptatus*, adjusting] **1.** Process of effectively adjusting to changing environments. **2.** In stuttering, a temporary reduction in the frequency or severity of behaviors resulting from repeated productions of the same or highly similar material.

adaptation effect See under stuttering.

adaptive behavior See under behavior.

ADD Attention deficit disorder.

addition See under articulation disorder.

adduction (ad-dək'shən) [L. *adduco*, to bring to] A drawing toward the midline of the body or a bringing toward each other, *e.g.*, the two vocal folds; opposite of abduction.

adductor (ad-dək'tėr) That which performs adduction, said of a muscle.

adductor paralysis See under laryngeal motor *paralysis*.

adenoid (ad'ə-noid) [G. *adēn*, gland + *eidos*, appearance] Lymphoid tissue located in the posterior wall of the nasopharynx; when inflamed, it is referred to as adenoids. Syn: pharyngeal tonsil.

adenoidectomy (ad'ə-noi-dek'tə-mē) [adenoid + G. *ektomē*, excision] Surgical removal of the pharyngeal tonsils. See also tonsillectomy.
> **lateral a.** Removal of the sides (external boundary) of the adenoids, leaving the midline bulk intact. Syn: lateral trim of the adenoid.

adhesive otitis media See under otitis.

adiadochokinesis (ə-dī'ə-dō-kō-ki-nē'-sis) [a- + G. *diadochos*, successive + *kinēsis*, movement] In speech, inability to perform rapid repetitive alternating movements of the articulators; the opposite of diadochokinesis. See also dysdiadochokinesia.

adjective See under parts of speech.

admittance (ad-mit′əns) Ease of flow of energy transmission through a system.

Adolescent Language Screening Test See *Language Tests and Procedures* in appendices.

adolescent voice See under voice.

adventitious (ad-ven-tish′əs) [L. *adventicius*, coming from abroad (foreign)] Not innate; having occurred after birth; acquired.

adventitious deafness See under deafness.

adverb See under parts of speech.

AERA Average evoked response audiometry.

aerodynamic analysis In speech, measurement of airflow and pressure below, at, and above the glottis.

aerodynamics (ār′ō-dī-nam′iks) [G. *aēr*, air + *dynamis*, force] Study of air and other gases in motion, forces setting them in motion, and results of such motion.

aerophagia (ār-ō-fā′jē-ə) [G. *aēr*, air + *phagein*, to eat] Swallowing of air, usually followed by belching; used in alaryngeal speech.

affect (a′fekt) [L. *affectus*, state of mind] Feeling, emotion, mood, and temperament associated with a thought.

affective function Listener's observable reactions to that said by the speaker.

afferent (af′ėr-ənt) [L. *afferens*, bringing to] Coming in, as opposed to efferent, going out; may be sensory or nonsensory.

afferent feedback Proprioceptive *feedback*.

afferent (kinesthetic) motor aphasia See under aphasia.

afferent nerve See under nerve.

affix (a′fiks) In linguistics, a bound morpheme attached either to the beginning or end of a base word; can be a prefix (*dis*-engage) or a suffix (engag*ed*).

affricate or **affricative** See under consonant, manner of formation.

affrication See under substitution, phonological processes.

after-glide Off-glide.

agenesis (ə-jen′ə-sis) [a- + G. *genesis*, production] Absence, failure of formation, or imperfect development of a body part.

agenitive See under parts of speech.

agent (ā′jənt) [L. *agens*, fr. *ago*, to put in motion] That which initiates or is responsible for an action or an effect.

agent-action See under semantic relations.

agent-object See under semantic relations.

agitolalia (aj′i-tō-lā′lē-ə) [L. *agito*, to hurry + G. *lalia*, talking] Excessive rate of speech in which sounds, words, or parts of words are omitted or distorted.

aglossia (ə-glo′sē-ə) [a- + G. *glōssa*, tongue] Partial or complete absence of the tongue; partial absence of the tongue is often referred to as dysglossia.

agnathia (ag-nā′thē-ə) [a- + G. *gnathos*, jaw] Partial or complete absence of the mandible.

agnosia (ag-nō′sē-ə, -shə) [a- + G. *gnōsis*, knowledge] Inability to recognize or attach meaning to sensory information, although the physiologic receptor mechanism is intact; usually associated with a central nervous system disorder.

    acoustic a. Disturbance of discriminative hearing, *i.e.*, defective analysis of the phonemic (speech-sound) system of a language; errors for speech-sound discrimination increase as differences between sounds decrease; *e.g.*, /t/, /d/.

    auditory a. 1. Impairment of the ability to comprehend auditory stimuli. **2.** Disturbance in the interpretation of language and/or nonlanguage sounds. Syn: auditory imperception;

dysacusis. See also Wernicke's *aphasia*.

auditory verbal a. Inability to understand spoken presentations. See also pure word deafness under pure *aphasia(s)*.

environmental a. Inability to recognize and navigate in familiar environments; often associated with nondominant hemisphere lesions.

finger a. Loss of finger recognition; one of five classic features of Gerstmann syndrome.

phonagnosia a. An inability to recognize familiar voices.

prosopagnosia a. An inability to recognize familiar faces; often associated with right hemisphere occipital lobe lesions.

simultagnosia a. An inability to visually synthesize components of a visual gestalt; often associated with nondominant hemisphere lesions.

tactile a. Impairment of the ability to differentiate objects through the sense of touch.

visual or **visual verbal a. 1.** Difficulty in the ability to differentiate visual stimuli. **2.** Inability to comprehend printed words. See also alexia. **3.** An inability to recognize or decode the written word. See also pure word blindness under pure *aphasia(s)*.

agonist (ag′ə-nist) [G. *agōn*, contest] A muscle in a state of contraction, with reference to its opposing muscle (antagonist); *e.g.*, in the closing of the glottis, the transverse arytenoid muscle is the agonist and the posterior cricoarytenoid muscle is the antagonist.

agrammalogia or **agrammatalogia** (ə-gram-ə-lō′jē-ə, ə-gram′ə-tə-lō′jē-ə) [G. *agrammatos*, unlearned + *ogos*, treatise] Agrammatism.

agrammaticia (ə-gram′ə-tə-sē′ə) [G. *agrammatos*, unlearned] Agrammatism.

agrammatism (ə-gram′ə-tizm) [G. *agrammatos*, unlearned] Impairment of the ability to produce words in their cor-

rect sequence; difficulty with grammar and syntax. Syn: agrammalogia, agrammatalogia, agrammaticia. See also syntactic *aphasia*.

agraphia (ə-gra′fē-ə) [a- + G. *graphō*, to write] Disorder of writing which may result from a central nervous system lesion or from lack of muscular coordination; in a less severe form, often referred to as dysgraphia.

pure a. See under pure *aphasia(s)*.

aided augmentative communication See under augmentative communication.

air-blade sound Friction sound emitted through an opening that is wide horizontally and narrow vertically; *e.g.*, /f/. See also consonant, manner of formation.

air-bone gap (ABG) Difference between a bone-conduction hearing threshold and an air-conduction hearing threshold for a given frequency in the same ear, as shown on an audiogram; it denotes conductive pathology when the difference averages 10 or more dB. See figure.

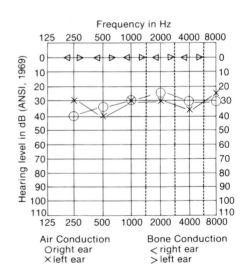

Air-Bone Gap

air conduction (AC) 1. See under conduction. **2.** See under pure-tone *audiometry*.

air-conduction hearing aid See under hearing aid.

air-conduction receiver See under receiver.

airflow management In stuttering, a clinical approach wherein the stutterer attempts to integrate a long, relaxed passive sigh with the slow initiation of the first syllable of a word in order to maintain airflow by reducing tension and pressure within the vocal tract.

air wastage Silent exhalation before or after phonation; may be associated with speaking with residual air.

ala, pl. **alae** (ā′lə, ā′lē) [L. wing] Any winglike or expanded structure.

alalia (ə-lā′lē-ə) [a- + G. *lalia*, talking] Inability to speak, characterized by complete absence of meaningful articulated speech. See also dyslalia.

alar (ālär) Denoting a winglike or expanded structure.

alar flutter Fluttering movement of the nasal alae, as observed in nasal respiration.

alaryngeal (ā-lə-rin′jē-əl, -jəl) Without a larynx.

alaryngeal speech. See under speech.

Albrecht syndrome [K. Albrecht, Ger. anatomist, 1851–1894] Heritable progressive high tone hearing loss developing in childhood, with increasing impairment suggestive of an increased rate of presbycusis.

alexia (ə-lek′sē-ə) [a- + G. *lexis*, word or phrase] Inability to read; may be the result of neurologic impairment; in a less severe form, often referred to as dyslexia. Syn: word blindness.

    auditory a. Difficulty in distinguishing similarities and differences in sounds, perceiving a sound within a word, and synthesizing sounds into words and dividing them into syllables; an individual so afflicted cannot learn to read via an alphabetic or phonic approach.

    pure a. Pure word blindness.

    visual a. Inability to differentiate, interpret, or remember printed words.

See also visual or visual verbal *agnosia*.

allergy (al′ėr-jē) [G. *allos*, other + *ergon*, work] Abnormal and individual hypersensitivity to substances that are ordinarily harmless.

alliteration (ə-li-tėr-ā′shən) Repetition of the same consonant, especially an initial one, in several words within the same sentence or phrase; a common device in poetry and slogans; *e.g.*, sister Susie smiled sweetly.

allomorph (a′lə-môrf) [G. *allos*, other + *morphē*, form] One of two or more forms that a given morpheme has at different points in a language, while making the same difference in meaning and having the same meaning wherever they are used; *e.g.*, plurals (cat*s*, rose*s*, child*ren*) and tenses (bak*ed*, skat*ed*, smil*ed*).

allophone (a′lə-fōn) [G. *allos*, other + *phonē*, sound] **1.** Nondistinctive variant of a phoneme. The following are the basic criteria by which phonetically different sounds in a language are classified together: (a) phonetic similarity, (b) complementary distribution or free variation differences, (c) similarity in manner or place of articulation. For example, three distinct versions of /k/: unaspirated in s*k*i, front aspirated in *k*ey, back aspirated in *c*aw. **2.** Phonetic variation caused by a phoneme's position in a word.

allusion See under figure of speech.

alogia (ə-lō′jē-ə) [a- + G. *logos*, speech] Inability to speak due to central nervous system dysfunction; in a less severe form, often referred to as dyslogia. See also aphasia.

alphabet (al′fə-bet) [G. *alphabētos* (α + β)] Letters of a language arranged in their proper sequential order.

    American Manual A. Specific positions of the hands and fingers used to symbolize the different letters of the alphabet; supplements sign language in deaf communication. See

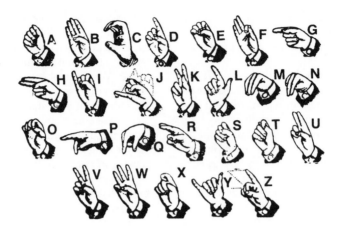

American Manual Alphabet

also finger spelling; unaided *augmentative communication*.

initial teaching a. Orthographic system, intended to teach the phonetic approach to reading, which consists of a modified alphabet that has a direct symbol for each phoneme; the individual is able to learn a specific sound for each symbol. It is used by some to teach speech and reading to hearing-impaired individuals.

International Phonetic A. (IPA) Alphabet designed to provide a consistent and universally understood system of symbols for writing the speech sounds of all languages; usually printed in a specific format.

International Standard Manual A. Alphabet used primarily in communicating with deaf-blind individuals; simple block letters are printed with the finger of the speaker on the palm of the listener.

alpha rhythm or **wave** See under electroencephalogram.

Alternate Binaural Loudness Balance (ABLB) See *Audiometric Tests and Procedures* in appendices.

alternate forms reliability coefficient See under reliability coefficient.

Alternate Monaural Loudness Balance

(AMLB) See *Audiometric Tests and Procedures* in appendices.

alternate motion rate (AMR) Alternating repetitive movements of the tongue, fingers, and toes.

alternating current (AC) See under current.

alternating pulse See under pulse.

alternative communication See augmentative and alternative communication.

alveolar (al-vē′ə-lėr) **1.** Denoting a small pit, cavity, or cell (alveolus), such as a tooth socket (alveolus dentalis). **2.** Relating to the alveolar process.

alveolar area See under consonant, place of articulation.

alveolar process or **ridge** Ridge on the mandible and maxilla that overlies the roots of the teeth; most commonly, that part directly behind the upper anterior teeth. See also consonant, place of articulation.

Alzheimer's disease [A. Alzheimer, Ger. neurologist, 1864–1915] Presenile dementia, usually beginning in middle or later life, characterized initially by slight defects in memory and behavior, with progressive mental deterioration marked by confusion, disorientation, agnosia, speech disturbances, and inability to carry out purposeful move-

PULMONIC CONSONANTS

	Bilabial	Labiodental	Dental	Alveolar	Postalveolar	Retroflex	Palatal	Velar	Uvular	Pharyngeal	Glottal
Plosive	p b			t d		ʈ ɖ	c ɟ	k g	q ɢ		ʔ
Nasal	m	ɱ		n		ɳ	ɲ	ŋ	N		
Trill	ʙ			r					R		
Tap or Flap				ɾ		ɽ					
Fricative	ɸ β	f v	θ ð	s z	ʃ ʒ	ʂ ʐ	ç ʝ	x ɣ	χ ʁ	ħ ʕ	h ɦ
Lateral fricative				ɬ ɮ							
Approximant		ʋ		ɹ		ɻ	j	ɰ			
Lateral Approximant				l		ɭ	ʎ	ʟ			

When symbols appear in pairs, the one to the right represents a voiced consonant. Shaded areas denote articulations judged impossible

CONSONANTS (NON-PULMONIC)

Clicks		Voiced Implosives		Ejectives	
ʘ	Bilabial	ɓ	Bilabial	'	Examples:
ǀ	Dental	ɗ	Dental/alveolar	p'	Bilabial
!	(Post)alveolar	ʄ	Palatal	t'	Dental/alveolar
ǂ	Palatoalveolar	ɠ	Velar	k'	Velar
ǁ	Alveolar lateral	ʛ	Uvular	s'	Alveolar fricative

Vowels	Front	Central	Back

OTHER SYMBOLS

ʍ	Voiceless labial-velar fricative	ɕ ʑ	Alveolo-palatal fricatives
w	Voiced labial-velar approximant	ɺ	Voiced alveolar lateral flap
ɥ	Voiced labial-palatal approximant	ɧ	Simultaneous ʃ and x
ʜ	Voiceless epiglottal fricative		
ʢ	Voiced epiglottal fricative	Affricates and double articulations can be represented by two symbols joined by a tie bar if necessary.	k͡p t͡s
ʡ	Epiglottal plosive		

SUPRASEGMENTALS

ˈ	Primary stress
ˌ	Secondary stress
	stress, e.g., foʊnəˈtɪʃən
ː	Long ... eː
ˑ	Half-long ... eˑ
̆	Extra-short ... ĕ
ǀ	Minor (foot) group
ǁ	Major (intonation) group
.	Syllabic break
	break, e.g., ɹi.ækt
‿	Linking (absence of a break)

DIACRITICS Diacritics may be placed above a symbol with a descender, e.g. ŋ̊

̥	Voiceless	n̥ d̥	̤	Breathy voiced	b̤ a̤	̪	Dental	t̪ d̪
̬	Voiced	s̬ t̬	̰	Creaky voiced	b̰ a̰	̺	Apical	t̺ d̺
ʰ	Aspirated	tʰ dʰ	̼	Linguolabial	t̼ d̼	̻	Laminal	t̻ d̻
̹	More Rounded	ɔ̹	ʷ	Labialized	tʷ dʷ	̃	Nasalized	ẽ
̜	Less Rounded	ɔ̜	ʲ	Palatalized	tʲ dʲ	ⁿ	Nasal release	dⁿ
̟	Advanced	u̟	ˠ	Velarized	tˠ dˠ	ˡ	Lateral release	dˡ
̠	Retracted	e̠	ˤ	Pharyngealized	tˤ dˤ	̚	No audible release	d̚
̈	Centralized	ë	~	Velarized or pharyngealized	ɫ			
̽	Mid-centralized	ĕ	̝	Raised	e̝ (ɹ̝ = voiced alveolar fricative)			
̩	Syllabic	n̩	̞	Lowered	e̞ (β̞ = voiced bilabial approximant)			
̯	Non-syllabic	e̯	̘	Advanced Tongue Root	e̘			
˞	Rhoticity	ɚ a˞	̙	Retracted Tongue Root	e̙			

TONES AND WORD ACCENTS

	Level			Contour	
e̋ or ˥	Extra high		ě or ˩˥	Rising	
é or ˦	High		ê or ˥˩	Falling	
ē or ˧	Mid		e᷄ or ˦˥	High-rising	
è or ˨	Low		e᷅ or ˩˨	Low-rising	
ȅ or ˩	Extra low		e᷈ or ˧˦˧	Rising-falling etc.	
↓	Downstep		↗	Global rise	
↑	Upstep		↘	Global fall	

International Phonetic Alphabet

Courtesy of the International Phonetic Association, c/o Department of Linguistics, University of Victoria, Victoria, British Columbia, Canada.

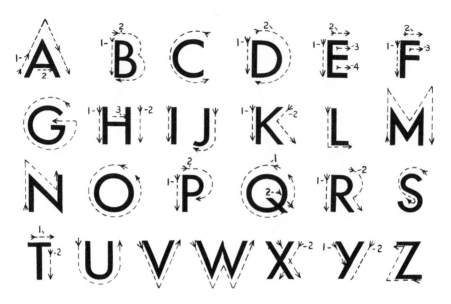

International Standard Manual Alphabet

Dotted lines, arrows, and numbers indicate proper direction, sequence, and number of strokes used in printing letters on the palm of the hand.

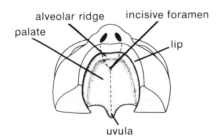

Alveolar Ridge

From Sadler, TW. *Langman's Medical Embryology,* 5th Ed. Baltimore: Williams & Wilkins, 1985.

ments; there is progressive neuronal degeneration and cerebral atrophy, with death occurring in 5 to 10 years.

AM Amplitude modulation.

ambidextrous (am-bi-dek'strəs) [L. *ambo*, both + *dexter*, right] Denoting the ability to use either hand with equal efficiency.

ambient noise See under noise.

ambiguous word See under word.

ambilaterality (am'bi-la-tèr-al'i-tē) [L. *ambo*, both + *latus*, side] Lack of marked dominance of ordinarily unilateralized structures; *e.g.*, hands, eyes.

ambisyllabic (am-bi-si-lab'ik) Intervocalic. See under consonant position.

ambivalence (am-biv'ə-ləns) [L. *ambo*, both + *valentia*, strength] Emotional attitude involving an individual's inability to determine a psychological direction; *e.g.*, love-hate, acceptance-rejection, denial-affirmation.

ambiversion (am-bi-vėr'zhən) [L. *ambo*, both + *verto*, to turn] Personality manifestation vacillating between introversion and extroversion.

amentia (ə-men'shē-ə) [L. madness] General term for mental impairment which may be a result of congenital or developmental factors.

American Association on Mental Deficiency (AAMD) Organization of specialists from many fields who are dedi-

CHARACTERISTICS OF COMMUNICATIVE BEHAVIOR IN EARLY, MIDDLE, AND LATE STAGES OF ALZHEIMER'S DISEASE

Stage	Phonology	Grammar	Words/Content	Usage
Early	Unimpaired	Generally correct	Omits meaningful word; reduced vocabulary; complains of problems thinking of the word	May have difficulty understanding humor or sarcasm
Middle	Unimpaired	Some sentence fragments and difficulty understanding complex sentences	Difficulty thinking of words within a category; impaired naming; reliance on automatisms	Rarely corrects a mistake; may be insensitive to conversational partners
Late	Generally correct; may have some phonological paraphasias	Sentence fragments and deviations are common; fails to comprehend grammatical forms	Marked anomia; jargon; bizarre content	Unable to produce a sequence of related ideas; inappropriate repetitive utterances

From Shadden, B. *Communication Behavior and Aging.* Baltimore: Williams & Wilkins, 1988.

cated to furthering the cause of the mentally retarded.

American Indian Sign Language (Amer-Ind) See under sign systems.

American Manual Alphabet See under alphabet.

American National Standards Institute (ANSI) Voluntary association of manufacturers and consumers which publishes standards for manufacturers of various types of measuring equipment, including audiometers; ANSI is presently the current standard for audiometry. Formerly known as American Standards Association (ASA), and for a brief period as United States of America Standards Institute (USASI).

American Sign Language (ASL, Ameslan) See under sign systems.

American Speech and Hearing Association (ASHA) Former name for American Speech-Language-Hearing Association.

American Speech-Language-Hearing Association (ASHA) Professional organization which represents speech and language pathologists and audiolo-

gists; formerly American Speech and Hearing Association (ASHA).

American Standards Association (ASA) Former name for United States of America Standards Institute (USASI).

Americans with Disabilities Act (ADA) Public Law 101–336 which defines disability as "a substantially limiting physical or mental impairment which affects basic life activities such as hearing, seeing, speaking, walking, caring for oneself, learning, or working." The law prohibits discrimination by employers, by any facility open to the general public, and by state and local public agencies that provide services such as transportation.

Amer-Ind American Indian Sign Language.

Ameslan American Sign Language.

amimia (ə-mim′ē-ə) [a- + G. *mimos*, mimic] Loss or impairment of the ability to use or understand gestures or signs. See also aphasia.

AMLB Alternate Monaural Loudness Balance.

amnesia (am-nē′sē-ə, -zhə) [G. *amnēsia*,

forgetfulness] **1.** Partial or total inability to recall or identify past experiences. **2.** Loss of memory.

> **localized a.** Amnesia restricted to a special time, place, or experience.

> **posttraumatic a. (PTA)** Period of time between sustaining a head injury and the return of full consciousness.

> **retroactive a.** Amnesia extending to events immediately preceding trauma or shock. Syn: retrograde.

amnesic or **amnestic** (am-nē′sik, am-nes′-tik) Relating to or affected with amnesia.

amnesic aphasia See under aphasia.

ampere (A) (am′pēr) [A. Ampère, Fr. physicist, 1775–1836] Practical unit of electric current.

amplification (am-pli-fi-kā′shən) [L. *amplifico*, to enlarge] Process of increasing the magnitude (current, power, or voltage) of a signal. See also gain.

> **compression a.** Limitation or compression of the amplification of a hearing aid to a definite maximum, to prevent waveform distortion and peak clipping; equivalent to a rapidly acting automatic volume control.

amplifier (am′pli-fi-ėr) [See amplification] Electronic device which increases the strength of electrical impulses; a component of hearing aids.

amplify (am′pli-fī) To perform amplification.

amplitude (am′pli-tud) [L. *amplitudo*, largeness] **1.** Range of intensity of sound, as measured from its mean position to an extreme. See also intensity; volume. **2.** Height of a wave, as measured from trough (valley) to crest (peak). **3.** In speech, energy with which the vocal folds vibrate during the production of a speech sound.

> **acoustic reflex a.** Magnitude of the change in acoustic immittance, associated with reflexive contraction of the stapedius muscle, when compared to quiescent acoustic immittance.

> **effective a.** Average height of a sound or wave throughout its phase; the primary determiner of loudness of a sound.

> **maximum a.** Highest point of a periodic sound or wave.

> **peak a.** Maximum momentary displacement obtained by a vibrating source; occurs twice in the cycle of a sine wave, once when a vibrator reaches its maximum displacement in one direction and once when the maximum displacement is reached in the opposite direction.

> **peak-to-peak a.** Amplitude of a vibrating source measured from the maximum positive peak to the maximum negative peak; the peak-to-peak amplitude of a sine wave is twice the peak amplitude.

> **zero a.** Area in a sound spectrograph which has little or no sound energy. Syn: antiresonance. See also phase.

amplitude distortion Harmonic *distortion.*

amplitude modulation (AM) 1. Variation of a radio carrier wave in accordance with the strength of the audio or other signal. **2.** Change in amplitude of a sound wave.

amplitude shimmer Shimmer (2).

AMR Alternate motion rate.

amusia (ə-myu′zē-ə, -zhə) [a- + G. *mousa*, music] Inability, total or partial, to produce or to comprehend musical sounds.

an- Privative prefix denoting without, not; equivalent of Latin *in-* and English *un-*.

anacusis or **anakusis** (an-ə-ku′sis) [an- + G. *kousis*, hearing] Total deafness; profound conductive or sensorineural dysfunction which cannot be corrected medically, surgically, or with prosthetic techniques.

analog A continuously varying audio signal whereby communication is transmitted by a sound wave. It is in contrast to a sequence of discrete values. See also digital.

analog-to-digital converter (A/D converter) An electronic device that converts a continuously varying electrical signal to a series of numeric values, which can then be processed by a computer.

analogy (ə-nal′ə-jē) [G. *analogos*, proportionate] Form of comparison in which a relation of likeness between two things consists in the resemblance not of the two things but of two or more of their structures and/or functions; *e.g.*, the heart as a pump.

analysis, pl. analyses (ə-nal′i-sis, -sēz) [G. a breaking up] **1.** Method of study that separates the object of study into smaller units. *Cf.* synthesis. **2.** Technique of psychoanalysis. See also auditory analysis.

analysis of homonymy See under phonological analysis.

analytic (an-ə-lit′ik) Denoting analysis.

analytic method See aural rehabilitation.

analyze (an′ə-līz) [See analysis] To examine critically to determine the essential elements.

anaphoric (an-ə-fôr′ik) [G. *ana*, up + *phoros*, bringing (back)] Exophoric.

anaphoric pronoun See pronoun, under parts of speech.

anaphoric reference See under cohesive devices.

anaptyxis, pl. anaptyxes (an-ap-tik′sis, -sēz) [G. act of unfolding] Excrescence.

anarthria (an-är′thrē-ə) [an + G. *arthron*, joint (of sound, disjointed)] Inability to articulate; may result from brain lesion or damage to peripheral nerves that innervate the articulatory muscles. See also dysarthria.

anatomic, anatomical (an-ə-tom′ik, -i-kəl) Relating to anatomy; structural. Syn: morphological (2).

anatomy (ə-nat′ə-mē) [G. *anatomē*, dissection] **1.** Structure of an organism. **2.** Science concerned with the structure of organisms.

anechoic chamber (an-ek′ō-ik) Specially built room designed with soft surfaces constructed of large wedges of sound-absorbing material on the walls, floor, and ceiling; its purpose is to provide an area of maximum sound absorption and minimum reverberation. Syn: dead room; free-field room; no-echo chamber. *Cf.* reverberation room.

anesthesia (an-es-thē′zē-ə, -zhə) [G. *anaisthēsia*, without sensation] State characterized by loss of sensation, whether as a result of neurologic disease or dysfunction or of pharmacologic depression of nerve function.

    laryngeal a. See under laryngeal sensory *paralysis*.

aneurysm (an-yu′rizm) [G. *aneurysma*] **1.** Circumscribed dilatation of an artery formed by a stretching of its walls; suggestive of a condition in which the weakened blood vessel may burst. **2.** A localized, balloon-like dilatation of a blood vessel caused by a weakened arterial wall or a genetic defect.

angular gyrus See under gyrus.

animate [L. *animatus*] **1.** (an′ə-mit). Alive, vital, capable of movement (usually said of man and animals); opposite of inanimate. **2.** (an′ə-māt). To give life, vitalize, endow with movement.

ankyloglossia (aŋ′ki-lō-glo′sē-ə) [G. *ankylos*, bent, crooked + *glōssa*, tongue] Limited movement of the tongue due to abnormal shortness of the lingual frenum; commonly referred to as tongue-tie.

ankylosis (aŋ-ki-lō′sis) [G. stiffening of joint] **1.** Abnormal immobility of a joint due to fusion of joint structures. **2.** In hearing, fixation of the stapes in otosclerosis.

    cricoarytenoid a. Injury, infection, or arthritic changes in the cricoarytenoid joint causing a weak voice and hoarseness, sometimes with pain.

anode (an′ōd) [G. *anodos*, a way up] Positive electrode in a vacuum tube which collects the free electrons released by the negative electrode (cathode). *Cf.* cathode.

anomalous (ə-nom′ə-ləs) [See anomaly] In speech, denotes an utterance which may be syntactically correct but is semantically incorrect; *e.g.,* The egg ate John.

anomaly (ə-nom′ə-lē) [G. *anōmalia,* irregularity] Structure or function deviating significantly from the norm.

anomia (ə-nō′mē-ə) [a- + G. *ōnoma,* name] Loss of the ability to identify or to recall and recognize names of persons, places, or things; in a less severe form, often referred to as dysnomia. See also anomic *aphasia.*

anomic (ə-nō′mik) Denoting anomia.

anomic aphasia See under aphasia.

anosognosia (an′ə-səg-nō′sē-ə) [a- + G. *nosos,* disease + *gnōsis,* knowledge] **1.** Impairment of an individual's ability to relate to his environment or the parts of his body to each other, due to trauma in the right cerebral hemisphere; ability to use language may be retained. **2.** Inability to perceive and recognize body parts.

anoxia (ə-nok′sē-ə) [a- + oxygen + G. *-ia,* condition] Deficiency of oxygen content of the blood.

    cerebral a. Lack of oxygen in the blood supply to the brain.

ANSI American National Standards Institute.

antagonist (an-tag′ə-nist) [G. *antagonisma,* fight against] A muscle whose contraction specifically opposes the action of its prime mover (agonist); *e.g.,* if the posterior cricoarytenoid muscles are prime movers, the antagonists of this movement are the lateral cricoarytenoid muscles.

antecedent (an-ti-sē′dent) [L. *antecedens,* going before] Noun or noun equivalent to which a pronoun refers; *e.g., Bobby* is smart and *he* gets good grades.

antecedent event Verbal or nonverbal stimulus that precedes and sets the occasion for a response; *e.g.,* verbal in-

structions given by the clinician to the client to evoke a specific response.

anterior (an-tēr′ē-ėr) [L.] **1.** Denoting before or in front of, or the front part of, an anatomical structure; opposite of posterior. **2.** See under distinctive features.

anterior partial laryngectomy See under laryngectomy.

anterior vertical canal See semicircular canals, under inner *ear.*

anthelix (ant′hē-liks) [anti- + G. *helix,* coil] Anatomical landmark of the auricle of the ear; also spelled antihelix. See auricle, under external *ear.*

anthropological (an′thrə-pō-loj′i-kəl) [G. *anthrōpos,* man + *logos,* treatise] Pertaining to anthropology, the science of the origins, physical and cultural development, racial characteristics, and social customs and beliefs of man.

anthropological linguistics See under linguistics.

anti- [G. *anti,* against] Prefix denoting against, opposing.

anticipatory and struggle behavior theories See under stuttering theories.

anticipatory behavior See under behavior.

anticipatory coarticulation Backward *coarticulation.*

anticipatory emotions In stuttering, those initial feelings, emotions, or attitudinal reactions that result from the stutterer's dread of feared sounds, words, situations, or interpersonal relationships.

antiexpectancy (an′ti-ek-spek′tən-sē) In stuttering, means by which a stutterer prevents or minimizes stuttering, or distracts himself from anticipation of stuttering; *e.g.,* the stutterer may appear overly serious, with slow and deliberate speech.

antihelix (an-ti-hē′liks) Alternative spelling of anthelix.

antiresonance (an-ti-rez′ə-nəns) Zero *amplitude.*

antitragus (an-ti-trā′gəs) [anti- + tragus] Anatomical landmark of the auricle of the ear. See auricle, under external *ear.*

antonym See under word.

anvil (an'vil) [so called because of fancied resemblance] Incus. See under middle *ear.*

anxiety (aŋ-zī'ə-tē) [L. *anxius,* distressed] **1.** Emotional disturbance with apprehension or worry as the more prominent component. **2.** In stuttering, a state of apprehension or fear pertaining to the anticipation of speaking.

apathy (ap'ə-thē) [G. *apatheia,* fr. *a-* priv. + *pathos,* suffering] Absence of feeling or emotion; indifference.

aperiodic (ā'pēr-ē-od'ik) Not periodic; irregular.

aperiodic wave See under wave.

aperture (ap'ĕr-chər) [L. *apertura,* an opening] An opening or orifice.

apex, pl. **apices** (ā'peks, āp'i-sēz) [L. summit or tip] Uppermost point of any structure. See also tongue.

Apgar Score [V. Apgar, U.S. anesthesiologist, 1909–1974] Evaluation of a newborn infant's physical status by assigning numerical values (0–2) to each of five criteria: heart rate, respiratory effort, muscle tone, response to stimulation, and skin color; a score of 10 indicates the best possible condition; usually performed one minute after birth. An infant with a score of 0–3 is considered to be in severe distress and in need of resuscitation; a score of 4–6 indicates moderate distress; and a score of 7–10 is normal, indicating a well baby.

aphasia (ə-fā'zē-ə, -fā'zhə) [G. speechlessness] Communication disorder caused by brain damage and characterized by complete or partial impairment of language comprehension, formulation, and use; excludes disorders associated with primary sensory deficits, general mental deterioration, or psychiatric disorders. Partial impairment is often referred to as dysphasia.

  acoustic-amnestic a. Impairment of the retention of speech; single words or digits may be repeated or written correctly, but as the amount of information increases, the disturbance becomes more apparent [Luria]. See also Wernicke's *aphasia.*

  afferent (kinesthetic) motor a. Articulation disorder resulting from a disturbance in the kinesthetic analysis of speech movements [Luria]. See also Broca's *aphasia;* apraxia.

  amnesic a. Disturbance of the ability to appropriately use words as names for objects, circumstances, characteristics, relationships, etc. [Weisenberg and McBride]. See also anomic *aphasia.*

  anomic a. 1. Fluent aphasia in which the predominant characteristic is the prominence of word-finding difficulties in the context of fluent, grammatically well-formed speech; auditory comprehension is fairly intact [Head, Geschwind, Goodglass and Kaplan]. **2.** Inability to recall or ex-

APGAR SCORE			
		Score	
Criteria	*0*	*1*	*2*
Skin color	Pale blue	Pink body, blue extremities	All pink
Heart rate	Absent	<100	>100
Respiratory effort	Absent	Irregular; slow	Good crying
Muscle tone	Limp	Some flexion of extremities	Active
Reflex response to nose catheter	Limp	Grimace	Sneeze, cough

press names for objects or proper names. See also amnesic, nominal, and semantic *aphasia*.

auditory a. Impaired ability to comprehend spoken words [Eisensen]. See also under pure aphasias, pure word deafness.

Broca's a. [P. Broca, Fr. neurologist, 1824–1880] Nonfluent, predominantly expressive aphasia characterized by problems with initiation of sound sequences in words and associated with a lesion in the third frontal convolution of the left or dominant hemisphere; grammar and vocabulary are restricted, so that speech is often limited to expression of high-frequency content words; auditory comprehension is relatively spared, allowing the individual to communicate information through yes-no or multiple-choice questions; writing is often affected [Geschwind, Goodglass and Kaplan]. See also afferent (kinesthetic), efferent (kinetic), executive, expressive, motor, subcortical motor, syntactic, and verbal *aphasia;* contiguity disorder, under aphasia.

callosal disconnection syndrome Aphasia resulting from partial isolation of the two cerebral hemispheres, due to injury or surgical section of the corpus callosum; behavior related to the nondominant side of the body is affected [Goodglass and Kaplan].

central a. Inner speech disturbance reflected in both receptive and expressive difficulties of a symbolic nature [Myklebust, Goldstein]. See also conduction *aphasia*.

childhood a. Developmental *aphasia*.

conduction a. Fluent aphasia characterized by impaired repetition in relation to the level of spontaneous speech; fluency may be limited to short bursts of speech; comprehension is good relative to the severity

of expressive disturbance; associated with a lesion in the arcuate fasciculus and also with a lesion deep to the supramarginal gyrus [Geschwind, Goodglass and Kaplan]. See also central, dynamic, expressive, receptive, and transcortical sensory *aphasia*.

contiguity disorder Aphasia characterized by difficulties with the production of speech [Jakobson]. See also Broca's *aphasia*.

developmental a. Any failure of the normal growth of language function when deafness, mental deficiency, motor disability, or severe personality disorder can be excluded [Eisensen, Myklebust, Osgood and Griffith]. Syn: childhood or infantile aphasia.

dynamic a. Disturbance of inner language manifested by a disruption of the ability to express one's thoughts or to transform another's speech into one's own thoughts [Luria]. See also conduction *aphasia*.

efferent (kinetic) motor a. Disturbance of the ability to analyze and sequence speech movements; individual sounds may be unaffected, but series of sounds requiring a sequential order are impaired [Luria]. See also Broca's *aphasia*.

executive a. Difficulty in transmitting meaningful messages through speech, writing, or gesturing [Van Riper]. See also Broca's *aphasia*.

expressive a. 1. Impairment of the production of speech, although comprehension and motor function are usually good; difficulties with writing are often present [Weisenberg and McBride, Myklebust]. **2.** Inability to recall the pattern of movements required to say words or sequences of words, even though the individual knows what he wants to say. See also Broca's *aphasia*.

expressive-receptive a. Aphasia in which both the comprehension and production of language functions are greatly disturbed [Weisenberg and McBride, Myklebust]. See also conduction *aphasia*.

fluent a. Aphasia in which speech flows smoothly, with a variety of grammatical constructions; paraphasias and circumlocutions may be numerous [Goodglass and Kaplan]. See also Wernicke's *aphasia*.

global a. Aphasia characterized by severe impairment of the production and comprehension of language; all sensory modalities may be impaired. The individual may be incapable of using any expressive speech, or, if communication is attempted, it is usually done with primitive gestures; responses may be automatic words and phrases which are rarely used in appropriate context [Schuell, Wepman and Jones].

infantile a. Developmental *aphasia*.

isolation a. Disturbance characterized by an inability to comprehend speech; ability to repeat phrases and sentences is retained, but naming of things is difficult [Geschwind, Goodglass and Kaplan]. See also anomic *aphasia*; Wernicke's *aphasia*.

jargon a. Disorder in which phonemes are produced in unintelligible, inaccurate sequences devoid of meaning; the individual appears to have a phonemic system which makes sense only to him [Wepman and Jones, Eisenson, Critchley]. See also Wernicke's *aphasia*; jargon.

motor a. Breakdown of speech production in which speech is articulated slowly and hesitantly, with numerous substitutions of one phoneme for another [Broca]. See also Broca's *aphasia*; apraxia.

nominal a. 1. Difficulty in uttering an appropriate term regardless of its part of speech; appears to occur most often with nouns because nouns comprise the bulk of most vocabularies [Head, Eisenson]. **2.** Ina-

bility to use names. See also anomic *aphasia*.

nonfluent a. Aphasia in which the flow of speech is interrupted by superfluous or insufficient motor involvement of the speech mechanism [Goodglass and Kaplan]. See also Broca's *aphasia*.

pragmatic a. Impairment of symbol formulation in which the difficulty is in conceptualizing from a given stimulus; little meaning is conveyed from the speech used [Wepman and Jones]. See also Wernicke's *aphasia*.

pure a.'s Term for rare types of aphasia which affect only a single input or output modality, leaving language intact in associated modalities [Goodglass and Kaplan].

  Pure agraphia is a disorder affecting writing and spelling; reading is only slightly affected.

  Pure alexia, word blindness, is an inability to read; visually presented objects may still be identified and acuity usually is not disturbed.

  Pure aphemia is a disorder of articulation in which the individual is unable to produce any speech sounds, either in imitation or spontaneously. See also Broca's *aphasia*; subcortical motor *aphasia*.

  Pure word deafness is the loss of auditory comprehension without any effect on speech output, reading, or writing; ability to repeat is severely impaired. See also subcortical sensory *aphasia*; Wernicke's *aphasia*.

receptive a. Disturbance in the perception and understanding of language, spoken or written [Weisenberg and McBride, Myklebust]. See also Wernicke's *aphasia*.

semantic a. 1. Difficulty in recognizing the full meaning of words and phrases. **2.** Disorder of formulation in which there is difficulty in recalling and evoking appropriate and meaningful verbal signs to previously acquired concepts [Luria, Wepman and Jones, Head]. See also Wernicke's *aphasia*.

sensory a. Defects in the comprehension and production of speech [Luria]. See also Wernicke's *aphasia*.

similarity disorders of a. Disorders in decoding [Jakobson]. See also Wernicke's *aphasia*.

simple a. Aphasia in which available language is reduced in all modalities, with no specific perceptual or sensory motor involvement and no dysarthria [Schuell].

speechreading a. Inability to associate meaning with movements of the lips [Johnson and Myklebust].

subcortical motor a. Isolated disorder of articulation in which auditory comprehension, reading, and writing are intact; the individual can speak in grammatically complete sentences and has no word-finding problems [Goodglass and Kaplan]. See also pure aphemia, under pure *aphasia(s)*; apraxia.

syntactic a. Disorder of symbol formation characterized by impairment of the individual's previously established grammatical structure; words may be produced, but their arrangement into coordinated phrases is defective [Head, Wepman and Jones]. See also Broca's *aphasia*.

transcortical motor a. Individuals with transcortical motor aphasia exhibit phonemic and global paraphasias, syntactic errors, perseveration, and difficulty initiating and organizing responses in conversation. Repetition appears to be intact but auditory comprehension is limited.

transcortical sensory a. Rare syndrome characterized by the inability to spontaneously initiate speech; when addressed, the individual may respond with well-articulated but irrelevant paraphasia [Goodglass and Kaplan]. See also conduction *aphasia*.

verbal a. Difficulty in forming words for speech [Head]. See also Broca's *aphasia*.

Wernicke's a. [C. Wernicke, Ger. neurologist, 1848–1905] Fluent, predominantly receptive aphasia characterized by varying degrees of impaired auditory comprehension, with circumlocutory or jargon speech; word-finding problems and paraphasias are common. As the amount of information presented increases, the disturbance usually becomes more apparent and the impairment may be so severe that the individual has difficulty even at the one-word level of comprehension. It is associated with a lesion of the posterior first temporal gyrus of the left or dominant cerebral hemisphere [Geschwind, Goodglass and Kaplan]. See also acoustic-amnestic, auditory, isolation, jargon, pragmatic, receptive, sensory, and subcortical motor *aphasia*; similarity disorders of *aphasia*.

CHARACTERISTICS OF THE APHASIC PATIENT

Short attention span	Problems with short-term memory
Impulsivity	Thought rigidity
Orderliness	Concretism
Euphoria	Perseveration
Withdrawal	Disorientation (confusion)
Vision problems (double, loss of peripheral field)	Lack of oral sensitivity (tongue, taste)
Swallowing problems	Receptive language problems (discrimination, comprehension)
Expressive language problems (thoughts, words, motor)	Catastrophic responses (emotional problems, mood swings)

Aphasia Clinical Battery I See *Language Tests and Procedures* in appendices.

Aphasia Diagnostic Profiles See *Language Tests and Procedures* in appendices.

Aphasia Language Performance Scales (ALPS) See *Language Tests and Procedures* in appendices.

Aphasia Screening Test, The See *Language Tests and Procedures* in appendices.

aphasic (ə-fā′sik) Pertaining to aphasia.

aphasic phonological impairment Faulty articulation viewed as a linguistic disturbance, as opposed to a motor disturbance [Martin]. See also apraxia.

aphasiologist (ə-fā-zē-ol′ə-jist) [G. *aphasia*, speechlessness + *logos*, treatise] One who studies language as it is manifested in the impaired verbal behavior of aphasic individuals.

aphasiology (ə-fā-zē-ol′ə-jē) [G. *aphasia*, speechlessness + *logos*, study] Study of language as it is manifested in the impaired verbal behavior of aphasic individuals.

aphemia (ə-fē′mē-ə) [a- + G. *phēmē*, speech] Obsolete term for an inability to speak, presently referred to as aphasia.

    pure a. See under pure *aphasia(s)*.

aphonia (ə-fō′nē-ə) [a- + G. *phōnē*, voice] Loss of voice. See also under voice disorders of phonation.

    conversion a. Loss of voice in the absence of physical factors, *e.g.*, disease, trauma; usually a result of psychogenic factors. Syn: functional or hysterical aphonia.

    functional a. Conversion *aphonia*.

    hysterical a. Conversion *aphonia*.

    intermittent a. Aphonic episode.

    syllabic a. See under voice disorders of phonation.

aphonic (ə-fon′ik, ā-) Pertaining to aphonia.

aphonic episode 1. Loss of voice that is not constant; voice may be reduced to a whisper or disappear, and then return to normal. **2.** Abnormal brief cessation of vocal-sound production. Syn: intermittent aphonia; phonation break.

aphrasia (ə-frā′zē-ə, -zhə) [a- + G. *phrasis*, speaking] Inability to speak or to comprehend words arranged in phrases; in a less severe form, often referred to as dysphrasia.

apical (āp′i-kəl) Related to or situated near or at an apex.

apicalization See under substitution, under phonological processes.

apices (āp′i-sēz) Plural of apex.

aplasia (ə-plā′zē-ə, -zhə) [a- + G. plasis, a molding] Congenital absence of an organ or tissue. See also dysplasia; hypoplasia.

    cochlear a. Defective development or congenital absence of the organ of Corti.

    a. of labyrinth Developmental anomaly of labyrinth structures as a result of dysplasia of petrous bone.

apnea (ap′nē-ə) [G. *apnoia*, lack of breath] Transient arrest or cessation of respiration. *Cf.* dyspnea.

aponeurosis, pl. **aponeuroses** (ap-ə-nu-rō′sis, -sēz) [G. fr. *apo*, from + *neuron*, sinew + *-osis*, condition] Expanded tendon which serves as a means of attachment for flat muscles at their origin or insertion, or as a fascia to enclose or bind a group of muscles.

apoplexy (ap′ə-plek-sē) [G. *apoplēxia*] Cerebral vascular accident.

apostrophe See under figure of speech.

apperception (ap-ėr-sep′shən) [L. *ad*, to + *perceptio*, perception] **1.** Adding of other mental acts to perception, as interpretation, recognition, and classification. **2.** Powers of intellect involved in the acquisition, conversation, and elaboration of knowledge.

applied linguistics See under linguistics.

applied phonetics See under phonetics.

appositive (ə-poz′ə-tiv) [L. *appositus*, placement at] Type of modifier, an identifying word or phrase (a noun or pronoun and its modifiers), usually set off by commas, which is considered grammatically equivalent to the noun or pronoun it modifies; *e.g.*, "We, the People of the United States, in order to form. . . . " See also parenthetical elements.

Appraisal of Language Disturbances (ALD) See *Language Tests and Procedures* in appendices.

approach-avoidance Conflicts produced when an individual is confronted by two opposing drives; *e.g.*, in stuttering, to speak or not to speak.

approach-avoidance theory See under learning theory, under stuttering theories.

approximation (ə-prok-sə-mā′shən) [L. *approximatus*, drawn near to] **1.** Act or process of drawing together, as of the vocal folds. **2.** In stuttering, a deliberate attempt by the stutterer to speak in a less abnormal manner, thereby achieving a closer resemblance to normal speech patterns. **3.** In articulation, the production of a misarticulated phoneme which approaches the standard production of that phoneme. See also shaping.

APR Auropalpebral reflex.

apraxia (ə-prak′sē-ə) [G. lack of action] **1.** Disruption in the ability to transmit or express a motor response along a specific modality; involves disruption of voluntary or purposeful programming of muscular movements while involuntary movements remain intact; characterized by difficulty in articulation of speech, formation of letters in writing, or movements of gesture and pantomime. **2.** In speech, a nonlinguistic sensorimotor disorder of articulation characterized by impaired capacity to program the position of speech musculature and the sequencing of muscle movements (respiratory, laryngeal, and oral) for the volitional production of phonemes. **3.** In a less severe form than above, apraxia is often referred to as dyspraxia. See also aphasic phonological impairment; *Diagnostic Differences* in appendices.

constructional a. Apraxia characterized by difficulty with visuospatial tasks; *e.g.*, drawing, block arrangements, assembling stick designs.

ideational a. A disorder of motor planning in which complex motor plans cannot be executed, although individual motor components of the plan can be performed.

ideomotor a. A motor disturbance in which there is inability to carry out motor acts on command. Some evidence is present that these motor acts can be carried out imitatively or automatically.

oral a. Some authorities differentiate between verbal and oral apraxia, maintaining that oral apraxia is a motor disturbance in volitional movement of the jaw, lips, or tongue in purposeful or imitative tasks for normal speech movements.

verbal or **speech a.** Some authorities differentiate between verbal and oral apraxia, maintaining that verbal apraxia is the inability or difficulty with the ability to carry out purposeful movements for speech in the absence of a paralysis of the speech musculature. In children, it may influence the development of phonology and language.

Apraxia Battery for Adults—Second Edition (ABA) See *Articulation Tests*

CHARACTERISTICS OF APRAXIA

Groping for articulatory postures	Halting, effortful sequencing of phonemes
Awareness of errors	Errors of phoneme substitution
Longer vowel and word duration	Automatic speech is better than novel utterances
Prosodic elements are unnatural	

See also *Diagnostic Differences* in appendices.

and Phonological Analysis Procedures in appendices.

apraxic (ə-prak′sik) Denoting apraxia.

aprosody (ə-pros′ə-dē, ā-) [a- + G. *prosōdia*, voice modulation] Loss of the melody of speech (prosody); in a less severe form, often referred to as dysprosody. Syn: hypoprosody.

aptitude (ap′tə-tud) Natural ability to acquire general or special types of knowledge or skills with a given amount of training, formal or informal.

aptitude test Set of tasks standardized to yield an estimate of an individual's ability to perform skills, such as art, music, and mathematics.

AQ Achievement quotient.

arcuate fasciculus (är′kyu-āt fə-sik′yu-ləs) [L. *arcuatus*, bowed + dim. of *fascis*, bundle] Nerve fiber pathway in the brain believed to relay impulses from Wernicke's area to Broca's area.

area (ār′ē-ə) [L. courtyard] Circumscribed space or surface, or part of an organ which has a specific function. For types of area, see specific term.

argument (är′gyu-mənt) In pragmatics, any of the various elements of a sentence that are set in relation to one another by the predicate, regardless of the traditional classification of these elements as subject or complement.

Arizona Articulation Proficiency Scale: Revised See *Articulation Tests and Phonological Analysis Procedures* in appendices.

arrest (ə′rest) In articulation, ending a syllable either by the action of chest muscles or by the production of a consonant at the end of a syllable.

arresting consonant See under consonant.

artery A vessel in which blood flows from the heart to body parts.

Arthur Adaptation of the Leiter International Performance Scale See *Psychological Measures and Tests* in appendices.

article (är′ti-kəl) Noun modifier that denotes specificity; *e.g.*, a, an, the. See also determiner.

articulate [See articulation] 1. (är-tik′yu-lāt). In speech, to execute the movements and adjustments of the speech organs necessary to utter a speech sound. 2. (är-tik′yu-lət). Able to satisfactorily express oneself with words; easy and fluent verbal expression of thoughts, attitudes, feelings, etc. 3. (är-tik′yu-lāt). To join or connect loosely enough to allow motion between the parts.

articulation (är-tik-yu-lā′shən) [L. *articulatus*, jointed (distinct)] 1. In speech, vocal tract movements for speech sound production; involves accuracy in placement of the articulators, timing, direction of movements, force extended, speed of response, and neural integration of all events. 2. Series of overlapping ballistic movements which places varying degrees of obstruction in the path of the outgoing air stream and simultaneously modifies the size, shape, and coupling of the resonating cavities. Syn: articulation-resonance. 3. The way phonemes are formed. 4. Joint or connection loose enough to allow motion between the parts.

articulation area Location in the speech mechanism where a particular consonant or vowel is primarily formed. For specific articulation areas, see under consonant, place of articulation. See also vowel and subentries.

articulation curve See under curve.

articulation disorder 1. Incorrect production of speech sounds due to faulty placement, timing, direction, pressure, speed, or integration of the movement of the lips, tongue, velum, or pharynx. 2. Abnormality in speech due to the presence of defective, nonstandard speech sounds. 3. A difficulty in speech-sound (phoneme) production that attracts negative attention, lessens intelligibility, or disturbs the speaker.

    Addition is the insertion of sound(s) not part of the word itself;

e.g., ani*ma*mal for animal, p*uh*lease for please.

Distortion is an approximation of a phoneme in some manner which renders it acoustically unacceptable.

General oral inaccuracy is the indistinct production of sounds, even though no specific omission, addition, substitution, or distortion is heard.

Omission is the absence of a phoneme that is not replaced by another sound; *e.g.*, a—le for apple.

Substitution is the replacement of one standard speech sound by another standard speech sound, such as θ for /s/, or the replacement of one standard speech sound by a nonstandard speech sound, *e.g.*, glottal stop.

    functional a. d. Incorrect production of standard speech sound(s) for which there is no known anatomical, physiologic, or neurologic basis. See also *Diagnostic Differences* in appendices.

    organic a. d. Inability to produce correctly all or some of the standard speech sounds of the language due to anatomical, physiologic, or neurologic causes.

articulation error Defective production of a specific phoneme.

    phonemic a. e. Error in which the individual is able to execute the motor gestures involved in a sound production, but does not use the sound correctly in some linguistic productions; *e.g.*, an individual may substitute /g/ for /k/ as in "gat" for "cat," yet may be able to produce /k/ in other syllables or words.

    phonetic a. e. Error in which the individual fails to plan or execute the proper motor gestures involved in the production of a speech sound; *e.g.*, "gat" for "cat," and the clinician is unable to elicit a correct production of /k/ in other syllables or words.

articulation-gain function Performance-intensity function.

articulation index Estimation of the severity of an articulatory disorder in which each sound is weighted to reflect its frequency in the language as a means of measuring therapeutic progress.

articulation programming Behavior modification procedures used in the remediation of defective speech sounds.

articulation-resonance Articulation (2).

articulation test 1. Evaluation which yields information about the nature, number, and characteristics of the articulatory errors as they occur in a person's speech. **2.** Test devised to measure the general phonetic ability of an individual. See also appendices.

    deep a. t. Test to identify the specific phonetic contexts in which misarticulations occur, as well as the specific phonetic contexts in which sounds are correctly produced; assesses each phoneme in a variety of phonetic contexts.

    diagnostic a. t. Test designed to determine which sounds are defective, and to what degree, so that a speech correction program can be tailored to the particular person's needs.

    screening a. t. Gross measure of an individual's articulatory abilities to determine whether further testing or intervention is warranted.

articulators (är-tik′yu-lā-tərs) [L. *articulatus*, distinct] Organs of the speech mechanism which produce meaningful sound by interrupting the flow of exhaled air or by narrowing the space for its passage; *i.e.*, lips, lower jaw, velum, tongue, and pharynx. Some authorities include the cheeks, fauces, hyoid bone, larynx, uvula, alveolar ridge, nose, teeth, and sinuses. See also speech mechanism.

articulatory (är-tik′yu-lə-tô-rē) Pertaining to articulation.

articulatory basis All the habits of sound

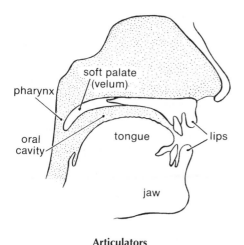

Articulators

pharynx

soft palate (velum)

oral cavity

tongue

lips

jaw

production which characterize a particular language.

articulatory phonetics See under phonetics.

artificial ear Standardized device utilized in audiometer intensity calibration which couples the earphone of the audiometer to a condenser microphone whose output is then led to a sound level meter. The coupler is so constructed that its volume approximates the volume of the external canal and middle ear, plus the air between the earphone diaphragm and the opening of the canal.

artificial larynx Mechanical device used to create alaryngeal speech.

    electrical or **electronic a. l.** Battery-powered, transistorized vibrator used to create a synthetic voice by producing a continuous buzzing sound; some models are capable of pitch variation. The device is placed snugly against the skin of the neck at a particular anatomical site, which varies with each individual. Syn: electrolarynx.

    pneumatic a. l. "U"-shaped appliance utilizing air pressure; one end is inserted into a tracheal tube and the other is inserted into the mouth

to serve as a bypass: expired air vibrates and is carried into the mouth where it is modified into speech sounds by the articulators.

    reed a. l. Any artificial larynx with a reed serving as the sound source.

artificial mastoid Device for calibration of bone-conduction vibrators; it consists of a resilient surface that simulates the vibrating properties of the mastoid process, an accelerometer, an amplifier, an attenuator, and a meter which reads either in dB or in dyne force.

artificial method Analytic method. See under aural rehabilitation.

aryepiglottic (ăr′ə-ep-i-glot′ik) Relating to the arytenoid cartilages and the epiglottis.

aryepiglottic folds Aryepiglottic muscles and the upper edge of the quadrangular membrane that together form the entrance to the larynx; they extend bilaterally from the sides of the epiglottis to the top and side surfaces of the arytenoid cartilages.

aryepiglottic muscle See *Muscles of the Larynx* table, under larynx.

arytenoid (ăr-i-tē′noid, ə-rit′ə-noid) [G. *arytanoeides*, ladle-shaped] Denoting especially the shape of the arytenoid cartilages; otherwise relating only to the arytenoid muscles.

arytenoid cartilages See under cartilage.

arytenoidectomy Surgical removal of an arytenoid cartilage. This procedure is sometimes used to improve vocal quality.

arytenoid muscle See *Muscles of the Larynx* table, under larynx.

ASA American Standards Association.

asapholalia (as′ə-fō-lā′lē-ə) [G. *asapheia*, obscure + *lalia*, talking] Indistinct speech; mumbling.

ascending pitch break See pitch break, under voice disorders of phonation.

ascending technique In audiometry, a method of establishing threshold of hearing by going from an inaudible to an audible stimulus; opposite of descending technique.

asemia or **asemasia** (ə-sē′mē-ə, as-ə-mā′sē-ə) [a- + G. *sēma*, sign, or *sēmasia*, signaling] Inability to use or understand symbols of any type for communication; *e.g.*, words, figures, gestures, signs. See also aphasia.

ASHA American Speech-Language-Hearing Association, formerly American Speech and Hearing Association; ASHA was retained for recognition and euphony.

ASL American Sign Language.

aspect (as′pekt) In grammar, a function of the auxiliary verb; it indicates the tense of the main verb; *e.g.*, He *is* eating. He *has been* eating.

Asperger's disorder Asperger's syndrome.

Asperger's syndrome (H. Asperger, German Doctor) (ahs′per-gerz) **1.** A pervasive developmental disorder characterized by severe and sustained impairment in social interaction and development of restricted and repetitive patterns of behavior, interests, and activities. These characteristics result in clinically significant impairment in social, occupational, or other important areas of functioning. There appear to be no significant delays in language, cognition, or self-help skills or in adaptive behavior, other than social interaction. Syn: Asperger's disorder, autistic psychopathy [DSM-IV]. **2.** A pervasive developmental disorder resembling autistic disorder, characterized by severe impairment of social interactions and by restricted interests and behaviors, but lacking the delays in development of language, cognitive function, and self-help skills that additionally define autistic disorder.

aspirate 1. (as′pėr-āt) To remove by aspiration (4). **2.** (as′pėr-it). See under consonant.

aspiration (as-pėr-ā′shən) [L. *aspiratus*, breathed upon] **1.** Generic term referring to the action of material penetrat-

ing the larynx and entering the airway below the true vocal folds; may occur (a) before the swallowing reflex is triggered when the airway has not elevated or closed, (b) during swallowing if the laryngeal valves are not functioning adequately, and (c) after the swallow when the larynx lowers and opens for inhalation. **2.** Food or liquid entering the lungs rather than the stomach after the swallow. **3.** Expelling of a noticeable amount of breath, as in pronouncing an aspirate. **4.** Removal by suction of air or fluid from a body cavity.

assessment (ə-ses′mənt) Evaluation.

Assessment Link Between Phonology and Articulation See *Articulation Tests and Phonological Analysis Procedures* in appendices.

Assessment of Children's Language See *Language Tests and Procedures* in appendices.

Assessment of Intelligibility of Dysarthric Speech See *Articulation Tests and Phonological Analysis Procedures* in appendices.

Assessment of Phonological Processes See *Articulation Tests and Phonological Analysis Procedures* in appendices.

assimilated nasality See under voice disorders of resonance.

assimilation (ə-sim-ə-lā′shən) [L. *assimilatus*, made alike] **1.** In cognition, the process of placing new events into existing categories; does not result in the development of new categories but does affect their growth. **2.** In speech, the effect one speech sound has on another when uttered in close sequence, such that the sounds become more like each other. **3.** Modification of a speech sound due to the influence of adjacent sounds. Syn: phonetics of juncture. See also coarticulation; phonological processes.

   alveolar a. See under assimilation *phonological processes*.

double a. Sound that has acquired the characteristics of the two surrounding sounds; a vowel tends to become nasalized when between two nasal consonants, *e.g.*, nanny.

labial a. See under assimilation *phonological processes.*

nasal a. See under assimilation *phonological processes.*

progressive a. Sound which is influenced by the sound preceding it; *e.g.*, nature.

progressive vowel a. See under assimilation *phonological processes.*

reciprocal a. Sounds that interact in such a way that they are combined in a single sound *e.g.*, gracious.

regressive a. Initial sound that is influenced by the second sound; *e.g.*, andiron.

velar a. See under assimilation *phonological processes.*

assistive listening devices In audiology, refers to systems that (a) improve the signal-to-noise ratio by transmitting amplified sound directly to the hearing-impaired listener, or (b) transform sound into a visual or tactile signal.

assistive technology device Any item, piece of equipment, or product system, whether acquired commercially, modified, or customized, that is used to increase, maintain, or improve the functional capabilities of individuals with disabilities.

association (ə-sō-sē-ā′shən) [L. *associatus*, joined to] Ability to establish connections between two or more symbols or concepts; *e.g.*, puppy/dog, hat/head, sound/symbol, quantity/numeral.

   auditory-vocal a. Ability to draw relationships from what is heard and then respond orally in a meaningful way; comprehension of auditory stimuli must occur before vocal expression can be utilized effectively. See also *Auditory Processes* table, under auditory processes.

assonance (as′ə-nəns) Similarity of vowel sounds in words which do not rhyme; *e.g.*, we, weep; like a diamond in the sky. *Cf.* consonance (1).

astereognosis (ə-stăr′ē-og-nō′sis) [a- + G. *stereos*, solid + *gnōsis*, knowledge] Inability to recognize by touch the form of solid objects. *Cf.* stereognosis.

astomia (ə-stō′mē-ə) [a- + G. *stoma*, mouth] Absence of a mouth opening. Syn: oral atresia. *Cf.* dystomia.

asymmetry (ə-sim′ə-trē) [G. *asymmetria*, lack of proportion] **1.** Lack of similarity of those parts of a structure that should be similar, as of facial features. **2.** Lack of correct proportion.

asynergia (ā-sin-ėr′jē-ə) Asynergy.

asynergic (ā-sin-ėr′jik) Denoting asynergy.

asynergy (ā-sin′ėr-jē) [a- + G. *syn*, with, + *ergon*, work] **1.** Faulty timing and coordination among parts or organs normally functioning in harmony, as of the articulators. **2.** In neurology, an abnormal state of muscle antagonism. Syn: asynergia.

ataxia (ə-tak′sē-ə) [a- + G. *taxis*, order] Disorder characterized by dyscoordination and tremors in fine and gross motor activity. See under cerebral palsy symptomatology. See also ataxic *dysarthria.*

ataxic (ə-tak′sik) Denoting ataxia.

ataxic dysarthria See under dysarthria.

athetosis (a-thə-tō′sis) [G. *athetos*, without position or place + *-osis*, condition] Disorder characterized by involuntary, primarily writhing movements usually occurring with, and blocking, volitional efforts. See under cerebral palsy symptomatology. See also hyperkinetic *dysarthria.*

athetotic (a-thə-tot′ik) Denoting athetosis.

atonia (ə-tō′nē-ə) [G. languor] Lack of muscle tone. See under cerebral palsy symptomatology.

atresia (ə-trē′zē-ə, -zhə) [a- + G. *trēsis*, hole] **1.** Congenital absence or pathologic closure of a normal orifice, passage, or cavity. **2.** In audiology, an abnormally small pinna; may be accompanied by occluded canals and/or anomalies of the middle ear.

aural a. Closure or absence of the external auditory meatus in the cartilaginous portion, in the bony portion, or in its entirety.

laryngeal a. Congenital failure of the laryngeal opening to develop, resulting in partial or total obstruction at or just above or below the glottis.

oral a. Astomia.

atrophy (a′trə-fē) [a- + G. *trophē*, nourishment] Withering or wasting away of tissues or organs, as may occur in paralysis.

attention (ə-ten′shən) Active selection of certain stimuli or aspects of experience, with consequent inhibition of all others. See also *Auditory Processes* table, under auditory processes.

auditory a. Ability to focus on specific sound units as significant stimuli; *e.g.*, noises, speech sounds, words, phrases, sentences.

attention deficit/hyperactivity disorder A persistent pattern of inattention and/or hyperactivity-impulsivity that is more frequent and severe than is typically observed in individuals at a comparable level of development. Some hyperactive-impulsive or inattentive symptoms that cause the impairment were present before the age of seven years. In addition, some impairment from the symptoms is present in two or more settings (*e.g.*, school and home). Finally, there must be clear evidence of clinically significant impairment in social, academic, or occupational functioning that is not accounted for by another mental disorder.

inattention Six or more of the following symptoms must have persisted to a degree that is maladaptive and inconsistent with the individual's developmental level: (a) often fails to give close attention to details or makes careless mistakes in schoolwork, or other activities; (b) often has difficulty sustaining attention in tasks or play activities; (c) often does not seem to listen when spoken to directly; (d) often does not follow through on instructions and fails to finish schoolwork, chores, or duties in the workplace (not due to oppositional behavior or failure to understand instructions); (e) often has difficulty organizing tasks and activities; (f) often avoids dislikes, or is reluctant to engage in tasks that require sustained mental effort (such as schoolwork or homework); (g) often loses things necessary for tasks or activities (*e.g.*, toys, school assignments, books, or tools); (h) is often distracted by extraneous stimuli; (i) is often forgetful in daily activities.

hyperactivity-impulsivity Six or more of the following symptoms have persisted for at least six months to a degree that is maladaptive and inconsistent with developmental level.

Hyperactivity (a) often fidgets with hands of feet or squirms in seat; (b) often leaves seat in classroom or in other situations in which remaining seated is expected; (c) often runs about or climbs excessively in situations in which it is inappropriate (in adolescents or adults, may be limited to subjective feelings of restlessness); (d) often has difficulty playing or engaging in leisure activities quietly; (e) is often "on the go" or often acts as if "driven by a motor;" (f) often talks excessively.

Impulsivity (g) often blurts out answers before questions have been completed; (h) often has difficulty waiting turn; (i) often interrupts or intrudes on others (*e.g.*, butts into conversations or games) [DSM-IV].

attention span Largest number of experiences that can be recalled after a limited exposure to them.

attenuation (ə-ten-yu-ā′shən) [L. *attenuatus*, thinned or weakened] In acoustics, a reduction in acoustic intensity; may be effected mechanically by the absorption of the energy of tones, or electronically by reducing the power input.

    interaural a. Loss of energy of a sound presented by either air conduction or bone conduction as it travels from the test ear to the nontest ear; number of decibels lost in cross-hearing. Often considered to be 40 dB for air-conducted sound and zero for bone-conducted sound.

attenuator (ə-ten′yu-ā-tèr) [See attenuation] **1.** Resistor or network of resistors used to reduce voltage, current, or power delivered to a load. **2.** Control for decreasing the intensity of a tone or signal, as in the hearing level dial of an audiometer.

attribute-entity See under semantic relations.

atypical clefts See under cleft.

audibility threshold Absolute *threshold.*

audible (ô′di-bəl) Capable of being heard.

audible range Span of acoustic frequencies which the normal human ear can perceive, generally from 20 Hz to 20,000 Hz.

auding (ô′diŋ) [L. *audio*, to hear] Integrative function involving the reception and comprehension of acoustic information; enables acoustic differentiation between similar sounding words; *e.g.*, lips and lisp.

audio- [L. to hear] Combining form relating to hearing.

audiogram (ô′dē-ə-gram) [audio- + G. *gramma*, a drawing] Standard graph used to record pure-tone hearing thresholds; air-conduction and bone-conduction thresholds are graphed by frequency and hearing level. Standard symbols for air conduction are ○ in the right ear and ✕ in the left ear (red

MODALITY	EAR⁺		
	RIGHT	BOTH	LEFT
AIR CONDUCTION - EARPHONES			
UNMASKED	○		✕
MASKED	△		☐
BONE CONDUCTION - MASTOID			
UNMASKED	<		>
MASKED	[		]
BONE CONDUCTION - FOREHEAD			
UNMASKED		⋁	
MASKED	⌐		⌐
AIR CONDUCTION - SOUND FIELD		S	

Recommended Symbols

MODALITY	EAR⁺		
	RIGHT	BOTH	LEFT
AIR CONDUCTION - EARPHONES			
UNMASKED	○		✕
MASKED	△		☐
BONE CONDUCTION - MASTOID			
UNMASKED	<		>
MASKED	[		]
BONE CONDUCTION - FOREHEAD			
UNMASKED		⋁	
MASKED	]		[
AIR CONDUCTION - SOUND FIELD		S	

Recommended "no response" Symbols

Audiometric Symbols

for right, blue for left). Although guidelines for audiometric symbols indicate < for right ear bone conduction and > for left ear bone conduction, some audiologists still utilize > for the right ear and < for the left ear. Symbols indicating masked bone conduction are [for the right ear, and] for the left ear.

audiogram configurations Categories based on the shape of the recorded hearing thresholds.

    Dipper curve. See saddle curve below.

    Flat indicates hearing loss approximately equal at all frequencies.

    Gradual falling or **gradual rising curve** indicates hearing loss that

AUDIOGRAM OF FAMILIAR SOUNDS

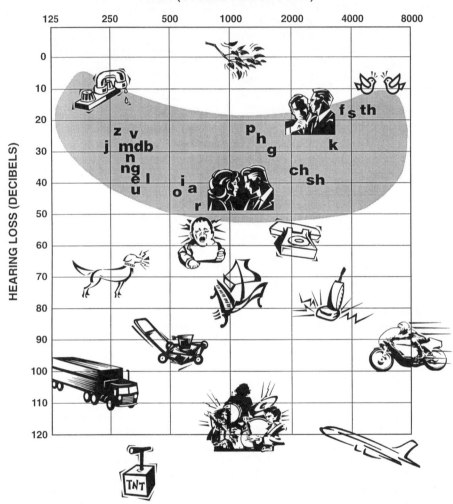

Audiogram of Familiar Sounds

Frequency spectrum of familiar sounds plotted on a standard audiogram. Shaded area represents the "speech banana" that contains most of the sound elements of spoken speech. From Northern JL, Downs MP. *Hearing in Children,* 5th Ed. Baltimore: Lippincott Williams & Wilkins, 2002.

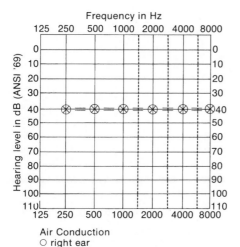

Flat

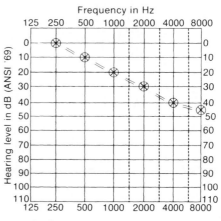

Gradual Falling Curve

falls or rises at approximately 5 to 10 dB per octave.

Marked falling curve. Sharply falling curve.

Saddle, dipper, trough, or **"U"-shaped curve** indicates less hearing loss at the low and high frequencies than in the middle range.

Saucer curve indicates equal loudness at all frequencies.

Sharply falling or **marked falling curve** indicates hearing loss that increases about 15 to 20 dB per octave at higher frequencies.

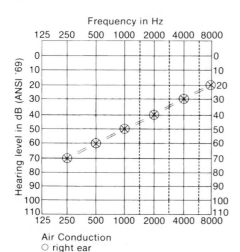

Gradual Rising Curve

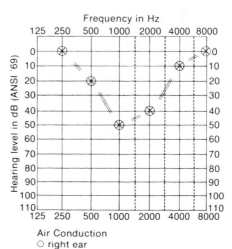

Saddle, Dipper, Trough, or "U"-Shaped Curve

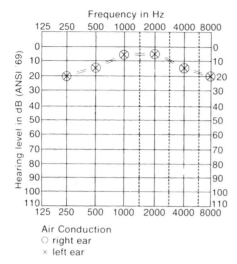

Air Conduction
○ right ear
× left ear

Saucer Curve

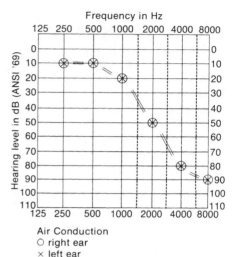

Air Conduction
○ right ear
× left ear

**Ski Slope, Steep Drop, Sudden Drop, or
Waterfall Curve**

Ski slope, steep or **sudden drop,** or **waterfall curve** usually indicates nearly normal hearing in lower frequencies, followed by a steep drop of 25 dB or more per octave.
Trough or **"U"-shaped curve.** See saddle curve above.
Waterfall curve. Ski slope curve.

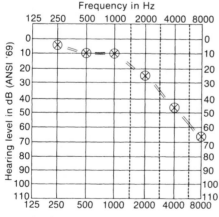

Air Conduction
○ right ear
× left ear

Sharply Falling or Marked Curve

audiologic, audiological (ô-dē-ə-loj′ik, -i-kəl) Pertaining to audiology.

audiological evaluation Procedures used to measure hearing ability. They include pure-tone and air- and bone-conduction thresholds; speech reception and discrimination scores; discrimination of speech in the presence of noise; case history; site of lesion testing (when present); and, if indicated, central test battery.

audiologic habilitation Aural rehabilitation.

audiologist (ô-dē-ol′ə-jist) One who holds a degree and/or certification in audiology, and whose specific interest is in identification, measurement, and rehabilitation of persons with hearing impairments.

audiology (ô-dē-ol′ə-jē) [audio- + G. *logos,* treatise] Study of hearing and hearing disorders; it is concerned with assessment of the nature and degree of hearing loss, hearing conservation, and rehabilitation of individuals with hearing impairments.

  clinical a. The practice of audiology concerned with hearing as the foundation of the learning and utilization of language skills; emphasis is placed upon understanding the social functions of hearing and increasing the ability of hearing-impaired persons to cope with the demands of communication.

educational a. Clinical audiology in an educational setting, such as the public school system.

experimental a. Aspect of audiology concerned with investigative study of the auditory system and its function in man and animals.

geriatric a. Aspect of audiology concerned with the hearing problems of the elderly.

pediatric a. Specialty of audiology concerned with hearing and hearing disorders in infants and young children.

rehabilitative a. Aural rehabilitation.

audiometer (ô-dē-om′ə-tėr) [audio- + G. *metron*, measure] Electronic instrument designed to measure the sensitivity of hearing; it is calibrated to register hearing loss in decibels.

automatic a. Audiometer which utilizes the client control principle to test hearing, an operator being needed only to start the machine; *e.g.*, Békésy and Rudmose audiometers.

Békésy a. [G. von Békésy, Hungarian biophysicist in U.S., 1899–1972] Automatic audiometer with which the client makes his own audiogram by pushing and releasing a button to indicate whether or not he hears pure tones at changing intensity levels; may be operated either at a fixed frequency or with steadily changing frequencies.

crib-o-gram a. Automatic neonatal screening audiometer which enables early detection of hearing; developed by F.B. Simmons. Responses are detected by a motion-sensitive transducer placed under the crib mattress and are registered on a strip-chart;

the transducer is sensitive to changes in respiration and to limb or almost any motor movement (excluding eye blinks or facial grimace).

group a. Audiometer designed to check the hearing of a number of persons at the same time, utilizing more than one pair of headsets; acoustic material, either pure tones or speech, is presented to a group of persons simultaneously by a procedure in which each individual can give reliable information as to the test items heard.

limited range a. Pure-tone audiometer designed to test restricted ranges of frequency and sound pressure; pure-tone frequencies of 500, 1000, 2000, 3000, 4000, and 6000 Hz are usually included, and sound pressures may be limited to 0 to 70 dB re standard reference level; facilities for bone conduction measurements and for masking may be omitted.

limited range speech a. Pure-tone audiometer restricted in its range of sound pressure level; facilities for masking need not be included.

narrow range a. Pure-tone audiometer more restricted than a limited range audiometer in its ranges of frequency and sound pressure levels; frequencies and levels are usually those appropriate for particular screening tests.

pure-tone a. Electroacoustical generator which provides pure tones of selected frequencies and calibrated output; a major classification of audiometers.

Rudmose a. [W. Rudmose (1957)] Automatic audiometer which uses the client control principle to test hearing at six frequencies in each ear.

speech a. Audiometer which provides spoken material at controlled sound pressure levels to obtain speech reception thresholds, tolerance for loud speech, and discrimination ability; input may be from a microphone for live voice testing or recorded and produced from a turntable or tape recorder; facilities for masking are included, and no facilities for bone conduction are required; a major classification of audiometers.

wide range a. Pure-tone audiometer which covers the major portion of the human auditory range in frequency and in sound pressure level; includes one or two air-conduction earphones, bone vibrator, tone switch, and masking facilities; used primarily for clinical and diagnostic purposes, or for determining hearing thresholds of children.

audiometric (ô′dē-ə-met′rik) Relating to audiometry.

audiometric tests Tests used to determine the nature and degree of hearing sensitivity. For specific audiometric tests, see appendices.

audiometric zero 1. Sound pressure level required to make any frequency barely audible to the average normal ear. Audiometers are calibrated to national standards based on studies of normal hearing subjects that specify the sound pressure levels for zero hearing level (audiometric zero) at each frequency for specific earphones. **2.** Hearing threshold level setting on an audiometer; identified as 0 dB.

audiometry (ô-dē-om′ə-trē) [audio- + G. *metron*, measure] The measurement of hearing. *Cf.* audiology.

ascending technique a. Method of establishing threshold of hearing by going from an inaudible to an audible stimulus.

auditory brainstem response a. (ABR) See under electrophysiologic *audiometry.*

automatic a. Technique of administering hearing tests by means of an automatic audiometer; the client tracks his own thresholds by control-

ling the intensity of the signal being presented to him, while the audiometer sweeps through the audible frequency range. See also Békésy *audiometry.*

average evoked response a. (AERA) Evoked response audiometry. See under electrophysiologic *audiometry.*

behavioral observation a. (BOA) Conditioning technique utilized to obtain hearing thresholds with infants and children through two years of age.

Three types of behavioral audiometry are **head turn technique,** a technique for studying speech-sound discrimination in infants, utilizing the head turn response of an infant; **high-amplitude sucking technique (HAS),** in which a speech sound is presented to an infant each time he produces a sucking response whose amplitude exceeds a criterion, so as to study his ability to discriminate speech sound pairs; and **startle technique,** in which an infant's startle reflex (Moro's reflex) in response to auditory stimuli is utilized.

Békésy a. [G. von Békésy, Hungarian biophysicist in U.S., 1899–1972] Automatic audiometry in which a Békésy audiometer is used to determine threshold of hearing; the client makes two threshold tracings, one in which the tone is rapidly turned on and off (interrupted tone) and one in which the tone is presented steadily (continuous tone); results may be classified into one of five types, and may suggest middle-ear, cochlear, or cranial nerve VIII lesions. See also Békésy tracing types; *Audiometric Tests and Procedures* in appendices.

brainstem evoked response a. (BSER) See under electrophysiologic *audiometry.*

brief tone a. (BTA) Procedure that examines the relative threshold dif-

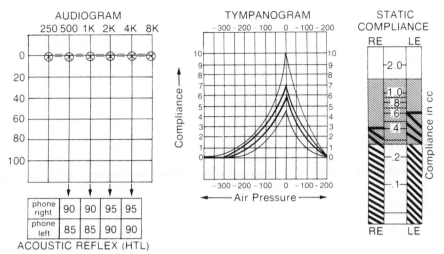

Normal audiogram, acoustic reflex, tympanogram, and static acoustic impedance.

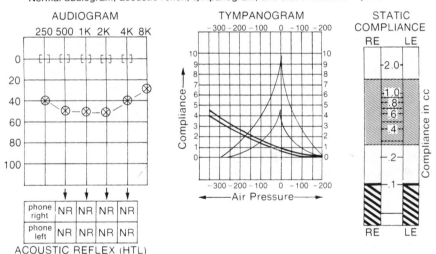

Acoustic Impedance

Abnormal configurations: audiogram shows conductive hearing loss, acoustic reflex shows no response of middle ear muscle, tympanogram shows a flat curve, and static acoustic impedance shows high impedance/low compliance. Such results can be found in cases of otitis media.

ferences among pulsed tones which vary in their duration; augments and supplements the findings of Békésy audiometry, and can be incorporated with it to achieve a degree of diagnostic accuracy greater than either alone provides.

cardiac evoked response a. (CERA)
See under electrophysiologic *audiometry*.

conditioned orientation reflex a. (COR) Procedure for assessing the auditory acuity of children two years of age and younger who cannot readily be conditioned to behavioral audiometry; based on the theory that a visual stimulus can reinforce auditory localization behavior in infants and young children.

delayed feedback a. (DFA) Procedure used to ascertain the presence of a functional hearing loss and an approximation of the true organic threshold by an experimentally imposed delay of auditory signals returning to the client's ears through headphones. Speech signals may be used in which the client, wearing earphones, reads aloud a measured passage in simultaneous feedback and then reads a matched passage in the delay condition; the signals also may be pure tones, using key tapping as a motor task. The client is instructed to tap a simple rhythmic pattern on an electromechanical key, which introduces bursts of pure tone to the client's ear with each tap; the pure-tone signal is then switched to the delay condition. This type of testing will cause the client to become dysfluent (during the testing procedures) or to forget the tapping pattern.

descending technique a. Method of establishing threshold of hearing by going from an audible to an inaudible stimulus.

diagnostic a. Measurement of hearing threshold levels to determine the nature and degree of hearing impairment; *e.g.*, conductive, sensorineural, or mixed.

electrodermal a. (EDA) See under electrophysiologic *audiometry.*

electrodermal response test a. (EDRA) Electrodermal audiometry. See under electrophysiologic *audiometry.*

electroencephalic a. (EEA) or **electroencephalic response a. (ERA)** See under electrophysiologic *audiometry.*

electrophysiologic a. Procedure using various types of objective audiometry designed to measure an individual's response to a sound stimulus.

Auditory evoked response (AER) is a type of electrophysiologic audiometry in which electrical activity evoked by sounds arising from the auditory portions of the peripheral or central nervous system are recorded with electrodes. AERs include **auditory brainstem response (ABR)**, in which electrical activity is evoked by very brief sounds from cranial nerve VIII and the brainstem; findings allow inference of hearing level and identification of site of lesion as the cochlea, cranial nerve VIII, or the brainstem. Syn: brainstem auditory evoked response (BAER), brainstem auditory evoked potential (BAEP), auditory brainstem evoked potential (ABEP), brainstem response (BSR), brainstem evoked response (BSER); **auditory middle latency response (AMLR)**, in which a series of waveforms occur from 10 to 80 ms after the onset of an auditory stimulus. It extends the assessment of the auditory system beyond the brainstem to the thalamocortical auditory pathway, and provides frequency-specific estimations of auditory sensitivity in older children and adults; **brainstem evoked response (BSER) audiometry** is a former term for auditory brainstem response (ABR) audiometry (see above). **Cardiac evoked response audiometry (CERA)** utilizes measurement of changes in heart activity that result from sound stimulus. **Electrocochleography (ECoG, ECochG)** measures electrical potential within the auditory system; as the auditory system is stimulated by an acoustic signal, it causes a change in the electrical potentials of the sensorineural mechanism that can be monitored through electrodes in place. It estimates hearing level and identifies cochlear, or occasionally eighth cranial nerve, site of lesion.

Electrodermal audiometry (EDA) is a method of determining hearing threshold by measuring changes in skin resistance, associated with a conditioned response to sound stimulus. Syn: electrodermal response test audiometry (EDRA); galvanic skin response audiometry (GSRA); psychogalvanic skin response audiometry (PGSRA).

Electroencephalic audiometry (EEA) or **electroencephalic response audiometry (ERA)** uses an electroencephalogram to measure and quantify changes in pattern resulting from sound stimulation; it is often used with young children.

Evoked response audiometry (ERA), electric response audiometry (ERA), or **average evoked response audiometry (AERA)** is a special type of electroencephalic audiometry considered by some to be a distinct variety of electrophysiologic audiometry; responses observed are electrical responses of the cerebral cortex which are recorded on the electroencephalograph. It does not require putting the subject to sleep.

evoked response a. (ERA) See under electrophysiologic *audiometry*.

galvanic skin response a. (GSRA) Electrodermal audiometry. See under electrophysiologic *audiometry*.

group a. Simultaneous testing of a group of persons in which the testing method, either pure tones or speech, is presented by a procedure in which each person may give reliable information as to the test items heard; usually used only in screening.

high-frequency a. Measurement, usually of thresholds, using tones of 10,000 Hz (frequencies above the range of conventional audiometers);

often used to monitor hearing levels of clients taking toxic drugs.

identification a. Screening *audiometry*.

industrial a. Audiometry to determine the effects of industrial noise exposure upon auditory abilities; involves testing, noise measurement, and protective device counseling.

live voice a. Presentation of a speech signal via a microphone for speech audiometric testing; the intensity of the examiner's voice is monitored visually by a VU meter. Syn: monitored live voice audiometry.

localization a. See visual reinforcement *audiometry*.

monitored live voice a. Live voice *audiometry*.

monitoring a. Periodic assessment of hearing sensitivity to determine whether any changes have occurred.

neonatal auditory response cradle a. Method that assesses the hearing of newborn infants; a narrow-band noise is presented to the ears via ear-insert devices and measurement of reflexive responses of the infant are recorded automatically.

play a. Any test in which a child is taught a play response to the stimulus, *e.g.*, dropping a block into a box when a tone is heard.

psychogalvanic skin response a. (PGSRA) Electrodermal audiometry. See under electrophysiologic *audiometry*.

pure-tone a. Audiometry utilizing tones of various frequencies and intensities as auditory stimuli to measure hearing; included are comparisons of results from testing air conduction and bone conduction.

Air conduction is tested by transmission of sounds, using earphones, through the outer and middle ears to determine auditory acuity; usually the first step in an audiological evaluation. See pure-tone air-conduction *threshold;* see also under conduction.

Bone conduction is tested by stimulation of the inner ear by placing a bone oscillator on the mastoid bone or forehead to determine whether the hearing loss is due to conductive and/or sensorineural factors. See pure-tone bone-conduction *threshold;* see also under conduction.

screening a. Rapid measurement of the hearing of groups of people against a predetermined limit of normalcy; auditory responses to different frequencies presented at a constant intensity level are tested, *e.g.,* 500, 1000, 2000, and 4000 Hz at 20 dB. Syn: sweep check test; identification audiometry.

Reduced screening audiometry uses 4000 Hz as a single monitor frequency to detect the beginning of hearing loss in hazardous noise exposure situations; a second frequency, usually 2000 Hz, is sometimes tested.

sound field localization a. See visual field localization *audiometry.*

speech a. Measurement of overall performance in hearing, understanding, and responding to speech for a general assessment of hearing and an estimate of the degree of practical handicap; earphones, bone oscillators, and sound field may be used.

Speech awareness is the hearing level at which the presence of a speech signal can be perceived. Syn: speech detection.

Speech discrimination (SD) is a measure of the ability to differentiate among various speech sounds; nonsense syllables, monosyllabic and multisyllabic words, and sentences may be presented to the client who is expected to repeat or point to them as an indicator of his ability to differentiate among sounds. The test is usually pre-

sented at 40-dB sensation level, at which the maximum discrimination ability should be obtained. The score is determined by the percentage of speech units repeated correctly. Syn: word discrimination score.

Speech reception (SR) is the minimum level at which one can repeat correctly 50% of the time a list of two syllable words presented with equal stress in each syllable (spondees).

sweep check test Screening *audiometry.*

tangible reinforcement operant conditioning a. (TROCA) Technique, used with mentally retarded or young children, that utilizes positive reinforcement (candy, cereal, toy) for appropriate responses and a mild punishment (time out) for false responses. The child's behavior is conditioned until he pushes a response button on a feeder box whenever he perceives a sound.

visual reinforcement a. Used with infants and young children (6 months to 2 years). The infant or child is conditioned to look for the movement of an object (*e.g.,* stuffed animal) after hearing a sound stimulus. Syn: sound field localization audiometry, localization audiometry.

audition (ô-di′shən) [L. hearing] The sense or act of hearing.

audito-oculogyric reflex See under reflex.

auditory (ô′-di-tôr-ē) Pertaining to the sense of hearing, as opposed to acoustic.

auditory acuity See under acuity.

auditory adaptation In audiology, an inability to maintain the audibility of a test tone. Syn: prestimulatory fatigue. See also tone decay.

auditory agnosia See under agnosia.

auditory alexia See under alexia.

auditory analysis Ability to separate a series of sounds that have been presented as a meaningful whole and to identify the component parts, *i.e.*, to perceive not only the auditory sequence but also the placement of sounds within the sequence. See also *Auditory Processes* table, under auditory processes.

Auditory Analysis Test See *Audiometric Tests and Procedures* in appendices.

auditory aphasia See under aphasia.

auditory area See temporal lobe, under cerebrum, under brain.

auditory attention See under attention.

auditory blending See under blending.

auditory brainstem evoked potential (ABEP) See under electrophysiologic *audiometry*, auditory brainstem response (ABR) audiometry.

auditory brainstem response (ABR) audiometry See under electrophysiologic *audiometry*.

auditory canal External auditory meatus. See under external *ear*.

auditory closure See under closure.

auditory cortex Auditory receiving area of the cerebral cortex located on the superior surface of the temporal lobe (transverse temporal gyri).

auditory cue Verbal expression used to aid communication; it may include stress, pitch, quality, intonation, and duration.

auditory differentiation Auditory figure-ground *discrimination*.

auditory discrimination See under discrimination.

Auditory Discrimination Test See *Auditory Tests and Procedures* in appendices.

auditory disorder Any difficulty, whether physical or psychological, in the reception or interpretation of sound stimuli.

auditory evoked potentials (AEP) The ability to record electrical potentials generated at various levels of the nervous system in response to acoustic stimulation.

auditory evoked response See under electrophysiologic *audiometry*.

auditory fatigue See under fatigue.

auditory feedback See under feedback.

auditory figure-ground See under figure-ground.

auditory figure-ground discrimination See under discrimination.

auditory flutter Awareness of a series of rapidly presented acoustic events as a series of events rather than as one continuous event.

auditory flutter fusion Perception of interrupted sound as one continuous sound.

auditory imperception Auditory *agnosia*.

auditory localization See under localization.

auditory memory See under memory.

auditory memory span See under memory span.

auditory method Acoustic method. See under aural rehabilitation.

auditory middle latency response See under electrophysiologic *audiometry*.

auditory modality Use of acuity, alertness, discrimination, memory, sequencing, and auditory-verbal ability to relate sound-symbol relationships.

auditory nerve See cranial nerves, VIII.

auditory pattern Order of speech sounds in syllables and words as determined by the rules of a particular language.

auditory perception See under perception.

auditory phonetics See under phonetics.

Auditory Pointing Test See *Auditory Tests and Procedures* in appendices.

auditory processes Specific skills such as discrimination, localization, auditory attention, auditory figure-ground, auditory closure, auditory discrimination, auditory blending, auditory analysis, auditory association, and auditory memory-sequential memory. Some authorities would include binaural fusion, binaural separation, and response to rapid transitions in acoustic signals. Syn: central auditory abilities, auditory skills, central auditory function, central auditory perception, central auditory processes.

AUDITORY PROCESSES IMPORTANT IN LANGUAGE AND LEARNING

Term	Process
Auditory analysis	Ability to identify phonemes or morphemes embedded in words
Auditory association	Ability to identify a sound with its source
Auditory attention	Ability to pay attention to auditory signals, especially speech, for an extended time
Auditory blending	Ability to synthesize isolated phonemes into words
Auditory closure	Ability to understand the whole word or message when part is missing
Auditory discrimination	Ability to discriminate among words and sounds that are acoustically similar Ability to differentiate among sounds of different frequency, duration, or intensity
Auditory figure-ground	Ability to identify a primary speaker from a background of noise
Auditory memory- 　sequential memory	Ability to store and recall auditory stimuli of different length or number in exact order
Binaural fusion	The ability to fuse into one sounds heard from two separate inputs
Binaural separation	Ability to attend to stimuli presented to one ear while ignoring stimuli presented to the opposite ear
Localization	Ability to localize the source of sound

auditory processing (AP) The ability to fully utilize what is heard. AP involves more than the perception of sound. It also involves a series of specific skills. See auditory processes.

auditory processing disorder 1. Impaired ability to attend, discriminate, recognize, or comprehend auditory information even though hearing and intelligence are within normal limits; more pronounced with distorted or competing speech, in noise, or in poor acoustic environments. Auditory processing abilities develop in parallel with language, and children with auditory processing disorders are a subset of those with receptive and/or expressive language disorders. **2.** Any breakdown in an individual's auditory skills that results in diminished learning through hearing, even though peripheral auditory sensitivity is normal.

auditory reflex Acoustic *reflex.*

auditory selective listening Auditory figure-ground *discrimination.*

auditory sequencing Ability to judge the proper order of sounds, syllables, and words; considered a fundamental auditory ability for understanding speech.

auditory skills Auditory processes.

auditory synthesis Cognitive integration of phonemes that have been presented separately, resulting in recognition of a syllable or a word; closely related to reading and spelling processes. Syn: phonemic synthesis, sound blending, vocal phonics.

auditory tests and procedures See appendices.

auditory training Process whereby the aurally handicapped person learns to take advantage of all acoustic cues available to him; designed to develop optimum use of residual hearing. See also aural rehabilitation.

auditory training units Specially designed hearing aids for training the hearing impaired in the use of hearing aids. The speaker's voice is fed into a nearby microphone, amplified, and directed to the listener through his receiver; the system provides high fidelity by producing a high signal-to-noise ratio.

Desk-type auditory trainer is a portable unit which contains a microphone, amplifier, and receiver; a major disadvantage of this type of unit is that as the speaker moves away from the receiving unit there is a reduction in the intensity of his voice, causing varying amplification levels for the listener.

Frequency-modulation (FM) auditory trainer is a commonly used classroom unit with which the speaker wears a microphone containing a transmitter; his voice is then broadcast by radio frequency to FM receivers worn by the listeners; it provides excellent mobility for both speaker and listener because neither is restricted by wires.

Hard-wire auditory trainer is a unit in which the listener's receiver is attached to a desk and the speaker's microphone is connected to an amplifier; mobility is restricted because the system is connected by wires.

Loop-induction auditory trainer is a unit in which the speaker uses a microphone connected to an amplifier; his voice is amplified and transferred to a telephone coil, and the listener receives the signal via a magnetic field; considerable mobility is provided for the listener, but he must remain within the magnetic field.

auditory tube Eustachian tube.

auditory verbal agnosia See under agnosia.

auditory-vocal association See under association.

auditory-vocal automaticity Ability to predict future linguistic events from past experience; implies automatic and correct responses to language; deficits in this ability are exhibited by difficulty with grammar, incorrect usage of small words, jumbled word order, and slowness with language processing skills.

augmentative and alternative communication (AAC) 1. Any approach designed to support, enhance, or supplement the communication of individuals who are not independent verbal communicators in all situations. Syn: alternative, nonoral, or nonvocal communication. **2.** An area of clinical practice that attempts to compensate (either temporarily or permanently) for the impairment and disability patterns of individuals with severe expressive communications disorders [ASHA, 1989]. **3.** The use of nonvocal instruments and approaches by those who cannot communicate vocally; includes picture boards and computer-assisted devices. Syn: nonoral or nonvocal communication.

aided a. c. Approaches that depend on a system or device of some kind, *e.g.*, Blissymbolics, rebus, communication boards, electronic devices.

unaided a. c. Approaches that rely on gestural communication, *e.g.*, American Manual Alphabet, American Sign Language, American Indian sign language, fingerspelling.

augmentative communication system Total communication system of an individual. It includes **communicative technique,** which serves to transmit information; **symbol set system,** which is the representational means through which information is conveyed; **communicative interaction,** which is the interindividual exchange necessary for the message to be transmitted and received.

aura (är′ə) [L. breeze, odor, glow] Subjective sensation which may precede an epileptic seizure.

aural (är′əl) [L. *auris*, ear] **1.** Pertaining

to the sensation of hearing. **2.** Pertaining to the ear.

aural atresia See under atresia.

aural rehabilitation Educational procedures used with hearing-impaired persons to improve the effectiveness of their overall communication ability. It includes the development and integration of existing receptive and expressive modalities (auditory, visual, tactile, and kinesthetic). Syn: audiologic habilitation, rehabilitative audiology. Although the communications techniques may be aural, visual, written, or oral, all are based on two methodologies: **1. Analytic method** stresses formal learning of the parts of the technique before assimilating the information into a whole or total picture. Syn: artificial, formal, logical, or systematic method. **2. Synthetic method** postulates that before a language principle is introduced formally, it should be used in natural (whole to part) situations through speech, reading, and writing. Syn: informal, mother, or natural method.

    Acoustic method is education in the use of the hearing mechanism, with or without amplified sound, for optimum effective utilization of residual hearing; procedures stress listening skills for differentiation of pitch, rhythm, accent, and inflection of sounds produced by voice or any sonorous instrument. Syn: auditory or acoupedic method. See also acoupedics.

    Grammatic method pertains to any one of a variety of specifically written programs to teach the hearing impaired the rules of grammar and syntax. Such systems categorize vocabulary items grammatically and syntactically, and offer continuity and consistency; rules may be applied orally or in writing. Some of these systems are Barry Five-Slate System, Bell's Visible Speech, Fitzgerald Key, Initial Teaching Alphabet, International Teaching Alphabet, Northampton Charts, Visual-Tactile System of Phonetic Symbolization, and Wing's symbol.

    Kinesthetic method is a technique used to develop an awareness of the movements of speech and to teach how these movements feel; it soon becomes a substitute for auditory awareness.

    Manual method is a means of nonverbal communication which includes fingerspelling and signs. Some authorities consider manual forms of communication to be part of aural rehabilitation; others do not. See also fingerspelling; French method; sign; sign *language*.

    Oral-aural method is the training of the hearing impaired to speak. They receive input through speechreading, kinesthesis, and amplification of sound, and express themselves through speech; gestures and signs are prohibited. Also referred to as oral communication (OC). Syn: bisensory method, German method.

    Simultaneous, combined, or **bimodal method** is the integration of the oral-aural and manual methods of aural rehabilitation for both expressive and receptive communication; communication simultaneously utilizes speech, sign, and/or fingerspelling. The Rochester method and cued speech are among specific techniques developed for implementation of this method.

    Speechreading or **lipreading** utilizes visual cues to determine what is being spoken, *i.e.*, comprehension of speech is accomplished through visual interpretation of lip and facial movements and of general body gestures.

    Analytic method teaches recognition of speech sounds in isolation, then in words, phrases, sentences, and paragraphs; proponents include Jena, Mueller-Walle, and

Bruhn (see their respective methods under the specific name).

Synthetic method teaches recognition of the meaning of whole paragraphs before breaking them into sentences, words, and sounds; proponents include Nitchie and Kinzie (see their respective method under the specific name).

Total communication (TC) is the philosophy of utilizing any or all communication methods (fingerspelling, sign, speech reading, oral, written, etc.) to enhance receptive and expressive communication.

auricle (är'i-kəl) [L. *auricula*] The most visible part of the ear; the concave elastic cartilaginous structure at-

tached to the surface of the skull. Syn: pinna. See under external *ear*.

auropalpebral (är-ō-pal′pē-brəl) Relating to the ear and eyelid (palpebra).

auropalpebral reflex (APR) See under reflex.

Austin Spanish Articulation Test See *Articulation Tests and Phonological Analysis Procedures* in appendices.

autism or **autistic disorder** (ô′ti-zəm) [G. *autos*, self] **1.** The essential features are the presence of markedly abnormal or impaired development in social interaction and communication and a markedly restricted repertoire of activity and interests. Manifestations of the disorder vary greatly depending on the developmental level and chrono-

---

DIAGNOSTIC CRITERIA FOR AUTISTIC DISORDER

A. A total of six (or more) items from (1), (2), and (3), with at least two from (1), and one each from (2) and (3):
   (1) Qualitative impairment in social interaction, as manifested by at least two of the following:
      (a) Marked impairment in the use of multiple nonverbal behaviors such as eye-to-eye gaze, facial expression, body postures, and gestures to regulate social interaction
      (b) Failure to develop peer relationships appropriate to developmental level
      (c) A lack of spontaneous seeking to share enjoyment, interests, or achievements with other people (*e.g.*, by a lack of showing, bringing, or pointing out objects of interest)
      (d) Lack of social or emotional reciprocity
   (2) Qualitative impairments in communication as manifested by at least one of the following:
      (a) Delay in, or total lack of, the development of spoken language (not accompanied by an attempt to compensate through alternative modes of communication such as gesture or mime)
      (b) In individual with adequate speech, marked impairment in the ability to initiate or sustain a conversation with others
      (c) Stereotyped and repetitive use of language or idiosyncratic language
      (d) Lack of varied, spontaneous make-believe play or social imitative play appropriate to development level
   (3) Restricted repetitive and stereotyped patterns of behavior, interests, and activities, as manifested by at least one of the following:
      (a) Encompassing preoccupation with one or more stereotyped and restricted patterns of interest that is abnormal either in intensity or focus
      (b) Apparently inflexible adherence to specific, nonfunctional routines or rituals
      (c) Stereotyped and repetitive motor mannerisms (*e.g.*, hand or finger flapping or twisting, or complex whole-body movement)
      (d) Persistent preoccupation with parts of objects
B. Delays or abnormal functioning in at least one of the following areas, with onset prior to age 3 years: (1) social interaction, (2) language as used in social communication, or (3) symbolic or imaginative play.
C. The disturbance is not better accounted for by Rett's disorder or childhood disintegrative disorder [DSM-IV].

logical age of the individual [DSM-IV].
2. Type of psychotic illness in children which is differentiated from childhood schizophrenia by virtue of early onset, and from mental deficiency by the evidence of isolated intellectual abilities [Kanner]. See infantile *autism* (Kanner's syndrome). See also childhood *schizophrenia;* aphasia.

    infantile a. Autism developing before three years of age and characterized by continual aloofness as opposed to withdrawal from reality, obsessive desire to maintain sameness, avoidance of eye contact with and lack of visual or auditory response to others, and marked preference for and facility with objects in contrast to interpersonal relationships and communication; although appearance, alertness, expressiveness, and motor coordination (with quick, skillful movements) seem normal, from infancy there is no physical reaching out, imitation of gestures or sounds, and use of speech to communicate; rate of occurrence is less than 1% in a general population. Syn: Kanner's syndrome. *Cf.* childhood *schizophrenia.*

    primary a. Autism considered to be psychogenic in origin and characterized by early onset, but with no apparent precipitating causes.

    secondary a. Autism regarded as organic in nature and characterized by a period of normal development, followed by an episode of great turbulence resulting in a period of withdrawal, regression, and rigidity, and finally a phase of partial recovery. See also childhood *schizophrenia.*

autistic (ô-tis′tik) **1.** Denoting a child with autism. **2.** Characteristic of autism.

autistic psychopathy Asperger's syndrome.

autistic spectrum disorder Pervasive developmental disorder.

auto- [G. *autos*, self] Prefix meaning self, name.

autoclitic (ô-tō-klit′ik) [auto- + G. *klino*, to make bend] Controlled within oneself.

autoclitic operant See under operant, verbal.

autogenic (ô-tō-jen′ik) [auto- + G. *genesis*, origin] Originating within oneself.

autoimmune Relating to an immune response by the body against one of its own tissue cells, or molecules.

autoimmune disease 1. A disease resulting from a disordered immune reaction in which antibodies are produced that damage parts of one's own body. **2.** In hearing, an injury to the inner ear and its neural elements that may occur as a result of inflammation in the absence of an identifiable infection: the body itself initiates the inflammatory process, attacking its own tissues as foreign so as to combat infection.

automatic audiometer See under audiometer.

automatic audiometry See under audiometry.

automatic gain control Automatic *volume control.*

automatic language See under language.

automatic speech See under speech.

automatic volume control (AVC) See under volume control.

automatism (ô-tom′ə-ti-zəm) [G. a happening of itself] Performance of an act without reflection of intent.

autonomic (ô-tō-nom′ik) [auto- + G. *nomos*, law] Denoting independence of external control, or control by cerebrospinal nerve centers.

autonomic nervous system See under nervous system.

autophonia (ô-tə-fō′nē-ə) [auto- + G. *phōnē*, sound] Condition produced by some middle ear or eustachian tube abnormalities in which an individual's voice seems to himself to be louder than normal.

auxiliary verb Any verb used with the main verb to show its voice and mood;

a verb form of *have*, *be*, or *do*. Syn: helping verb. See also modal, aspect.

AVC Automatic volume control.

Avellis syndrome [G. Avellis, Ger. laryngologist, 1864–1916] Ipsilateral paralysis of the vocal cords and soft palate, with loss of pain and temperature sensibility in the contralateral leg, trunk, arm, and neck, and in the skin over the scalp; results from lesion involving the origin of motor fibers of the vagus and glossopharyngeal nerves (cranial nerves X and IX), and the accessory nerves.

average (av′ėr-ij) **1.** General term applied to the various measures of central tendency *(q.v.)*. The three most widely used averages are the arithmetic mean (mean), the middle score in a distribution (median), and the score or value that occurs most frequently in a distribution (mode). When the term "average" is used without designation as to type, the most likely assumption is that it is the arithmetic mean. **2.** Typical or ordinary; sometimes used imprecisely to indicate a mean *(q.v.)*.

average evoked response audiometry (AERA) Evoked response audiometry. See under electrophysiologic *audiometry*.

avoidance (ə-voi′dəns) In stuttering, device(s) employed by the stutterer prior to the moment of stuttering in an attempt to prevent its occurrence; may include postponements, reformulations, use of synonyms, circumlocutions, vocalized or unvocalized pauses, or the complete refusal to speak. See also nonavoidance therapy.

axioversion See under teeth malpositions.

axon (aks′on) [G. *axon*, axis] See neuron.

β Second letter of the Greek alphabet, beta.

babbling (bab′liŋ) **1.** Prelinguistic verbal conduct of infants during the second half of the first year of life. **2.** Deliberate, volitional play and experimentation with sound by infants which begins about 4 months of age.

> **nonreduplicated b.** Babbling in which vowel, consonant-vowel, and even consonant-vowel-consonant syllables appear, and the consonants as well as the vowels may be different from one syllable to another; usually occurs between 9 and 18 months of age.

> **reduplicated b.** Production of series of consonant-vowel syllables in which the consonant is the same in every syllable; usually occurs between 25 and 50 weeks of age; *e.g.*, /ən ən ə/. Syn: canonical.

> **social b.** Utterances produced by an infant in response to similar sounds or speech stimulation from others; usually begins about 6 to 9 months of age.

Babinski reflex See under reflex.

baby talk Infantile perseveration.

back See under distinctive features.

background noise See under noise.

backing, backing to velars See under substitution, under phonological processes.

back phoneme See under phoneme.

back vowel See under vowel.

backward coarticulation See under coarticulation.

backward masking See under masking.

balance (bal′əns) **1.** Normal state of action and reaction between two or more body parts or organs; *e.g.*, upright posture is maintained by harmonious interreactions of muscles against gravity. **2.** Emotional equilibrium. See also equilibrium.

balance mechanism See inner *ear*.

ballistic movement 1. In articulation, a rapid skilled movement by which a consonant or vowel is produced with resonator adjustments and obstructions. **2.** Rapid movement of a body part, such as a hand, arm, or leg; a "throwing" in a certain direction by a muscular contraction that ceases before the excursion is completed, the full excursion being completed by momentum.

band A range of frequencies. For types of band, see specific term. See also band *frequency.*

band frequency See under frequency.

band-pass filter See under filter.

band spectrum Graphic representation of sound. See also sound spectrogram.

bandwidth 1. Range of frequencies within which a device will respond effectively; *e.g.*, in speech, the range of frequencies important for high-quality speech is about 100 to 10,000 Hz, roughly a bandwidth of 10,000 Hz. **2.** Frequencies included between specified cutoff frequencies. See also filter, and its subentries.

Bankson Language Screening Test—Second Edition See *Language Tests and Procedures* in appendices.

bar Measure referring to the pressure of one dyne per square centimeter.

barium swallow Evaluates the structure and the function of the esophagus and stomach. Barium is placed in the esophagus either by oral feeding or via nasogastric tube. Esophageal motility can be evaluated as the barium flows into the stomach. Fluoroscopy is used to view the images. See also swallow.

> **modified b. s.** The use of videofluoroscopy to evaluate the pharyngeal swallow. Used to determine whether or not aspiration is occurring; also shows the reason for the aspiration

and the point at which it occurs. Differs from the barium swallow in that the normal feeding situation is simulated and the area of interest is the pharynx. Syn: videofluoroscopic swallow study (VSS). See also swallow.

barotrauma (bār′ə-trä-mə) [G. *baros*, weight + *trauma*, wound] Injury to the middle ear caused by reduction of air pressure in the middle ear as a result of exposure to abnormal atmospheric pressure.

Barrett's Classification See under tongue thrust classifications.

Barry Five Slate System [Katherine E. Barry, 1899, Colorado School for the Deaf] In aural rehabilitation, a simple method of teaching the hearing impaired the grammatical and syntactic principles of language by analyzing the relationships among the parts of a sentence. Slates are provided to represent the five principal parts of a sentence: subject, verb, direct object, preposition, and object of the preposition. See also grammatic method, under aural rehabilitation.

basal (bā′səl) **1.** Denoting the lowest point; the point from which progress is recorded. **2.** In testing, denoting the level at which an individual passes all of the items on a test.

basal age The highest level, on tests standardized in mental age units, at which a subject passes all the items assigned to that level; it is then assumed that the subject could pass all of the items at lower levels; *e.g.*, with all items at a 24-month level passed, credit is given for the items preceding that level, even though the subject has not performed those items.

basal fluency See under fluency.

basal ganglia See cerebrum, under brain.

basal pitch See under pitch.

base component Categorical part which defines a sentence and the basic grammatical relations in that sentence; includes a lexical component with sub-

categorization rules within which are marked contextual constraints. See also sentence.

baseline (bās′līn) **1.** Starting point or level of functioning, obtained at the beginning of a treatment program, from which future progress and assessments are measured. **2.** Rate or frequency of a specified behavior prior to training or conditioning procedures. Syn: operant level.

base rule In transformational grammar, an ordered law which generates the terminal string of a sentence. See also deep *structure*.

base structure Deep *structure*.

base word See under word.

Basic Language Concepts Test See *Language Tests and Procedures* in appendices.

basic skill In education, a fundamental activity, mastery of which is necessary to allow progression to higher levels; such achievement also is deemed fundamental for functioning in everyday life; *e.g.*, speaking, reading, writing, arithmetic.

basilar membrane See under membrane.

basilect (bā′sə-lekt) Dialect that is significantly different from standard English; often found in subcultural groups who are not frequently exposed to standard English; *e.g.*, Black English, English spoken in ethnic settlements.

battery (bat′ėr-ē) **1.** Combination of materials for producing an electrical effect; may be composed of a single cell or a group of two or more cells which furnish electric current. **2.** Specific group of diagnostic tests.

Bayley Scales of Infant Development See *Psychological Measures and Tests* in appendices.

BC Bone conduction.

BCL Békésy comfortable loudness.

BD Behavior disorder; brain dysfunction.

beat 1. Acoustic phenomenon occurring when two sound waves pass through the same medium simultaneously at different frequencies, intensities, and phases, resulting in a third type of wave; the ear perceives as many beats per second as the frequency cycles of difference between the two tones; *e.g.*, similar frequencies of 2000 Hz and 2003 Hz reaching the ear simultaneously will produce three pulsations (beats) per second, the difference between the tones. **2.** Production of throbs of pulsations resulting from the summation and interference of sound waves. **3.** In electricity, the periodic variation in the amplitudes of some physical or electrical quantity (force, voltage, current, etc.) as a result of the interference between two waves of different frequency.

Bedside Evaluation Screening Test—Second Edition See *Language Tests and Procedures* in appendices.

behavior (bē-hā′vyėr) **1.** Any observable response by an individual viewed in terms of stimuli, response, and consequence. **2.** Any response emitted or elicited from an individual; may be nervous, muscular, or emotional. For types of behavior not listed below, see the specific term.

> **aberrant b.** Behavior that departs from what is considered normal.
>
> **adaptive b.** Effectiveness of the individual in adjusting to the natural and social demands of his environment; may be reflected in maturation, learning, or social development.
>
> **anticipatory b.** In stuttering, those beginning feelings, emotions, or attitudinal reactions that result from the stutterer's dread of feared sounds, words, situations, or interpersonal relationships.
>
> **incompatible b.** A response which cannot exist at the same time with another response; *e.g.*, flexing and extending the arm at the same time.
>
> **learned b.** Behavior that results from experience or interaction with others.

ADAPTIVE BEHAVIOR

Infancy and Early Childhood
  Sensorimotor skills development
  Communication skills (including speech and language)
  Self-help skills
  Socialization (development of ability to interact with others)
Childhood and Early Adolescence
  Application of basic academic skills in daily life activities
  Application of appropriate reasoning and judgment in mastery of environment
  Social skills (participation in group activities and interpersonal relationships)
Late Adolescence and Adult Life
  Vocational and social responsibilities and performance

> **operant b.** See operant *conditioning.*
>
> **random b.** Behavior that occurs without purpose, reason, or pattern.
>
> **social b.** Conduct which is influenced by the presence of others, *e.g.*, peers, society. See also *Developmental Sequences of Social Behavior* in appendices.
>
> **terminal b. 1.** Observable conduct or response acceptable as an indicator that a previously determined objective has been achieved; *e.g.*, speech and language skills demonstrable at the completion of therapy. **2.** Identification and naming the observable act that will be accepted as evidence that an objective has been achieved. **3.** The final act or achievement.

behavioral criterion 1. Standard or test by which terminal responses are evaluated. **2.** Method of defining the important characteristics of performance accuracy.

behavioral objective Performance objective.

behavioral observation audiometry (BOA) See under audiometry.

behavioral semantics See under semantics.

behaviorism (bē-hā′vyėr-izm) Theoretical view of behavior that relies on directly observable events and resists inferring underlying processes.

behavior modification 1. Procedure used to change an individual's response either by removing or reducing undesirable responses or by producing desirable ones; responses to be studied are carefully defined, observed on a regular schedule, recorded according to a planned system, and analyzed in terms of their environment. **2.** Theory which considers a maladaptive response as the problem rather than as a symptom of some underlying cause or need; overt behavior is to be changed rather than restructuring of the personality.

Békésy Ascending-Descending Gap Evaluation (BADGE) See *Audiometric Tests and Procedures* in appendices.

Békésy audiometer See under audiometer.

Békésy audiometry See under audiometry.

Békésy comfortable loudness (BCL) In audiometry, comparison of comfort levels for pulsed and continuous tones tracked on a Békésy audiometer. See also Békésy Comfortable Loudness Procedure in *Audiometric Tests and Procedures* in appendices.

Békésy Forward-Reverse Tracings See *Audiometric Tests and Procedures* in appendices.

Békésy tracing types [G. von Békésy, Hungarian biophysicist in U.S., 1899–1972] Threshold tracings recorded automatically by the individual in response to continuous and interrupted (pulse) tones; the interrupted tracing should normally parallel air-conduction thresholds. An interpretation of swing width (difference between audibility and inaudibility) and interweaving of the two tracings may yield any of five types of tracings.

Type I Interrupted and continuous tone tracings interweave with an allowed swing width of about 10 dB; typical of subjects with normal hearing or with a conductive impairment.

Type II Interrupted and continuous tracings interweave in the lower frequencies, but at about 1000 Hz the continuous tone tracing drops (becomes more difficult to hear) 5 to 20 dB below the interrupted tracing; swing width is narrower in the high frequencies, indicating that the subject is able to identify sharp distinctions between audibility and inaudibility with small intensity changes; typically seen with cochlear lesions.

Type III Less commonly found tracing in which the continuous tone tracing drops 40 to 50 dB below that for the interrupted tracing, even in low frequencies, and the interrupted tone tracing follows the pattern of the conventional audiogram; seen with lesions of the acoustic nerve (cranial nerve VIII).

Type IV Similar to Type II except that the continuous tone drops 5 to 20 dB below the interrupted tone throughout the frequency range; typically seen with lesions of the acoustic nerve (cranial nerve VIII).

Type V Continuous tone tracing appears to be more easily heard than the interrupted tone; indicative of a nonorganic hearing loss.

bel [Alexander Graham Bell, U.S. inventor, 1847–1922] **1.** Unit used to express the ratio of acoustic or electrical power. **2.** Logarithmic unit which serves as the basic reference for the precise measurement of intensity; the number of bels is the logarithm to the base 10 of the power ratio; *e.g.*, 10 decibels equal 1 bel.

belch 1. Method utilizing air expelled from the stomach to create alaryngeal speech. **2.** Audible escape of gas from the stomach through the mouth. Syn: burp.

bell-shaped curve Normal *distribution.*

Bell's palsy [Sir C. Bell, Scottish physician, 1774–1842] Unilateral paralysis

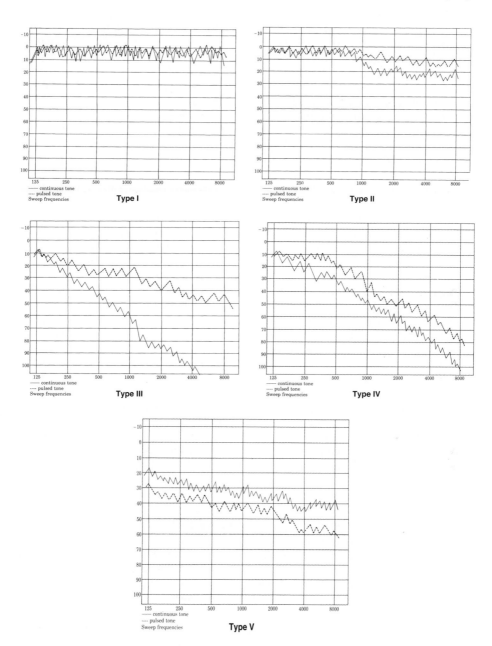

Békésy Tracings

of the face due to a lesion of the facial nerve (cranial nerve VII); characteristics include distorted speech, excessive lacrimation, and distorted features; adults are most commonly affected, and spontaneous recovery usually occurs within several weeks.

Bell's Visible Speech [A.G. Bell, 1891] In aural rehabilitation, a grammatical method in which consonants are represented by four fundamental curves that relate to various positions of the tongue and lips. Insertion of an additional mark indicates voicing of a consonant (*e.g.*, a′ for /k/, **ȧ** for /g/); vowels are represented by fundamental symbols. See also grammatic method, under aural rehabilitation.

benign (bə-nīn′) [L. *benignus*, kind] Denoting a nonmalignant neoplasm (tumor); *i.e.*, one which may displace neighboring tissue but does not invade and destroy it, and is not likely to recur after removal.

Bernoulli effect [D. Bernoulli, Swiss mathematician, 1700–1782] In voice, a consequence which, when applied to phonation, states that vibrations and closure of the vocal folds are the result of an inward sucking movement caused by a rapid flow of air moving through the vocal fold margins; produces a negative pressure and causes the folds to be pulled together.

Bernoulli's law or **principle** [D. Bernoulli, Swiss mathematician, 1700–1782] Velocity of flow of a gas or fluid through a tube is inversely related to its pressure against the side of the tube; *i.e.*, velocity is greatest and pressure lowest at a point of constriction.

beta rhythm or **waves** See under electroencephalogram.

bi- [L.] Prefix denoting two, both, double.

bibliotherapy (bib′lē-ō-thăr′ə-pē) [G. *biblion*, book + *therapeia*, medical treatment] Training exercise which utilizes reading; it is used (a) in stuttering therapy to allow the patient some freedom from stuttering and to allow concentration on various control techniques being utilized, and (b) in voice and articulation therapy to aid in carryover.

BICROS Bilateral contralateral routing of signals.

bicuspid teeth See under teeth.

bifid (bī′-fid) [L. *bifidus*] Divided into two parts; e.g., as a cleft of the uvula.

bifid tongue Diglossia.

bifurcation (bī-fėr-kā′shən) [bi- + L. *furca*, forked] Division or forking into two branches as of the trachea into the two bronchi.

bilabial (bī-lā′bē-əl) [bi- + L. *labia*, lips] Pertaining to the two lips.

bilabial area See under consonant, place of articulation.

bilateral (bī-lat′ėr-əl) [bi- + L. *latus*, side] Pertaining to two sides.

bilateral abductor paralysis See abductor paralysis, under laryngeal motor *paralysis.*

bilateral adductor paralysis See adductor paralysis, under laryngeal motor *paralysis.*

bilateral cleft lip See under cleft lip.

bilateral cleft palate See under cleft palate.

bilateral contralateral routing of signals (BICROS) See contralateral routing of signals (CROS), under hearing aid.

bilateral laryngeal paralysis See under paralysis.

bilingual (bī-liŋ′gwəl) Denoting bilingualism.

bilingualism (bī-liŋ′gwəl-ism) [bi- + L. *lingua*, tongue] Ability to utilize two languages with equal facility, especially speaking each with fluency and with a native-speaker accent.

    active b. Speaking, reading, writing, and understanding two languages, with both utilized.

    passive b. Speaking, reading, writing, and understanding one language while having knowledge of and understanding another language but not utilizing it.

Bilingual Syntax Measure (BSM) See

Language Tests and Procedures in appendices.

bimodal method Simultaneous method. See under aural rehabilitation.

binary (bī′när-ē) [L. *binarius*, consisting of two] **1.** Compounded of two elements. **2.** Separating into two branches.

binary principle A (+) or (−) value system which indicates that in a particular phoneme a feature may require more articulatory or perceptual effort than it does in a phoneme in which it is unmarked; a feature is a function of other features in a grouping and involves the effect of features on each other within the context of various phonemes in which they are present; *e.g.*, labial-nonlabial, nasal-oral. Syn: markedness theory. See also distinctive features; consonant; phoneme; vowel.

binaural (bī-nä′rəl) [L. *bini*, pair + *auris*, ear] **1.** Pertaining to the two ears. **2.** Pertaining to the two ears functioning together, as in normal hearing.

binaural CROS See contralateral routing of signals (CROS), under hearing aids.

binaural fusion Phenomenon by which a single sound is heard for two separate inputs; *e.g.*, in normal listening, the signals reaching the ears are similar but not quite identical, yet are heard as one sound. Syn: binaural integration or resynthesis. See also *Auditory Processes* table.

binaural hearing aid See under hearing aid.

binaural integration Binaural fusion.

binaural resynthesis Binaural fusion.

binaural separation Attending to stimuli presented to one ear while ignoring stimuli presented to the opposite ear. See also *Auditory Processes* table.

binaural summation **1.** Cumulative effect of sound reaching both ears which results in a threshold of about 3 dB lower than that of the better ear alone. **2.** Process of fusing two parts of a message, each part delivered to one ear and each insufficient for understanding, into a meaningful whole.

Bing Test See *Audiometric Tests and Procedures* in appendices.

bio- [G. *bios*, life] Combining form denoting life.

biofeedback See under feedback.

biolinguistic theory Nativist theory. See under language theories.

biological act Behavior of adaptation to the physical environment and its organization.

birth cry Reflexive vocalization of a newborn baby; may resemble a nasalized /ae/ sound.

bisensory method Oral-aural method. See under aural rehabilitation.

bisyllable (bī′sil-ə-bəl) **1.** Word with two syllables. **2.** Word with two syllables having equal stress on each syllable. Syn: disyllable. See also spondee, under word.

bite The forcible closure of the lower teeth against the upper teeth; to seize or grasp with the teeth.

   mature b. The teeth close easily on food, biting through it gradually. This is followed by an easy release of the food for chewing. Syn: sustained bite, controlled bite.

   phasic b. 1. A rhythmic bite and release pattern seen as a series of jaw openings and closings occurring when the gums or teeth are stimulated. Present at birth and continues at an automatic level until 3 to 5 months of age in the normal infant when it is gradually replaced by a more controlled bite. **2.** A term used to describe primitive movements found in the young infant and retained in many children with cerebral palsy or developmental delays.

   tonic b. 1. A forceful or tense biting pattern that interferes with all aspects of feeding. **2.** A strong closure of the jaw when the teeth or gums are stimulated. It is often difficult to release the bite and open the mouth after the tonic bite has been elicited. **unsustained b.** A closing of the teeth on food, followed by a hesitation and a new attempt to bite through the food. Biting through the food in a smoothly graded fashion does not occur.

Black English Ebonics.

blade of the tongue See tongue.

blending 1. The way speech flows from word to word within phrases. **2.** In stuttering, a technique used by stutterers to gradually shift from one part of the sound to the next.

> **auditory b.** Capacity to combine the phonemes of a word produced with pauses/hesitations between them into the entire word, *e.g.*, t-e-l-e-ph-o-n, d-o-g. See also *Auditory Processes* table.

blends See *consonant* cluster.

Blissymbolics (blis'sim-bol'iks) [C. Bliss] Graphic, meaning-based communica-

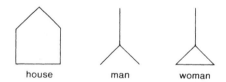

house   man   woman

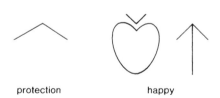

protection   happy

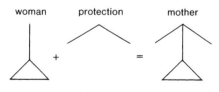

woman   protection   mother

Blissymbolics

tion system capable of conveying aspects of human experience; basic symbol elements, pictographs and ideographs, can be used to construct compound symbols, giving the system the potential to provide a large vocabulary. See also aided *augmentative communication.*

> **ideographs** Symbols representing ideas.

> **pictographs** Symbols that look like the things they represent.

block In stuttering: **1.** Stoppage or obstruction at one or several locations—larynx, lips, tongue, etc.—experienced by the stutterer when trying to talk which temporarily prevents smooth sound production. **2.** Speech behavior that occurs at the moment of stuttering; may be clonic or tonic.

> **clonic b.** In stuttering, a block characterized by repetitions.

> **tonic b.** In stuttering, a block characterized by complete fixation, prolongations, or hesitations.

Blom-Singer tracheoesophageal prosthesis [E. D. Blom, U.S. speech clinician, *1945; M. I. Singer, U.S. otolaryngologist, *1945] Surgical procedure during laryngectomy in which a plastic tube is fitted into the upper throat to serve as the new vocal sound source.

BOA Behavioral observation audiometry.

Bobath method [K. and B. Bobath, 1950] **1.** A form of therapy utilized with individuals who have central nervous system disorders resulting in abnormal movement. The treatment approach attempts to initiate or refine the normal stages and processes in the development of movement. **2.** Technique of rehabilitation based on resistance-traction; reflexive movements are inhibited by changing the message transmitted through the feedback system; attempts are made to eliminate inaccurate sensory motor signals, correct distorted movements, shut out excess motion, and elaborate useful patterns of posture and movement. Syn: neuro-development treatment (NDT).

body baffle effect Change in the response of a body-level hearing aid when worn on the body, as opposed to its response when not on the body.

body hearing aid See under hearing aid.

body image 1. Mental picture one has of his own body derived from internal sensations, postural changes, contact with outside objects and people, emotional experiences, and fantasies; how one sees oneself. **2.** Awareness of one's own body and the relationship of the body parts to each other and to the outside environment. **3.** In voice, the acquisition of a vocal quality and pitch that reflects an individual's self-image; *e.g.*, a young man imagines himself to be older and lowers the pitch of his voice to reflect this image.

body language See under language.

body of the tongue See tongue.

Boehm Test of Basic Concepts—Third Edition See *Language Tests and Procedures* in appendices.

Boehm Test of Basic Concepts, Pre-school—Third Edition See *Language Tests and Procedures* in appendices.

bolus 1. Food which, having been masticated and mixed with saliva and mucus, passes into and through the digestive tract. **2.** The rounded mass of food prepared by the mouth for swallowing.

bombarding Simultaneously utilizing more than one modality to present a stimulus; *e.g.*, using auditory, tactile, and visual channels together to teach a speech sound.

bone [A.S. *bān*] A type of connective tissue that constitutes the majority of the skeleton. It is composed of an organic component (cells and matrix) and an inorganic component (primarily calcium phosphate and carbonate) which gives rigidity to the structure. For various bones, see specific terms. For bones of the skull, see under skull.

bone conduction 1. See under conduc-tion. **2.** See under pure-tone *audiometry.*

bone-conduction hearing aid See under hearing aid.

bone-conduction oscillator Device for conveying mechanical vibration to the mastoid process or other parts of the head in a bone conduction test. Syn: bone-conduction vibrator.

bone-conduction receiver See under receiver. See also bone-conduction *hearing aid.*

bone-conduction vibrator Bone-conduction oscillator.

bonelet A small bone; often used to refer to the ossicles of the middle ear.

bony labyrinth See under labyrinth.

bore Hole made in the earmold of a hearing aid which allows passage of amplified sound into the ear canal. See also vent.

borrowing In linguistics, a process whereby one language absorbs words and expressions (sometimes also sounds and grammatical forms) from another language, and adapts them into its own use; may be with or without phonetic or semantic adaptation; *e.g.*, Eng. mother from L. mater.

Boston Assessment of Severe Aphasia See *Language Tests and Procedures* in appendices.

Boston Diagnostic Aphasia Examination See *Language Tests and Procedures* in appendices.

Boston University Speech Sound Discrimination Test See *Auditory Tests and Procedures* in appendices.

Bo-Tox botulinum toxin.

botulinum A powerful toxic agent which causes botulism in humans.

Botulinum (Bo-Tox) injection The use of Bo-Tox injections as a treatment, not a cure, for adductor and abductor spasmodic dysphonia. Bo-Tox is injected into the thyroarytenoid muscle as a treatment procedure for adductor spasmodic dysphonia. This treatment may last up to three months with a gradual return of spasmodic symptoms. Abductor spasmodic dysphonia is more difficult to treat. It has been reported that Bo-Tox has been injected into the posterior cricoarytenoid muscle or into the cricothyroid muscle. Success of the treatment for abductor spasmodic dysphonia is unreliable.

botulism Food poisoning.

bounce In stuttering: **1.** Easy, voluntary repetition of the first sound or syllable of a word; *e.g.*, b-b-b-b-baby. **2.** Technique used to modify a stuttering pattern.

bound morpheme See under morpheme.

bowed vocal folds See under vocal folds.

bradykinesia (bra-di-ki-nē′zē-ə, -zhə) [G. *bradys*, slow + *kinēsis*, movement] A specific impairment of motor activity distinguished from weakness or paresis in that (a) once initiated, motor movements attain full strength and (b) under certain conditions, including surprise or fright, movements are normal in terms of speed and agility.

bradykinesthetic (bra-di-kin-es-thet′-ik) **1.** Characterized by slow movement. **2.** Relating to bradykinesia.

bradylalia (bra-di-lā′lē-ə) [G. *bradys*, slow + *lalia*, talking] Abnormally slow utterances.

brain [A.S. *braegen*] That portion of the central nervous system composed of soft spongy nerve tissue occupying the cranial cavity; there are three basic subdivisions: cerebrum, cerebellum, and brainstem. It contains the nerve centers for correlation and integration of stimuli from sensory and motor impulses and for regulation of body system functions.

    brainstem The smallest portion of the brain composed of the midbrain, pons, and medulla oblongata; the diencephalon is included by some authorities. It serves as the connection between the spinal cord and the cerebrum.

        Diencephalon (dī-en-sef′ə-lon) [G. *dia*, through + *enkephalon*, brain]

is located between the cerebral hemispheres beneath the corpus callosum; it serves as a relay and integration center for sensory impulses (except that of smell) to cortical areas and is also concerned with regulating visceral, endocrine, metabolic, and autonomic functions as well as various body cycles, rhythms, and reflexes.

        Medulla oblongata (mə-dəl′ə ob-loŋ-gä′tə) [L. marrow, fr. *medius*, middle] tapers from the pons to the spinal cord. Here the sensory and motor trunk nerves cross over (decussate) from right to left and left to right, which explains the right cerebral hemisphere's control of the left side of the body and the left cerebral hemisphere's control of the right side of the body. It also has centers activating the cardiovascular and respiratory systems, and from it emerge the glossopharyngeal, vagus, spinal accessory, and hypoglossal nerves (cranial nerves IX, X, XI, and XII).

        Midbrain, connecting the diencephalon and pons, is a short narrow pillar containing a center for visual reflexes.

        Pons (ponz) [L. bridge] is a bulbous structure which connects the midbrain and medulla oblongata, and from which the trigeminal, abducens, facial, and vestibulocochlear nerves (cranial nerves V, VI, VII, and VIII) emerge.

    cerebellum (sār-ə-bel′əm) [L. dim. of *cerebrum*, brain] That portion of the brain located at the posterior base of the cranial cavity beneath the occipital and temporal lobes of the cerebrum, from which it is separated by a membrane (tentorium). It is attached to the medulla, pons, and midbrain of the brainstem by three pairs of tracts that connect it with the cerebrum, brainstem, and spinal cord and enable it to coordinate body motor func-

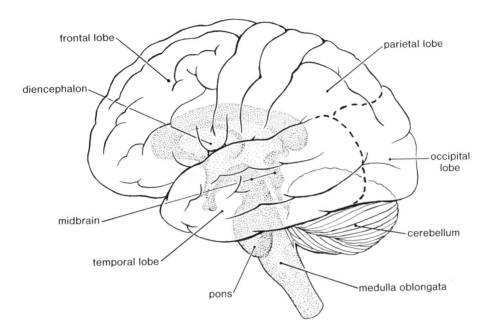

Brain and Brainstem

tion initiated by the cerebrum and to maintain muscle tone and equilibrium.

cerebrum (sa-rē′brəm, săr′ə-) [L. brain] Largest portion of the brain, consisting of paired right and left *hemispheres* united by the corpus callosum beneath the longitudinal fissure. Each hemisphere consists of an outer, highly convoluted, gray cortex, an underlying medullary mass of white matter, and a collection of deeply buried neuronal masses (basal ganglia). The **cortex** is divided by sulci and gyri into four lobes, each of which has areas with specific sensory or motor activities; it is the thinking and reasoning part of the brain that receives sensory input and directs conscious body responses. The **white matter** contains numerous fibers that convey impulses to and from the cortex to other areas, that interconnect various cortical regions of the same hemisphere,

and that interconnect corresponding cortical regions of both hemispheres. The **basal ganglia** and related nuclei play an important role in conducting motor function as mediated by cortical neurons. The **lobes** of each hemisphere of the cerebral cortex, frontal, occipital, parietal, and temporal, are named after the overlying bones of the skull and are demarcated by sulci and gyri; each lobe has areas with specific sensory or motor activities.

Frontal lobe is the largest lobe, at the front of the cerebral hemisphere bounded posteriorly by the central sulcus and laterally by the lateral sulcus. Its precentral gyrus and anterior bank of the central sulcus constitute the primary motor area for all parts of the body; Broca's area in the inferior frontal gyrus of the dominant (usually left) hemisphere is concerned with motor mechanisms of speech production.

Occipital lobe is the smallest lobe, at the rear of the cerebral hemisphere posterior to the occipitoparietal sulcus; it contains the primary visual area on its medial aspect.

Parietal lobe is the medial and upper lateral aspects of the cerebral hemisphere bounded anteriorly by the central sulcus, posteriorly by the occipitoparietal sulcus, and laterally by the lateral sulcus; its postcentral gyrus and posterior bank of the central sulcus constitute the primary somesthetic area, responsible for reception and integration of tactile and kinesthetic (proprioceptive) sensory impulses from all parts of the body.

Temporal lobe is the lower lateral aspect of the cerebral hemisphere bounded anteriorly and laterally by the lateral sulcus; the transverse temporal gyri (Heschl's gyri) on its inner bank of the lateral sulcus constitute the primary auditory area (Brodmann's area 41) concerned with the sensations and meaning of hearing.

brainstem See under *brain.*

brainstem auditory evoked potential (BAEP) See under electrophysiologic *audiometry*, auditory brainstem response (ABR).

brainstem auditory evoked response (BAER) See under electrophysiologic *audiometry*, auditory brainstem response (ABR).

brainstem evoked response (BSER) See under electrophysiologic *audiometry*, auditory brainstem response (ABR).

brainstem response (BSR) See under electrophysiologic *audiometry*, auditory brainstem response (ABR).

branches In transformational grammar, lines used in a branching tree diagram, *q.v.*

branching steps In programmed therapy,

a series of optional procedures which are decided upon on the basis of an individual's performance during an earlier part of the program.

branching tree diagram [semblance to inverted tree without a trunk] Graphic representation of a derivation of a sentence, similar to diagramming in traditional grammar; structurally consists of **branches** (lines that connect the nodes) which represent the rewrite rules and **nodes** (dots connecting the branches) which represent the constituent parts of the sentence. See also derivation of a sentence.

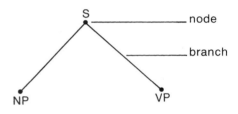

Branching Tree Diagram
S, sentence; NP, noun phrase; VP, verb phrase.

breakdown theory See under stuttering theories.

breaking See under phonological processes.

breath chewing Therapy technique which combines vocalizations with free chewing movements; movements, overt at first, are replaced with only the thought of the motion. It stresses relaxation of the oral musculature, and is used in stuttering therapy to ease stuttering blocks and in voice therapy to help change the pitch. Syn: chewing method.

breathiness See under voice disorders of phonation.

breathing (brēTH'iŋ) Respiration (1). For types of breathing, see specific terms. See also entries under respiration.

breathing disorder See respiration disorder.

breathing method Inhalation method. See

under speech, methods of esophageal speech.

breath stream Current of exhaled air released from the lungs and used to activate the vocal folds.

Brief Test of Head Injury See *Language Tests and Procedures* in appendices.

brief tone audiometry See under audiometry.

Briquet's syndrome [P. Briquet, Fr. physician, 1796–1881] Aphonia and shortness of breath due to hysterical paralysis of the diaphragm.

Brissaud-Marie syndrome [E. Brissaud, Fr. physician, 1852–1909; P. Marie, Fr. physician, 1853–1940] Unilateral spasm of the tongue and lips, of a hysterical nature.

broad transcription Phonemic *transcription*.

Broca's aphasia See under aphasia.

Broca's area [P. Broca, Fr. neurologist, 1824–1880] Motor speech area in the inferior frontal gyrus of the dominant (usually left) cerebral hemisphere; concerned with the elaboration and organization of motor speech patterns. Syn: Brodmann's area 44.

Brodmann's area 41 [K. Brodmann, Ger. neurologist, 1868–1918] Transverse temporal gyri in the parietal temporal area of the cerebral cortex; it is associated with auditory perception.

Brodmann's area 44 Broca's area.

bronchi, sing. **bronchus** [broŋ'kē, -kəs] [G. *bronchos*, windpipe] Primary divisions of the trachea which divide opposite the third dorsal vertebra and penetrate the lungs, one for the right lung and the other for the left lung; serve to convey air to and from the lungs.

bronchial respiration See under respiration.

brownian motion or **movement** [R. Brown, Eng. botanist, 1773–1858] **1.** Movement of air particles as they are affected by heat in the environment. **2.** Constant colliding movement of mole-

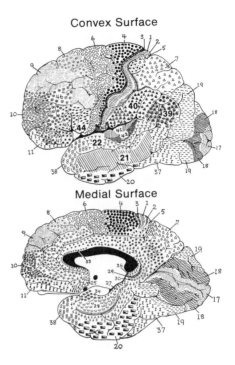

Convex Surface

Medial Surface

Brodmann's Areas
Cytoarchitectural map of the human cortex (after Brodmann, 1909). Note Brodmann's area 41, 44 (Broca's area), and 22, 39, and 40 (Wernicke's area). From Carpenter, MB, and Sutin, J. *Human Neuroanatomy,* 8th ed. Baltimore: Williams & Wilkins, 1982.

cules in a solid, liquid, or gaseous medium.

Bruhn method [M. Bruhn, 1902] In aural rehabilitation, analytic method of speechreading based on close observation of the movements of the lips from one sound position to another. See also speechreading, under aural rehabilitation.

bruxism (brəks'izm) [G. *brucho*, to grind the teeth] Clenching of the teeth associated with forceful lateral or protrusive jaw movements, resulting in rubbing, gritting, or grinding together of the teeth; usually occurs during sleep.

BSER Brainstem evoked response audiometry.

BTA Brief tone audiometry.

buccal (bə′kəl) [L. *buccus*, cheeks] Pertaining to or adjacent to the cheek.

buccal cavity Irregular space between the teeth and cheeks; distinct from the oral cavity, which is bounded externally by the teeth.

buccal speech See under alaryngeal *speech*.

buccal whisper See under whisper.

buccolabial (bək-ə-lā′bē-əl) Pertaining to the cheek and the lip.

buccoversion Facioversion. See under teeth malpositions.

bulbar (bəl′bėr) [L. *bulbus*, a bulbous root] Relating to or resembling a bulb; especially with reference to the medulla oblongata.

bulbar paralysis See under paralysis.

burp Belch.

AaBbCcDdEeFfGgHhIiJjKk
kLlMmNnOoPpQqRrSsTtUu
UuVvWwXxYyZzAaBbCcDd
EeFfGgHhIiJjKkLlMmNnOo

C Cathode; Celsius; Centigrade.

CA Chronological age.

Ca Cathode.

calibrate (kal′ə-brāt) **1.** Process of adjusting the values of the readings given by an instrument, in terms of a known standard. **2.** In audiology, reconciliation of the intensity levels of an audiometer to correspond with the levels of its headphones. **3.** Adjustment of a hearing aid to a predetermined response slope of intensity.

California Consonant Test See *Auditory Tests and Procedures* in appendices.

callosal disconnection syndrome See under aphasia.

Caloric Test See *Audiometric Tests and Procedures* in appendices.

canal (kə-nal′) [L. *canalis*] A duct, channel, or tubular structure.

anterior vertical c. See semicircular canals, under inner *ear.*

auditory c. External auditory meatus. See under external *ear.*

ear c. External auditory meatus. See under external *ear.*

horizontal c. See semicircular canals, under inner *ear.*

internal auditory c. Internal auditory meatus. See under inner *ear.*

lateral c. See semicircular canals, under inner *ear.*

posterior vertical c. See semicircular canals, under inner *ear.*

semicircular c.'s See under inner *ear.*

vestibular c. Scala vestibuli. See cochlea, under inner *ear.*

canal caps Semiaurals. See under hearing protection device.

canal hearing aid See under hearing aid.

cancellation (kan-sə-lā′shən) In stuttering: **1.** Method used by a stutterer to respond to the moment of stuttering; a deliberate pause is followed by a second utterance of the word in which a different and more fluent form of stuttering is attempted. This method does not ensure fluency on the second attempt; rather, it produces a method of attacking the block. This procedure may be referred to as "post-block" correction. **2.** Deliberate pause after a stuttered word, and then a reproduction of that word before proceeding to the next word. **3.** In acoustics, the reduction of the amplitude of a sound wave to zero; this results when two tones of the same frequency and amplitude are introduced 180 degrees out of phase.

cancer (kan′sėr) [L. crab] Any malignant tumor, including carcinoma and sarcoma.

canine teeth See under teeth.

cannula (kan′yə-lə) [L. dim. of *canna*, reed] **1.** Tube for surgical purposes, usually with a cutting instrument at one end. **2.** Tracheotomy tube fitting through the open stoma and extending into the trachea.

CANS Central auditory nervous system.

capacitance (kə-pas′i-təns) **1.** Quantity of electric charge that may be stored on a body per unit electric potential. **2.** Ability to store energy in the form of an electric charge.

capacitor (kə-pas′i-tėr) **1.** Device consisting of two electrodes, or sets of electrodes in the form of plates, separated from each other by a dielectric; used to store and control electrical energy, or as part of a frequency filter system. **2.** Device for holding a charge of electricity. Syn: condenser.

capacity (kə-pas′i-tē) [L. *capax*, able to contain] Potential volume of a cavity or receptacle. For types of capacity, see specific term.

carcinoma (kär-si-nō′mə) [G. *karkinos*, cancer + *-oma*, tumor] Any of various types of malignant tumors derived from epithelial tissue.

cardiac evoked response audiometry (CERA) See under electrophysiologic *audiometry.*

cardinal vowels See under vowel.

Cargot ear (kā-gō′) [a people in the Pyrenees, among whom physical defects are common] Absence of the lobule of the auricle.

Carhart notch [R. Carhart, 1950] Dip on a bone conduction audiogram of 5 dB at 500 and 4000 Hz, 10 dB at 1000 Hz, and 15 dB at 2000 Hz; observed in otosclerosis; not attributed to cochlear impairment but to the inability of fluids to move freely in the cochlea when the footplate of the stapes is firmly fixed in the oval window.

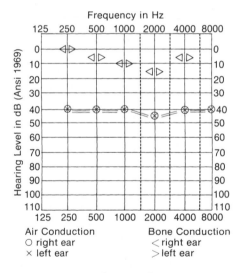

Carhart Notch

caries (kār′ēz) [L. dry rot] Molecular destruction of teeth; tooth decay.

Carrell Discrimination Test See *Auditory Tests and Procedures* in appendices.

carrier phrase Phrase which precedes the stimulus word during speech audiometry; designed to prepare the client for the test word and to assist the clinician (if monitored live voice is used) in controlling the input loudness of the test word; *e.g.,* "Now say . . . "

Carrow Auditory-Visual Abilities Test See *Auditory Tests and Procedures* in appendices.

Carrow Elicited Language Inventory (CELI) See *Language Tests and Procedures* in appendices.

carryover In speech, the habitual use of newly learned speech or language techniques in everyday situations. Syn: habituation (3).

carryover coarticulation Forward *coarticulation.*

cartilage (kär′tə-lij) [L. *cartilago*, gristle] Firm fibrous connective tissue that does not contain blood vessels.

   arytenoid c.'s Paired laryngeal cartilages, somewhat pyramidal in shape, that rest on the upper border of the cricoid cartilage and are attached to the posterior end of the vocal folds; the vocal folds are approximated by muscles attached to these cartilages.

   corniculate c.'s Paired laryngeal cartilages which appear as small horn-like nodules at the apex of each arytenoid cartilage; they assist in reducing the laryngeal opening during swallowing.

   cricoid c. Ring-shaped cartilage which lies directly below the thyroid cartilage and forms a complete ring around the larynx below the vocal folds; regarded as the foundation or base of the larynx.

   cuneiform c.'s Paired wedge-shaped laryngeal cartilages located in the aryepiglottic folds anterior to the corniculate cartilages; serve to tense or stiffen the aryepiglottic folds.

   thyroid c. Largest of the laryngeal cartilages which forms an anterior wall for the larynx and protects its interior; consists of two halves united at an angle called the laryngeal prominence.

case 1. Property of nouns, pronouns, or adjectives shown by changes in the form of the words, whether they are

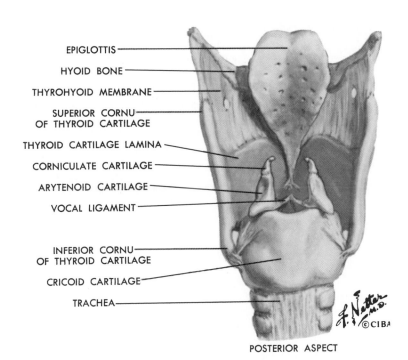

EPIGLOTTIS

HYOID BONE

THYROHYOID MEMBRANE

SUPERIOR CORNU
OF THYROID CARTILAGE

THYROID CARTILAGE LAMINA

CORNICULATE CARTILAGE

ARYTENOID CARTILAGE

VOCAL LIGAMENT

INFERIOR CORNU
OF THYROID CARTILAGE

CRICOID CARTILAGE

TRACHEA

POSTERIOR ASPECT

Cartilages of the Larynx

functioning as subjects (**nominative** or **subjective case**), as complements (**accusative** or **objective case**), or as modifiers (**possessive or genitive case**); *e.g.*, He hit Billy's ball. *He* is the subject in the nominative case, *Billy's* is the modifier in the possessive case, and *ball* is the direct object in the objective case. **2.** A particular instance of disease, injury, surgery, rehabilitation, therapy, etc.; often used incorrectly to identify the patient with the instance.

case grammar See under grammar.

case relations In case grammar, the effect one semantic category has on another; *e.g.*, the agenitive on the dative: John (agenitive) hit Bill (dative).

case study Questioning process, as part of the diagnostic procedure, to obtain information about a patient; may be obtained from the patient or from someone able to answer for him.

catalogia (ka-tə-lō′jē-ə) [G. *kata*, down + *logion*, declaration] Incoherent repetitions of meaningless words and sentences. Syn: verbigeration.

cataphoric reference See under cohesive devices.

catarrh (kə-tär′) [G. *katarrheō*, to flow down] Inflammation of any mucous membrane.

catarrhal deafness See under deafness.

catastrophic response 1. Psychobiological breakdown of an individual when successful performance does not seem possible, characterized by vascular changes, irritability, evasiveness, and aggressiveness which may precede or accompany the response; an extreme reaction may take the form of loss of consciousness; often associated with aphasia. **2.** Sudden change in behavior typified by irritability, flushing or fainting, withdrawal, or random movements.

cat cry syndrome Cri du chat syndrome.

catenative (kə-ten′ə-tiv) [L. *catenna*, chain] Type of verb, such as wanna (want to), gonna (going to), etc.

cathode (C or **Ca)** (kath′ōd) [G. *kathodos*, a way down] Negative electrode or element which releases electrons when heated in a vacuum tube. *Cf.* anode.

CAT scan Common term for image from or procedure of computed tomography.

Cattel Scales See *Psychological Measures and Tests* in appendices.

caudal (kô′dəl) [L. *cauda*, tail] Away from the head; toward the tail.

causality (kô-zal′i-tē) [L. *causa*, cause] **1.** Relation between a cause and its effect or between regularly correlated events or phenomena. **2.** Awareness of cause and effect relationships; occurs in language development during the sensorimotor period (Piaget's Period I).

cavity (kav′ə-tē) [L. *cavus*, hollow]. A hollow space; *e.g.*, the mouth. For types of cavity, see specific term.

ceiling In testing, denoting the highest item of a sequence in which a certain number of items has been failed. It is assumed that all items above this level are incorrect.

cell [L. *cella*, chamber] Smallest unit of life; the living active basis of all plant and animal organization; it is composed of a mass of protoplasm containing a nucleus and enclosed in a membrane (cell wall); cells vary in form according to their functions.

cell body See neuron.

central aphasia See under aphasia.

central auditory abilities Auditory processes.

central auditory disorder See central *deafness*.

central auditory function Auditory processes.

central auditory nervous system (CANS) See under nervous system.

central auditory perception Auditory processes.

central auditory processes Auditory processes.

central deafness See under deafness.

central hearing Ability of the central mechanism of hearing (the brain) to analyze and interpret messages meaningfully.

central incisor teeth See incisor *teeth.*

Central Institute for the Deaf (CID) Private residential school for the deaf founded in 1914 by Max Goldstein, an American otologist.

central language disorder (CLD) Inability to understand what is heard; the term specifies language functions as the major area of disability and localizes the dysfunction as central, not peripheral, but does not imply known organic involvement; organic involvement may, however, be present. Syn: central language imbalance. See also aphasia.

central language imbalance Central language disorder.

central masking See under masking.

central nervous system (CNS) See under nervous system.

central speech range See speech *frequencies.*

central sulcus See under sulcus.

central tendency Middle value between the extremes of a set of measures. There are many different kinds of central tendency measures, each of which has a somewhat different meaning. Among the more common are the mean, median, and mode *(q.v.)*, which, even when based on the same scores, need not yield identical values.

central vowel See under vowel.

centration (sen-trā′shən) [L. *centrum*, center] Child's limited perceptual aspect of a stimulus; inability to explore all aspects of the stimulus or to decenter visual inspection which results in assimilating only the superficial aspects of an event. See also Period II, under cognitive development stages.

cephalic (sə-fal′ik) [G. *kephalē*, head] Pertaining to or near the head.

CERA Cardiac evoked response audiometry.

cerebellar (săr-ə-bel′ėr) Relating to the cerebellum.

cerebellum See under brain.

cerebral (săr′ə-brəl, sə-rē′brəl) Relating to the cerebrum.

cerebral anoxia See under anoxia.

cerebral cortex Outer layer of the cerebrum.

cerebral dominance See under dominance.

cerebral dominance and handedness theory See breakdown theory, under stuttering theories.

cerebral localization See under localization.

cerebral palsy Term for a group of neurologic disorders with etiology in the central nervous system, particularly at motor control centers; may occur prenatally, perinatally, or postnatally before basic muscular system coordination is achieved. It is of a chronic nature, and may result in a range of disabilities including abnormal muscle tone, faulty coordination, or abnormal positioning; supplemental involvement may occur in intellectual, perceptual, auditory, speech and language, or emotional functioning. See also dysarthria.

  Cerebral palsy classifications include several systems of categorization: (a) *neuroanatomical characteristics*, based on the presumed site of the lesion; (b) *programming/ function*, based on therapy requirements or functional capacities; (c) *topography*, based on the part of the body affected (monoplegia to quadriplegia); (d) *symptomatology*, based on the external manifestations of the disorder.

cerebral palsy symptomatology Overt characteristics of the disorder; may be mixed, as in athetosis with mild spasticity. See subentries below.

ataxia Disorder characterized by dyscoordination and tremors in both fine and gross motor activity; speech is characterized by inconsistent articulatory errors and difficulty with the normal speed of conversation.

athetosis Disorder characterized by involuntary, primarily writhing, movements usually occurring with, and blocking, volitional efforts. Speech is characterized by varying degrees of a pattern of irregular, shallow, and noisy breathing; whispered, hoarse, or ventricular phonation; and mild to severe articulatory disorders.

atonia Lack of muscle tone; speech is characterized by difficulty with phonation, articulation, and prosody.

choreoathetosis Slow, writhing movements with quick movements on initiation of a volitional action; speech is characterized by explosive outbursts, variations in rate, prolongation of intervals, and episodes of hypernasality, harshness, or breathiness.

clonus Series of rapid, alternating extension and flexion movements of muscle on sudden stretch; speech is characterized by lack of vocal inflection, uncontrolled volume, and articulatory problems.

flaccidity Inability of a muscle to contract volitionally when it can do so reflexively and is not atrophied; speech is characterized by marked hypernasality coupled with nasal emission, continuous breathiness during phonation, and audible inspiration of air (stridor on inhalation).

rigidity Muscular resistance to passive motion from simultaneous agonist and antagonist muscle group contractions; speech is characterized by short bursts of verbalization and by a rapid rate which increases in speed from the beginning to the end of an utterance.

spasticity Hypertonicity of muscle, characterized by hyperactivity of the stretch reflex; speech is characterized by a slow, labored rate, lack of vocal inflection, guttural or breathy quality of voice, uncontrolled volume, and severe articulatory problems.

tremor Rhythmic, repetitive, involuntary contractions of flexor and extensor muscles, a generalized trembling of the extremities; speech is characterized by vocal arrests resembling spastic dysphonia, monopitch, intermittent strained or strangled harshness, pitch-breaks, and tremulous or quavering speech.

cerebral thumb Clenched fingers with the thumb inside the palm, a characteristic often associated with cerebral palsy; may also be associated with severe emotional withdrawal.

cerebral vascular accident (CVA) 1. Interruption of blood flow to the brain; may result from an aneurysm, embolism, or a thrombosis. **2.** Sudden onset of vascular accident in the brain; may produce symptoms such as loss of sensations, motor function, speech disturbance, visual difficulty, and intellectual or emotional disorders. Syn: apoplexy; stroke (1).

cerebrum See under brain.

cerumen (se-ru′mən) [L. *sera*, wax] Waxlike secretion of the lining of the external auditory meatus; functions as a trap for foreign particles. Syn: earwax.

cervical (sėr′və-kəl) [L. *cervix*, neck] Pertaining to the neck region, particularly the vertebrae and nerves in that area.

chaining 1. Teaching an entire behavior by conditioning and reinforcing each step separately, and then bringing the steps together. **2.** Putting words together to make phrases or sentences.

chamber (chām′bėr) [L. *camera*, vault] Compartment or enclosed space. For types of chamber, see specific term.

character (kăr′ək-tėr) **1.** Attribute, trait, or definite and distinct structural feature of an animal or plant. **2.** In speech,

often refers to a symbol of the International Phonetic Alphabet.

chest pulse Movements during respiration that produce the air pressure required to activate the vocal folds. See also respiration.

chest voice See under voice.

chewing Process of using the jaw, teeth, or tongue in a movement designed to break up or pulverize solid pieces of food in preparation for swallowing.

chewing method Breath chewing.

CHI Closed head injury.

childhood aphasia See under aphasia.

childhood psychosis Childhood *schizophrenia*.

childhood schizophrenia See under schizophrenia.

Children's Articulation Test See *Articulation Tests and Phonological Analysis Procedures* in appendices.

Children's Language Battery See *Language Tests and Procedures* in appendices.

chiloschisis (kī-los′kə-sis) [G. *cheilos*, lip + *schisis*, cleft] Cleft lip.

chink In alaryngeal speech, sound produced by esophageal speakers, with an audible air intake into the esophagus.

cholesteatoma (kə-les-tē-ə-tō′mə) [G. *chole*, bile + *stear*, tallow + *-oma*, tumor] Tumorlike mass resulting from a marginal perforation of the middle ear or from chronic otitis media, causing an ingrowth of skin which invades the middle ear and the mastoid spaces. Syn: keratoma (2).

choral reading Reading aloud in unison with others; sometimes used in stuttering therapy.

choral speaking Speaking in unison by two or more individuals; sometimes used in stuttering therapy.

chorditis See under laryngeal anomaly.
    c. nodosa or **tuberosa** Vocal nodules. See under laryngeal anomaly.

chorea (kô-rē′ə) [L. fr. G. *choreia*, choral dance] Disorder characterized by irregular, spasmodic, involuntary move-

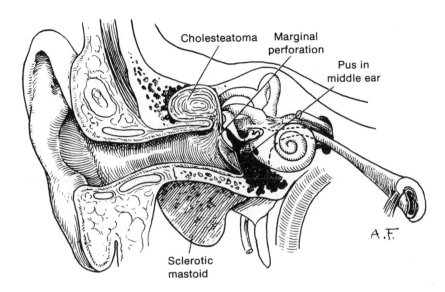

Cholesteatoma
From Davis, H, and Silverman, SR. *Hearing and Deafness,* 3rd Ed. New York: Holt, Rinehart and Winston, 1970.

ments of the limbs or facial muscles. See also hyperkinetic *dysarthria*.

choreoathetosis (kôr′ē-ō-ath-ə-tō′sis) [G. *choreia*, choral dance + *athetos*, unfixed, + *-ōsis*, condition] Slow writhing movements with quick movements on initiation of a volitional action. See under cerebral palsy symptomatology.

chromosome 21-trisomy syndrome Down's syndrome.

chronaxie (krō-nak′sē) [G. *chronos*, time + *axia*, value] Time characteristic; a measurement of excitability of nervous or muscular tissue.

chronic (kron′ik) [G. *chronos*, time] Of long duration with slow progress, usually said of a disease. *Cf.* acute.

chronic laryngitis See laryngitis.

chronic suppurative otitis media See under otitis.

chronological age (CA) Actual age of an individual, derived from date of birth; usually expressed in years, months, and days.

chunking (chəŋk′iŋ) **1.** Segment of expe-

rience determined by how previous experiences have been categorized. **2.** Arranging adjacent elements into meaningful groups for understanding and recall; *e.g.*, 7743477 chunked as 774–34–77.

CID Central Institute for the Deaf.

cinefluorography (sin′ə-flu-rog′rə-fē) Cinefluoroscopy.

cinefluoroscopy (sin′ə-flu-ros′kə-pē) [G. *kineō*, will move + L. *radius*, ray + G. *graphō*, to write] Motion picture recording of physiologic or pathologic speech activity observed by fluoroscopy. It is useful in the study of respiratory, swallowing, and vocal fold movements, and in determining the adequacy of velopharyngeal closure. Syn: cineradiography, cinefluorography, cineroentgenography. *Cf.* radiography; tomography; fluoroscopy. See also electrical measurement of speech production; x-ray.

cineroentgenography (sin′ə-rent-gen-og′ rə-fē) Cinefluoroscopy.

circuit (sėr′kit) [L. *curcuitus*, going

around] Complete path for the flow of an electric current. For types of circuit, see specific term.

circumaural (sėr-kəm-är'əl) Around the ear; describing an earphone or earmuff cushion that presses against the head and encircles the pinna.

circumaural hearing protection devices Earmuffs. See under hearing protection device.

circumflex (sėr'kəm-fleks) [L. a bend (around)] A diacritic, as in ûrge.

circumlocution (sėr'kəm-lō-kyu'shən) [L. *circum*, around + *locutio*, speaking]. **1.** Description by use or by definition due to an inability to recall the name; *e.g.*, cup: drink from; ball: that round thing. **2.** In stuttering, an attempt to avoid feared words by rephrasing the original thought, using different words.

classical conditioning See under conditioning.

classifications of cleft palate See table under cleft palate.

class word Content *word*.

clause Group of words containing a subject and predicate, and functioning as a member of a complex or compound sentence.

> **constituent, dependent,** or **embedded c.** Subordinate *clause.*
> **independent c.** Main *clause.*
> **main c.** Clause containing a subject and verb, and expressing a complete thought; it can stand alone. Syn: independent or principal clause; matrix. See also sentence classifications.
> **principal c.** Main *clause.*
> **subordinate c.** Clause acting as a subject, complement, or modifier, but having a subject and verb of its own; usually introduced by a subordinating word stated or understood; *e.g.*, The book *you sent for* is here. This is the book *that I want.* Syn: constituent, dependent, or embedded clause. See also sentence classifications.

clause terminal Terminal *juncture.*

clavicular (klə-vik'yu-lėr) [L. *clavicula*, small key] Relating to the clavicle (collar bone).

clavicular respiration See under respiration.

CLD Central language disorder.

cleft 1. Fissure, a space or opening made by splitting. **2.** Partially split or divided.

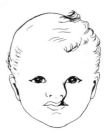

Unilateral
cleft lip

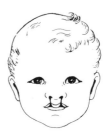

Bilateral
cleft lip

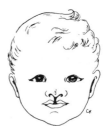

Median
cleft lip

Cleft Lip
From Sadler, TW. *Langman's Medical Embryology*, 6th Ed. Baltimore: Williams & Wilkins, 1990.

atypical or **rare c.'s** Orofacial anomalies which occur infrequently; *e.g.*, clefts of the mandibular process, those naso-ocular in direction and oro-ocular (oblique); submucous clefts not associated with clefts of the prepalate or palate; congenital pits in the lower lip; cleft lip nose; congenital palatal insufficiency; and transverse facial clefts.

labial c. Cleft lip.

nose c. See atypical *clefts.*

rare c.'s Atypical *clefts.*

cleft lip Congenital deformity of the upper lip which varies from a notching to a complete division of the lip; the alveolar process and palate may or may not be involved. Syn: chiloschisis; harelip; labial cleft.

bilateral c. l. Cleft lip in which the cleft extends from the vermillion border of the upper lip toward both the right and left nostrils.

median c. l. Vertical cleft through the center of the upper lip.

unilateral c. l. Cleft lip in which the cleft is either on the right or left side of the upper lip and extends from the vermillion border toward the nostril.

cleft palate Congenital fissure in the median line of the palate which may extend through the uvula, soft palate, and hard palate; cleft lip may or may not be involved. Syn: uranoschisis. See also *Cleft Palate Classifications* table.

bilateral c. p. Failure of the palate on the right and left sides to fuse to the nasal partition or septum.

complete or **total c. p.** Cleft palate in which the cleft extends from the lip through the alveolar process, hard palate, and soft palate.

incomplete, partial, or **subtotal c. p.** Cleft palate in which the cleft can be limited to the lip, alveolar process,

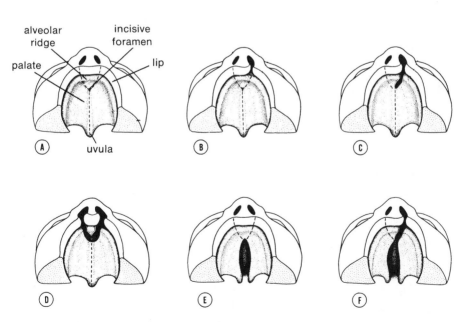

Cleft Palate

A, normal; B, unilateral cleft lip; C, unilateral cleft involving the lip and primary palate; D, bilateral cleft involving the lip and primary palate; E, incomplete cleft of the hard and soft palates; F, complete unilateral cleft of the palates and lip. From Sadler, TW. *Langman's Medical Embryology,* 5th Ed. Baltimore: Williams & Wilkins, 1985.

CLEFT PALATE CLASSIFICATIONS
Categories and Terminology Used to Identify and Locate Various Types of Clefts
(Palate and Lip)

American Cleft Palate Association	Davis and Ritchie	Kernahan and Stark	Veau
Based on current embryological theory concerning the development of the face; utilizes the positions of the cleft relative to the incisive foramen as the dividing point between the prepalate and the palate.	Based on the position of the cleft relative to the alveolar process.	Based on current embryological theory concerning the development of the face; utilizes the position of the cleft relative to the incisive foramen as the dividing point between the prepalate and the palate.	Used the anatomical structures affected as a method of classifying clefts.
Cleft of prepalate (lip and alveolar process)	Prealveolar cleft (lip only, alveolar process complete)	Clefts of primary palate only	

Cleft lip
  Unilateral
    Right, left
    Extent in thirds
      (1/3, 2/3, 3/3)
  Bilateral
    Right, left
    Extent in thirds
  Median
    Extent in thirds
	Unilateral
	  Right, left
	
	Bilateral
	
	Median
		Unilateral
		  Right, left
		  Complete
		  Incomplete
		Bilateral
		  Complete
		  Incomplete
		Median
		  Complete (pre-maxilla absent)
		  Incomplete (pre-maxilla rudimentary)	

Prolabium
  Small, medium, large
Congenital scar
  Right, left, median
Cleft of alveolar process
Unilateral
  Right, left
  Extent in thirds
Bilateral
  Right, left
  Extent in thirds
Median
  Extent in thirds
  Submucous
    Right, left, median
Any combination of foregoing types
Prepalate protrusion
Prepalate rotation
Prepalate arrest (median cleft)			

(Continued)

CLEFT PALATE CLASSIFICATIONS—*Continued*

American Cleft Palate Association	Davis and Ritchie	Kernahan and Stark	Veau
Cleft of palate	Postalveolar cleft (palate only, alveolar process complete)	Clefts of secondary palate only	Soft palate only
Cleft soft palate Extent	Soft palate only, or part thereof	Complete Incomplete	Soft and hard palate

Postanterior in thirds
      Width (maximum in mm)
    Palatal shortness
      None, slight, moderate, marked
    Submucous cleft
      Extent in thirds
Cleft hard palate
  Extent
    Postanterior in thirds
    Width (maximum in mm)
    Vomer attachment
    Right, left, absent
    Submucous cleft
      Extent in thirds
Cleft of soft and hard palate
	Soft and hard palate, or part thereof
	
	Submucous cleft
		Submucous	Soft and hard palate extending forward along one side of the premaxilla and continuing through the lip and alveolar arch on the side (complete unilateral)

Clefts of prepalate and palate	Alveolar clefts (cleft may be complete or incomplete and is usually associated with a cleft of the lip and palate)	Clefts of primary and secondary palate	Soft and hard palate continuing forward along both sides of the premaxilla and through the lip and alveolar arch on two sides (complete bilateral)

Any combination of clefts described under clefts of prepalate and clefts of palate	Unilateral
	  Right, left
	
	Bilateral
	
	Median
		Unilateral
		  Right, left
		  Complete
		  Incomplete
		Bilateral
		  Complete
		  Incomplete
		Median
		  Complete
		  Incomplete	

Facial clefts other than prepalatal and palatal			

hard palate, or soft palate, or a combination of these structures.

occult c. p. Submucous *cleft palate.*

partial c. p. Incomplete *cleft palate.*

submucous c. p. Condition in which the surface tissues of the hard or soft palate unite but the underlying bone or muscle tissues do not; may occur alone or in structures adjacent to incomplete clefts. Syn: occult cleft palate.

subtotal c. p. Incomplete *cleft palate.*

total c. p. Complete *cleft palate.*

unilateral c. p. Fusion of the palate to the vertical nasal septum only on one side.

cleft palate, prosthetic management Utilization of artificial materials (prostheses) to provide a separation of the oral cavity from the nasal cavity or to replace missing or extracted teeth.

cleft palate, speech and language characteristics Characteristics described as (a) hypernasal; (b) indistinct, with inaccurate articulation and frequent substitutions of the glottal stop; (c) nasal emission during production of fricative sounds; and (d) delayed development of language skills. Speech is often accompanied by undesirable facial distortions or mannerisms, such as a constriction of the nasal alae.

cliche (klē-shā′) [Fr.] Trite or stereotyped term, expression, idea, or observation lacking in originality or ingenuity because of excessive commonplace usage; *e.g.*, sings like a bird; sadder but wiser.

click Brief sound used primarily in evoked response audiometry; early brainstem responses are elicited only by signals with rise times less than or equal to 2.5 ms.

clinical (klin′i-kəl) **1.** Denoting diagnosis and treatment on the basis of observation of the person's symptoms and not on the basis of membership in a stereotyped group. **2.** Denoting a program or curriculum which emphasizes therapy and rehabilitation.

clinical audiology See under audiology.

Clinical Evaluation of Language Functions (CELF) See *Language Tests and Procedures* in appendices.

Clinical Probes of Articulation Consistency (C-PAC) See *Articulation Tests and Phonological Analysis Procedures* in appendices.

clinical psychology See under psychology.

clip In audiology, to control intensity by limiting output of a hearing aid or amplifier.

clipped word See under word.

clonic (klon′ik) Denoting or of the nature of clonus.

clonic block See under block.

clonus (klō′nəs) [G. *klonos*, tumult] Series of rapid, alternating extension and flexion movements of a muscle on sudden stretching. See under cerebral palsy symptomatology.

closed bite Supraversion. See under teeth malpositions.

closed class Syntactic classes that are small and closed; any one class has few members, and new members are not readily added. Classes include inflections, auxiliary verbs, articles, prepositions, and conjunctions.

closed head injury (CHI) Term used to indicate cases in which the primary source of brain injury is one of blunt trauma to the skull, excluding brain injury secondary to penetrating head wounds, cerebral vascular insults, and tumors. The injury may be so mild as to result in only a brief period of unconsciousness or so severe as to result in prolonged unconsciousness and abnormal neurologic signs.

closed juncture See under juncture.

closed-set test Tests in which the listener is limited to one of a fixed number of possible responses. See also open-set tests.

closed syllable See under syllable.

close transcription Phonetic *transcription*.

close vowel High *vowel*.

closure (klō′zhèr) **1.** Ability to recognize a whole when one or more parts of the whole are missing, or when there are gaps in continuity. **2.** Principle of Gestalt psychology; subjective closing of gaps, or completion of incomplete forms, so as to constitute wholes. **3.** In speech, a closing of the vocal folds, lips, etc., such that there is complete stoppage of airflow. The duration of the closures may range from extremely brief to many seconds.

    auditory c. Ability to integrate auditory stimuli into a whole; *i.e.*, completion of a word or words by filling in the parts omitted when the word or words are spoken. See also *Auditory Processes* table.

    grammatic c. Comprehension of syntactic as well as grammatic structures, even though those structures are missing in an utterance; *e.g.*, the (girl/girls) plays; the (girl/girls) play; he (have/has) candy; they (have/has) candy.

    visual c. Recognition of objects, shapes, or words from an incomplete visual presentation; *e.g.*, ⌐ = □; (= ○; ∠ = △.

clot A coagulation of blood.

cluster See *consonant* cluster.

cluster reduction See under syllabic structuring, under phonological processes.

cluttering (klət′ėr-iŋ) **1.** Speech disorder characterized by a short attention span, disturbances in perception, articulation, and formulation of speech, and often by excessive speed of delivery; individual is usually unaware of the disorder. **2.** Rapid utterances with many elisions, transpositions, and omissions of significant speech sounds; lapse of syntax may also occur. Speech is generally jerky and word groups are spoken in rapid spurts, making the utterance difficult to understand; often confused with stuttering. **3.** Disorder of the thought processes preceding speech; the verbal manifestation of central language imbalance, which affects all channels of communication.

CMV cytomegalovirus.

CNS Central nervous system.

CNT "Could not test."

co- See con-.

coalescence (kō-ə-les′ens) Combination of phonemes from two syllables into one syllable. See also under phonological processes.

coarticulation (kō′är-tik-yu-lā′shən) [co- + L. *articulatio*, place of union (joint)] **1.** Articulatory movements for one phone which are carried over into the production of previous or subsequent phones, but which do not affect the primary place of articulation, as occurs when assimilation affects the place of articulation. **2.** Influence of one phoneme on another in perception or production.

    anticipatory c. Backward *coarticulation*.

    backward c. Right to left influences in which earlier phonetic activity replaces forthcoming phonetic activity. Syn: anticipatory coarticulation.

    carryover c. Forward *coarticulation*.

    forward c. Left to right influences in which forthcoming phonetic activity replaces earlier phonetic activity. Syn: carryover coarticulation.

cochlea (kōk′lē-ə) [L. snail shell] That part of the inner ear containing the sensory mechanism of hearing. See under inner *ear*.

cochlear (kōk′lē-ėr) Relating to the cochlea.

cochlear aplasia See under aplasia.

cochlear duct Scala media. See cochlea, under inner *ear*.

cochlear implant 1. An electromagnetic device, surgically implanted into the ear, designed to stimulate sensory

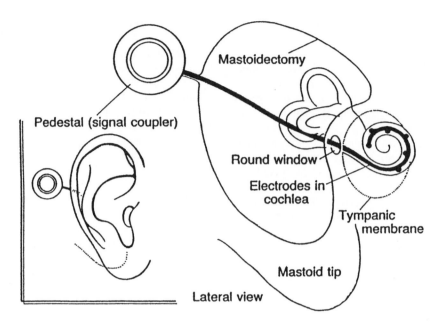

Cochlear Implant

components remaining in the cochlea of persons with severe or profound hearing impairment who cannot use hearing aids effectively. An electrode array is inserted into the inner ear by a mastoidectomy through the round window. An externally worn signal processor interfaces with the cochlear implant at the signal coupler. **2.** An auditory system designed to directly activate the auditory nerve.

cochlear microphonic (kōk'lē-ėr mī-krō-fon'ik) Electrical potential that can be recorded from various places in the cochlea and closely resembles the waveforms of the sounds that enter the ears. It is thought that it originates in the hairs of the hair cells and serves to stimulate the auditory nerve fibers which innervate the hair cells.

cochlear nerve Anterior branch of the acoustic nerve; arises from the nerve cells of the spiral ganglion of the cochlea and terminates in the dorsal and ventral cochlear nuclei in the brain stem. See also *Cranial Nerves* table.

cochlear nuclei Cell bodies of second-order neurons within the auditory pathway, only three of which appear to be of importance: the anterior and posterior ventral cochlear nuclei, and the dorsal cochlear nuclei.

cochlear reflex Acoustic *reflex*.

cochlear window Round window. See under middle *ear*.

cochleoorbicular (kōk'lē-ō-ôr-bik'yu-lėr) Relating to the cochlea and orbit of the eye.

cochleoorbicular reflex Auropalpebral *reflex*.

cochleopalpebral (kōk'lē-ō-pal'pǝ-brǝl) Relating to the cochlea and eyelid (palpebra).

cochleopalpebral reflex (CPR) Auropalpebral reflex.

code 1. Set of unambiguous rules whereby information is converted from one representation to another. **2.** System of signals used in communication; may consist of characters or symbols with arbitrary conventionalized meanings.

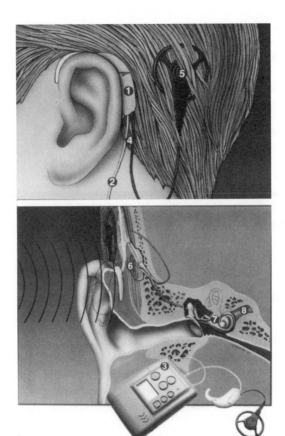

Cochlear Implant Operation
(1) Directional microphone; (2) sound is carried to speech processor worn on belt or pocket; (3) processor filters, analyzes, and digitizes sound into coded signals and sends it (4) to transmitting coil (5). Coil sends coded signals as FM radio signals to the cochlear implant inserted under the skin. Cochlear implant (6) delivers energy to electrodes surgically inserted into cochlea (7). Electrodes stimulate the remaining auditory nerve fibers (8), and sound information is sent to the brain for interpretation. Photograph provided by Cochlear Corporation, Englewood, CO. From Northern JL, Downs MP. *Hearing in Children,* 5th Ed. Baltimore: Lippincott Williams & Wilkins, 2002.

coefficient (kō-ə-fish′ənt) [co- + L. *efficio,* to accomplish] **1.** In mathematics, the constant by which a variable is multiplied. **2.** In statistics, an index of the degree in which some characteristic or relation appears in a given case of measurement, as in coefficient of correlation, of variability, of reliability, of validity.

coefficient of correlation Measure of the degree of relationship between two sets of measures for the same group of individuals. See also correlation (3); reliability coefficient.

  product moment (r) Coefficient of correlation most frequently used in test development and educational research to determine the relationship between paired sets of measures; the range in value or relationship is from

−1.00 for perfect negative relationship, through 0.00 for none or pure chance, to + 1.00 for perfect positive relationship; commonly used when N (number) is relatively large.

rank order Coefficient of correlation based on a comparison of the ranks of individuals on two sets of scores; usually used when N (number) is relatively small (15–20).

cognate(s) (kog′nāt) **1.** Consonants produced in the same place and manner, except that one is voiceless and the other voiced; usually written in pairs, with the voiceless sound given first; e.g., /p-b/, /hw-w/, /f-v/, /θ-ð/, /t-d/, /s-z/, /ʃ-ʒ/, /tʃ-dʒ/, /k-g/. **2.** Similarities among words in various languages; e.g., mother (English), *meter* (Greek), *mater* (Latin), *mat′* (Russian), *mutter* (German).

cognate confusion Substitution of the voiced sound for its voiceless cognate, or vice versa.

cognition (kog-ni′shən) [L. *cognitio*, knowing] **1.** General concept embracing all of the various modes of knowing: perceiving, remembering, imagining, conceiving, judging, and reasoning. **2.** Act or process of knowing.

cognitive (kog′nə-tiv) Relating to cognition.

cognitive development 1. Progressive and continuous growth of perception, memory, imagination, conception, judgment, and reason; the growth of "thinking" skills. **2.** Intellectual counterpart of biological adaptation to the environment.

cognitive development stages Progression of four periods or stages from early perceptual motor functioning (infancy) to formal operations at about 12 years of age; consists of four broad factors: (a) maturation, (b) physical experience, (c) social interaction, and (d) general progression of equilibrium [Piaget]. See also *General Outline of Language Development From Birth to 11 Years* in appendices.

Period I Sensorimotor intelligence (0–2 years): behavior is primarily motor; there is no conceptual thinking, although the infant's reflexive behavior gradually grows into intellectual behavior.

Period II Preoperational thought (2–7 years): characterized by the development of language and rapid conceptual development; intellectual behavior moves to a conceptual level, and by the end of this period the child's thought is prelogical.

Period III Concrete operations (7–11 years): child develops the ability to apply logical thought to concrete problems; logical operations of reversibility, seriation, and classification are developed, but logical thinking cannot yet be applied to verbal and hypothetical problems.

Period IV Formal operations (11–15 years): thought structures reach their greatest level of development, and logic is able to be applied to all classes of problems, verbal and scientific; during this time the adolescent tries to see human behavior as what is logical rather than what is real; he possesses egocentric ideals.

cognitive dissonance Conflict between what one knows and perceives in a meaning; may result in a distortion of information.

cognitive distancing 1. Behavior or events which separate the individual from his environment; e.g., father and son discussing a baseball game to be played in the future. **2.** Behavior or events which require the individual to attend to or react in terms of the nonpresent, e.g., a child searching in his closet for shoes he knows are there.

cognitive mapping Ability to organize and construct mental pictures of the environment; aids in predicting and organizing responses to the environment.

cognitive style Person's characteristic approach to problem-solving and cognitive tasks.

cohesive devices Lexical items and syntactic constructions that tie utterances together.

    anaphoric reference c. d. The use of pronouns or definite articles that refer to a previously established entity; *e.g.*, Mike is sick. *He* has a cold. See also parts of speech, pronoun.

    cataphoric reference c. d. The use of pronouns or demonstratives that direct the listener to coming events; *e.g.*, After *she* eats, Linda will go home.

    ellipsis c. d. The deletion of information available in an immediately preceding portion of the discourse; *e.g.*, John, close the door. I will (close the door).

    lexical cohesion c. d. The use of synonyms that refer to a previously noted referents; *e.g.*, The dog barked. The *animal* was frightened.

cold-running speech See under speech.

Cold-Running Speech Test See *Audiometric Tests and Procedures* in appendices.

collective monologue Nonconversation; even though a child speaks to others, there is no communication. See also egocentric *language.*

Collet-Sicard syndrome [F. J. Collet, Fr. laryngologist, *1870; J. A. Sicard, Fr. neurologist, 1872–1929] Anesthesia of the larynx, pharynx, soft palate, and posterior third of the tongue, hemiatrophy of the tongue, and paralysis of the sternocleidomastoideus and trapezius muscles, with hoarseness, difficulty in swallowing, and nasal regurgitation; results from lesions of the glossopharyngeal, vagus, spinal accessory, and hypoglossal nerves (cranial nerves IX, X, XI, and XII).

colloquial (kə-lō′kwē-əl) Familiar and informal, as in conversation.

colloquialism (kə-lō′kwē-əl-izm) [L. *colloquium,* conversational] Local or regional dialect expression; *e.g.*, tote (carry) the bag.

Coloured Progressive Matrices See *Psychological Measures and Tests* in appendices.

Columbia Mental Maturity Scale See *Psychological Measures and Tests* in appendices.

columella, pl. **columellae** (kol-yu-mel′ə, -ē) [L. dim. of *columna,* column] Fleshy anterior portion of the nasal septum between the nostrils.

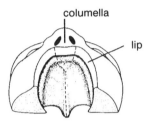

Columella

After Sadler, TW. *Langman's Medical Embryology,* 5th Ed. Baltimore: Williams & Wilkins, 1985.

com- See con-.

combined method Simultaneous method. See under aural rehabilitation.

commentary (kom′en-tär-ē) See subvocal *speech.*

commissure (kom′is-shur) [L. *commissura,* a joining together, seam] Nerve fibers connecting similar structures on both sides of the brain.

communication (kə-myu-nə-kā′shən) [L. *communicatio*] **1.** Any means by which an individual relates experiences, ideas, knowledge, and feelings to another; includes speech, sign language, gestures, writing. **2.** Process by which meanings are exchanged between individuals through a system of symbols.

communication board Apparatus upon which is represented the alphabet, numbers, and commonly used words; used when oral expression is difficult or cannot be obtained. Syn: conversa-

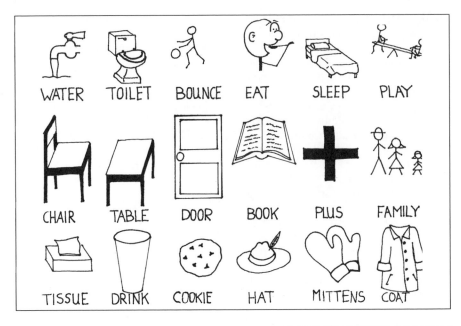

Communication Board

Top, demonstrating the use of pictures. Bottom, using letters to represent words, numbers, and concepts.

tion board. See also aided *augmentative communication.*

direct selection c. b. Techniques in which the message sender indicates elements of his message by directly pointing to them in some manner; there is a one to one correspondence.

encoding c. b. Communication board which uses various input techniques which the user must learn before the device can be used; input scheme may resemble a Morse code telegraphic operation or may utilize sucking, pausing, and blowing on a tube; requires some dexterity by the user.

scanning c. b. Technique that presents message elements (*e.g.*, pictures, words) or groups of elements one at a time to the individual and requires only a minimum amount of physical control by the user; in most cases, the individual merely indicates by a prearranged signal (*e.g.*, movement of arm, leg, head, eyes) when the desired message element has been presented.

communication disorder Communicative disorder.

communication failure theory See under anticipatory and struggle behavior theory, under stuttering theories.

communication sciences Study of the various aspects of communication; includes speech, hearing, gestures, and language (oral, written, and sign).

communication skills of the hearing impaired See *Hearing Impairment Degrees* table.

Communicative Abilities in Daily Living (CADL) See *Language Tests and Procedures* in appendices.

communicative competence Speaker's ability to effectively communicate an intentional message so as to alter the listener's attitudes, beliefs, or behaviors. A very young child could, therefore, be communicatively competent with a minimal development of linguistic skills.

communicative disorder Impairment in the ability to (a) receive or process a symbol system; (b) represent concepts or symbol systems; or (c) transmit and use symbol systems. The impairment may be observed in disorders of hearing, language, or speech processes. Syn: communication disorder. See also language impairment, speech impairment.

communicative interaction See augmentative communication system.

communicative stress The perception that a given speaking situation (speaking to authority figures or large groups of people, formulating linguistically complex utterances, reading difficult material, speaking on the telephone, or talking under the pressure of having a lot to say in a limited amount of time) will be difficult.

communicative technique See augmentative communication system.

communicologist (kə-myu-nə-kol′ə-jist) Speech and language pathologist.

communicology (kə-myu-nə-kol′ə-jē) Speech and language pathology.

compact phoneme See under phoneme.

comparable forms reliability coefficient Alternate forms *reliability coefficient.*

comparative (kəm-par′ə-tiv) See under comparison.

comparative linguistics See under linguistics.

comparative research Animal research, with application for humans.

comparison (kəm-par′ə-sən) In grammar, the name given to the change in the form of adjectives and adverbs when they are used to demonstrate the qualities of the words they modify.

comparative Comparison made between only two items; *e.g.*, He is the tall*er* of the two men.

positive Ordinary form of the adjective or adverb, without any suggestion of comparison between two or more items; *e.g.*, He is a *tall* man.

superlative Comparison made among

three or more items; *e.g.*, He is the tall*est* of the three men.

compensation (kom-pen-sā′shən) [L. *compensatus*, weighing together, counterbalancing] Adjustment intended to counteract the effect of some anomaly, dysfunction, disability, or social deficiency (real or imagined); may be neural, physical, neuromotor, or psychological.

compensatory movement In articulation, the production of a sound utilizing alternative placement of the articulators rather than the usual placement; may be necessary because of paralysis or other disorders.

competence (kom′pə-tens) See linguistic competence.

competing messages Dichotic listening.

competing messages integration Auditory figure-ground *discrimination*.

Competing Sentence Test (CST) See *Audiometric Tests and Procedures* in appendices.

complement (kom′plə-ment) [L. *complimentum*, that which completes] Word or words used to complete the sense of the verb, subject, or object; may be predicate noun or nominative (Bob was a good *boy*.), predicate adjective (The boy was *good*.), or predicate object or objective complement (He called the man *a hero*.).

complemental air Inspiratory reserve volume. See under respiratory volume.

complementary distribution See under distribution.

complete cleft palate See under cleft palate.

complete predicate See predicate.

complete recruitment See under recruitment.

complete subject See subject (1).

complex noise See under noise.

complex sentence See under sentence classification, traditional grammar.

Complex Speech Sound Discrimination Test See *Auditory Tests and Procedures* in appendices.

complex syllabics Diphthong. See under vowel.

complex tone See under tone.

complex wave See under wave.

complex word See under word.

compliance (kəm-plī′əns) **1.** Ease with which a structure may be distended or deformed. **2.** In audiology, the ease with which the tympanic membrane and middle ear mechanism function. See also impedance.

compound-complex sentence See under sentence classification, traditional grammar.

compound consonant See under consonant.

compound sentence See under sentence classification, traditional grammar.

compound word See under word.

comprehension (kom-prē-hen′shən) [L. *comprehensus*, comprehending] **1.** Knowledge or understanding of an object, situation, event, or verbal statement. **2.** In speech, understanding of spoken utterances, as distinguished from producing utterances.

comprehension span Greatest number of events, things, and processes of human experiences which an individual can perceive (as judged by response) in a spatial-temporal sequence of stimuli.

Comprehensive Assessment of Spoken Language See *Language Test and Procedures* in appendices.

Comprehensive Receptive-Expressive Vocabulary Test-Adult See *Language Test and Procedures* in appendices.

Comprehensive Test of Nonverbal Intelligence See *Psychological Measures and Tests* in appendices.

Comprehensive Test of Phonological Processing See *Articulation Tests and Phonological Analysis Procedures* in appendices.

compressed speech See under speech.

compression (kəm-presh′ən) [L. *compressus*, pressing together] In acoustics: **1.** A pushing together resulting in a more compact condition of particles in a sound wave. **2.** Part of the sound wave cycle in which the particles are forced against each other. Syn: condensation. See also wave (2).

compression amplification 1. See under amplification. **2.** See automatic *volume control.*

compression bone conduction See under conduction.

Compton-Hutton Phonological Assessment See *Articulation Tests and Phonological Analysis Procedures* in appendices.

Compton Speech and Language Screening Evaluation See *Language Tests and Procedures* in appendices.

compulsion (kəm-pəl'shən) [L. *compulsus,* driven together] An irresistible impulse to perform an act, often repetitive, contrary to the conscious will.

computed tomography (CT) See under tomography.

computerized axial tomography (CAT) See under tomography.

computer language See under language.

con- Prefix from Latin meaning with, together; appears as com- before p, b, or m, and as co- before a vowel; corresponds to Greek *syn-.*

concatenation (kon'kat-ə-nā'shən) [L. *concatenatus*] Linking together in a series or chain.

concept (kon'sept) [L. *conceptum,* something understood] **1.** General idea or meaning usually mediated by a word, symbol, or sign. **2.** Idea which combines several elements from different sources into a single notion.

    abstract c. Characteristic, such as number, goodness, or quality, which cannot be attributed to a specific object or event but which refers to an infinite number of objects or events.

    concrete c. Characteristic attributed to a particular instance or object, as opposed to a general instance or quality of many objects.

conceptual disorder Disturbance in thinking processes, cognitive activities, or ability to formulate concepts.

conceptualization (kon-sep'chyu-əl-i-zā'-shən) **1.** Process of thinking or imagining. **2.** Ability to abstract and to categorize. **3.** Formation of a concept or ideal.

concha, pl. **conchae** (kon'kə, -kē) [L. shell] Anatomical landmark of the auricle of the ear. See auricle, under external *ear.*

concrete operations period See Period III under cognitive development stages.

concretism (kon-krēt'izm) Approach to thinking and behavior in which a person tends to regard each situation as essentially new and unique, with a failure to see essential similarities between situations which others accept as similar or even identical.

concurrent validity See criterion-related *validity.*

condensation (kon-den-sā'shən) [L. *condensatus,* making thick] Compression.

condenser (kon-den'sėr) [L. *condenso,* to make thick] Capacitor (2).

conditioned disintegration theory See under learning theory, under stuttering theories.

conditioned orientation reflex audiometry (COR) See under audiometry.

conditioned reinforcer See under reinforcer.

conditioned response See under response.

conditioned stimulus See under stimulus.

conditioning (kən-di'shən-iŋ) Process of acquiring, establishing, learning, or training new responses in animals or man. Used to describe both respondent and operant behavior; in both usages it refers to a change in the frequency or form of behavior as a result of the influence of the environment.

    classical c. Stimulus substitution; a form of learning, as in Pavlov's experiments, in which a previously learned neutral stimulus becomes a conditioned stimulus when presented together with an unconditioned stimulus; called stimulus substitution because the new stimulus evokes the response in question. Syn: respondent conditioning; Pavlovian conditioning; reflex conditioning.

counter c. Any of a group of specific behavior therapy techniques in which a second conditioned response is instituted for the express purpose of counteracting or nullifying a previously conditioned or learned response. Syn: deconditioning; nonreinforcement.

instrumental c. Operant *conditioning.*

operant c. Method of changing behavior in which an experimenter waits for the response to be conditioned to occur spontaneously, immediately after which the subject is given a reinforcer (reward); after this procedure is repeated many times, the frequency of target response emission should have significantly increased over its preexperiment base rate; also referred to as operant behavior, learning, procedures, or therapy. Syn: instrumental conditioning; Skinnerian conditioning.

respondent c. Classical *conditioning.*

conductance (kon-dək′təns) [L. *conductus*, leading] Measure of conductivity; the ratio of the current flowing through a conductor to the difference in potential between the ends of the conductor.

conduction (kon-dək′shən) [L. *conductus*, leading] **1.** Act of transmitting or conveying certain forms of energy (heat, sound, electricity) from one point to another, without evident movement in the conducting body. **2.** In audiology, transmission of sound waves from one point to another.

air c. (AC) Transmission of sound to the inner ear through the external auditory canal and the structures of the middle ear. See also under pure-tone *audiometry.*

bone c. (BC) Transmission of sound to the inner ear through vibration applied to the bones of the skull; allows determination of the cochlea's hearing sensitivity while bypassing any outer or middle ear abnormalities. See also under pure-tone *audiometry.*

compression bone c. Vibratory energy that reaches the cochlea and causes alternate compressions and expansions of the cochlear shell; the cochlear fluid cannot be compressed and must yield, which produces displacement of the basilar membrane. Syn: distortional bone conduction.

distortional bone c. Compression bone *conduction.*

inertial bone c. Stimulation of the inner ear caused by the lag or inertia of the ossicular chain when the bones of the skull are set into motion, resulting in relative movement between the stapes and the oval window.

osseotympanic bone c. That part of hearing by bone conduction created when the vibrating skull causes vibration on air in the external ear canal, causing sound waves to be generated in the canal, striking the tympanic membrane and thus being conducted through the middle ear to the inner ear.

conduction aphasia See under aphasia.

conductive (kon-dək′tiv) Pertaining to conduction.

conductive deafness See under deafness.

conductivity (kon-dək-tiv′ə-tē) Power of transmission or conveyance of certain forms of motion, such as heat, sound, and electricity, without perceptible motion in the conducting body.

cone of light Triangular reflection from the tympanic membrane of the external light source used by an examiner while examining the external auditory meatus.

configuration (kon-fig-yu-rā′shən) In articulation therapy, the patterning of sounds in proper sequence.

confused language See under language.

congenital (kon-jen′ə-təl) [L. *congenitus*, born with] Denoting a disease, deformity, or deficiency existing at or dating from birth; may be the result of heredity or of a pathologic condition following conception of the embryo; may be genetic (endogenous) or acquired (exogenous) following the conception of the embryo. *Cf.* hereditary.

congenital deafness See under deafness.

conjoiner See under parts of speech.

conjunction See under parts of speech.

connected speech See under speech.

connective See conjunction, under parts of speech.

connective tissue Supporting or framework tissue of the body which includes blood and lymph, bone, cartilage, fat, membrane, and tendon. See also tissue.

connotation (kon-ə-tā′shən) [L. *con-* + *notatus*, designating] Word or words that have special meaning for the user based on associational, emotional, or other factors; *e.g.*, pig: animal, sloppy person, unsavory individual.

consequence (kon′sə-kwens) [L. *consequens*, following logically] **1.** Result of an antecedent condition; the effect of a cause. **2.** Event that follows a response; may be planned (use of a verbal reinforcement following a desired response in an effort to strengthen the desired response) or unplanned (inappropriate speech behavior, followed by amused or negative reactions from the listeners).

conservation (kon-sėr-vā′shən) [L. *conservatio*, preservation] In cognitive development, the conceptualization that the amount of quantity of matter stays the same regardless of any changes in shape or position.

consistency effect See under stuttering.

consonance (kon′sə-nəns) **1.** In linguistics, the repeated use of the same consonant sounds before and after vowels; *e.g.*, pep-pop. *Cf.* assonance. **2.** In acoustics, an auditory sensation re-sulting from the frequencies of a simultaneous tone in a musical chord; the overtones are harmonious. *Cf.* dissonance.

consonant (kon′sə-nənt) **1.** Conventional speech sound made, with (voiced) or without (voiceless) vocal fold vibration, by certain successive contractions of the articulatory muscles which modify, interrupt, or obstruct the expired air stream so that its pressure is raised. **2.** Speech sound element articulated by either stopping the outgoing breath stream or creating a narrow opening of resistance against the energy of the breath stream; consonant sounds are separated from vowel sounds on this physiologic basis, and may also be defined according to manner of formation (mode of articulation) and place of articulation (point of articulation).

  abutting c.'s Adjacent consonants that are different sounds, one of which stops the first syllable and the other which releases the following syllable; *e.g.*, /st/ in hi*st*ory. *Cf.* compound *consonant*.

  arresting c. Consonant that closes a syllable.

  aspirate (as′pėr-it) Phonetic unit whose prominent characteristic is the sound generated by the passage of breath through a relatively open channel; *e.g.*, /h/ or a sound followed by or combined with /h/.

  c. blend Consonant cluster.

  c. cluster Two or more consonant sounds appearing next to each other with no vowel separation; *e.g.*, /tr/, /str/. Syn: consonant blend.

  compound c. Group of two or more consonants functioning as a single consonant to release or arrest a syllable; *e.g.*, /st/ in *st*op, po*st*. *Cf.* abutting *consonants*.

  double c. Abutting consonants in which the arresting consonant of the first syllable and the releasing consonant of the second syllable are the

CONSONANTS

Letter	Phonetic Symbol	Ways in Which Sound Is Spelled
p	p	*p*ull, su*pp*er, ho*p*e, hiccou*gh*
b	b	*b*ig, ra*bb*it, ro*b*e
m	m	*m*ove, pal*m*, lam*b*, ta*m*e, phleg*m*, sole*mn*
t	t	*t*ie, *Th*omas, le*tt*er, bi*t*e, talk*ed*, tau*ght*, recei*p*t, de*b*t, indi*c*t, ya*ch*t
d	d	*d*ay, su*dd*en, ti*d*e, mow*ed*, woul*d*, Bu*ddh*a
n	n	*n*ow, su*nn*y, *kn*ife, *gn*at, *pn*eumonia, li*n*e, ha*n*dsome, We*d*nesday, demes*n*e, *mn*emonic, champag*ne*
k	k	*k*ind, *c*at, pa*ck*, taba*cc*o, *ch*emist, a*ch*e, tal*k*, smo*k*e, cli*qu*e, li*qu*or, la*cqu*er, *kh*aki
g	g	*g*one, e*gg*, *gh*astly, *gu*ide, ro*gu*e, bla*c*kg*u*ard
ng	ŋ	si*ng*, ta*n*k, ton*gue*
h	h	*h*ow, *wh*o, mo*j*ave
f	f	*f*ew, co*ff*ee, *ph*otograph, cal*f*, kni*f*e, cou*gh*
v	v	*v*iew, ga*v*e, hal*v*e, o*f*, Ste*ph*en
th	θ	*th*in
th	ð	*th*en, ba*th*e
s	s	*s*o, gue*ss*, *c*ity, *sc*issors, *p*salm, has*t*le, fa*c*e, cour*s*e
z	z	*z*one, bu*zz*, posse*ss*, boy*s*, lo*s*e, sei*z*e, *cz*ar, Win*d*sor, *x*enia
sh	ʃ	*sh*ut, ti*ss*ue, ten*s*ion, o*c*ean, na*t*ion, *Ch*icago
zh	ʒ	sei*z*ure, oc*c*asion, rou*ge*
hw	hw	*wh*ite
w	w	*w*as, q*u*eer, one, *J*uanita
l	l	*l*ow, sha*ll*, who*l*e, ki*l*n
r	r	*r*ed, *w*rite, a*rr*ive, *rh*yme
y	j	*y*ou, law*y*er, hallelu*j*ah
ch	tf	*ch*aire, wa*tch*
j	dʒ	*j*ob, *g*em adjourn, hed*ge* ca*ge*

same consonant repeated; *e.g.*, /s/ in mi*ss*ing.

flap c. 1. Sound produced by the rapid vibration of an articulator; often equal to a single vibration or a single bounce of the tip of the tongue against the hard palate. **2.** Phoneme produced which involves closure of the vocal tract, such closure being so rapid that not enough pressure can build up to produce a sharp burst upon release; *e.g.*, /t/ in Be*tt*y, /r/ in ve*r*y.

fortis c. [L. strong] Plosive sound that is strongly pronounced and is strongly aspirated; *e.g.*, voiceless stops /p/, /t/, /k/; voiceless spirants /f/, /s/, /ʃ/. *Cf.* lax or lenis *consonant*.

lax or **lenis c.** [L. gentle] Phoneme that is weakly articulated and there-

fore weakly aspirated; *e.g.*, /b/, /d/, /g/, /v/, /z/, /ʒ/. See also lax or lenis *phoneme*.

releasing c. Consonant that begins a syllable.

syllabic c. A consonant which acts like a vowel in forming a syllable nucleus; *e.g.*, The final sounds in the words *battle* /b æ tl/ and *button* /b ʌ tn/.

velarized c. Dark lateral. See lateral, under consonant, manner of formation.

vibrant c. See trill, under consonant, manner of formation.

voiced c. Consonant produced with vibration of the vocal folds: /b/, /d/, /g/, /l/, /m/, /n/, /ŋ/, /r/, /ð/, /v/, /w/, /j/, /z/, /ʒ/, /dʒ/.

voiceless c. Phoneme pronounced

without any vibration of the vocal folds: /f/, /h/, /ʍ/, /k/, /p/, /t/, /s/, /ʃ/, /θ/, /tʃ/.

consonant, manner of formation or **manner of articulation** or **mode of articulation** Refers to (a) direction of air or voice emission from the vocal tract, or (b) degree of narrowing of the vocal tract. See also distinctive features.

  affricate or **affricative** (af'ri-kət, ə-frik'ə-tiv) Consonantal sound beginning as a stop but expelled as a fricative; *e.g.*, /tʃ/, /ʤ/.

  continuant (kon-tin'yu-ənt) Speech sound in which the speech organs are held in position during the period of production; vowels may also be considered as belonging to this group; *e.g.*, /s/, /m/, /f/. See also under distinctive features.

  fricative (frik'ə-tiv) **1.** Sound formed by directing the breath stream with adequate pressure against one or more surfaces, principally the hard palate, alveolar ridge behind the upper teeth, teeth, and lips; the breath stream is continuously flowing but restricted. **2.** Any sound made by forcing the air stream through a narrow opening, resulting in audible high-frequency sounds: /f/, /v/, /θ/, /ð/, /s/, /z/, /ʃ/, and /ʒ/. Syn: spirant.

    Groove fricative is formed by placing the tip of the tongue directly behind the teeth, with the blade of the tongue under the alveoli and being slightly grooved so that the air stream escapes only through this central channel: /s/, /z/, /ʃ/, /ʒ/.

    Slit fricative is formed by forcing the air stream through a narrow opening between the upper teeth and the lower lip: /f/, /v/, /θ/, /ð/.

  frictionless (frik'shən-les) Glide (see below).

  glide Speech sound which consists primarily of the movement of an articulator, in contrast to sounds produced with the articulators in a rela-

tively static position: /r/, /w/, /j/, /ʍ/. Syn: frictionless.

  implosive (im-plō'siv) Stop sound made when the release of air pressure is achieved by lowering the velum and allowing air to flow through the nasal cavity; *e.g.*, /t/ in shoo*t*ing.

  lateral (lat'ėr-əl) Sound produced by the air stream passing through the mouth, but around the sides of the tongue; the tip of the tongue is placed against the gum ridge, restricting the airflow to the sides of the tongue: /l/.

    Dark lateral is a sound resulting from the raising of the back of the tongue toward the soft palate: /l/ as in ca*ll*. Syn: velarized consonant.

    Light lateral is a weak sound caused by friction of the air current against the side edges of the tongue: /l/ as in *l*it.

  liquid (lik'wid) Sound made with the soft palate raised: /r/, /l/.

  nasal (nā'zəl) Sound resulting from the closing of the oral cavity, preventing air from escaping through the mouth, with a lowered position of the velum or soft palate and a free passage of air through the nose; usually voiced but may lose its voicing in combination with voiceless consonants: /n/, /m/, /ŋ/.

  nonsonorant (non-son'ər-ənt) Sibilant (see below).

  obstruent (ob-stru'ənt) Sound in which the flow of breath is partially or totally obstructed; *e.g.*, /p/, /b/, /f/, /v/, /θ/, /ð/, /t/, /d/, /k/, /g/, /s/, /z/, /ʃ/, /ʒ/, /tʃ/, /ʤ/.

  plosive (plō'siv) Stop sound produced when the impounded air pressure in the portion of the vocal tract behind the constriction is released through the oral cavity; *e.g.*, /t/ in shor*t*.

  retroflex (re'trō-fleks) Sound produced with the tongue tip turned backward to touch the palate: /r/. Syn: rhotic.

semivowel Sound produced by keeping the vocal tract briefly in the vowel-like position, and then changing to the position required for the following vowel in the syllable; usually followed by a vowel in whatever syllable it is used: /w/, /j/, /r/.

sibilant (sib′ə-lənt) Fricative sound whose production is accompanied by a hissing noise: /s/, /z/, /ʃ/, /ʒ/, /tʃ/, /ʤ/. Syn: nonsonorant.

sonorant or **sonant** (son′ər-ənt, so-n′ənt) Sound produced with a relatively unobstructed flow of air between the articulator and the point of articulation: /m/, /n/, /ŋ/, /l/, /r/, /j/, /w/.

spirant (spi′rənt) Fricative (see above).

stop Sound made by blocking the air pressure in the mouth and then suddenly releasing it; the airflow can be blocked momentarily by pressing the lips together (labial) or by pressing the tongue against either the gums (alveolar) or soft palate (velar): /p/, /d/, /t/, /b/, /k/, /g/.

trill Series of very short occlusions separated by small vocalic elements, the articulator being either the tip of the tongue or the uvula: /r/; sometimes referred to as a vibrant consonant.

consonant, place or **point of articulation** That location along the length of the vocal tract from the anterior (bilabial) portion to the posterior (glottal) point where the tract is occluded or narrowed to produce a specific consonant phoneme; includes the lips, teeth, alveolar ridge, palate, and glottis. See also distinctive features.

    alveolar or **lingua-alveolar area** Articulation area where sound is produced with the tongue contacting the upper alveolar ridge; *e.g.*, /t/, /d/, /n/, /s/, /z/, /l/, and sometimes /r/.

    bilabial area Articulation area where

a sound is produced using both lips; *e.g.*, /p/, /b/, /m/, /w/, /ʍ/.

    glottal area Articulation area where a sound is produced at the level of the vocal folds; the air is impeded at the glottis, but not sufficiently to produce vocal fold vibration; *e.g.*, /h/ - who.

    labiodental area Articulation area where a sound is produced which involves the contact of the lower lip with the upper teeth; *e.g.*, /f/, /v/.

    lingua-alveolar area Alveolar area (see above).

    linguadental area Articulation area where a sound is produced with the tongue between the upper and lower front teeth; *e.g.*, /θ/, /ð/. Syn: interdental.

    palatal area Articulation area where a sound is produced by the tongue contacting or approximating the hard palate; *e.g.*, /ʃ/, /ʒ/, /ʤ/, /tʃ/, /j/, and sometimes /r/.

    velar area Articulation area where a sound is produced when the point of contact is farthest back in the vocal tract; *e.g.*, /k/, /g/, /ŋ/.

consonantal (kon-sə-nən′təl) See under distinctive features.

consonant blend See under consonant.

consonant cluster See under consonant.

consonant-injection method See injection method, under speech, methods of esophageal speech.

consonant position Location of a consonant in a word or syllable.

    final c. p. Term used by some speech and language pathologists to indicate the last sound in a word or utterance; *e.g.*, /s/ in bu*s*.

    initial c. p. Term used by some speech and language pathologists to specify a sound that appears in the first position of a word or utterance; *e.g.*, /s/ in *s*un.

    intervocalic c. p. Consonant or consonant cluster that occurs between two vowels or syllabic segments and functions both to end one syllable and to begin the next; *e.g.*, /p/ in pa*p*er; /nd/ in ca*nd*le; /ns/ in pe*n*cil. Syn: ambisyllabic.

medial c. p. Middle sound in a word; *e.g.*, /p/ in dia*p*er.

postvocalic c. p. Consonant or consonant cluster that occurs after a vowel at the end of a word *(e.g.*, /g/ in pi*g)* or before a syllable boundary *(e.g.*, /θ/ in ba*th*/tub*)*.

prevocalic c. p. Consonant or consonant cluster that appears before a vowel at the beginning of a word *(e.g.*, /p/ in *p*ig, *p*encil) or after a syllable boundary *(e.g.*, /m/ in to/*m*ato, /t/ in bath/*t*ub).

consonant voicing See voicing.

consonant-vowel (CV) See under syllable.

consonant-vowel-consonant (CVC) See under syllable.

consonant-vowel preference Deletion of final consonant. See under syllabic structure, under phonological processes.

constancy (kon′stən-sē) Perception of objects or words as essentially the same regardless of differences in their occurrence or production.

constituent (kən-stich′yu-ənt) [L. *constituens*, set up] Morpheme, word, or construction that participates in some larger construction.

constituent clause Subordinate *clause.*

constituent sentence See under sentence classification, transformational grammar.

constricted vocal production Tight inefficient voice produced with excessive effort.

construction (kən-strək′shən) [L. *construction*, a putting together] In linguistics, the arrangement of noun phrases and verb phrases within a sentence.

    absolute c. Word or phrase that does not grammatically affect the sentence in which it appears; *e.g.*, interjections, transitional words or phrases, nouns of address, nomina-

tive absolutes, adverbs of affirmation, negatives.

    endocentric c. Syntactic arrangement that has a center and is capable of being expanded by words which modify, explain, or describe the center; *e.g.*, green fat frog (*frog* is the center; *green* and *fat* are the expansions). *Cf.* exocentric *construction.*

    exocentric c. Linguistic structure that does not have a center, and neither of the members can be considered an expansion (description or explanation) of the other; both of the constituents must be present or there is no construction; *e.g.*, frogs croak (neither part is expanded from the other). *Cf.* endocentric *construction.*

constructional apraxia See under apraxia.

construct validity See under validity.

contact ulcer See under laryngeal anomaly.

content or **contentive word** See under word.

content validity See under validity.

context (kon′tekst) In pragmatics, the immediate environment of the speaker and listener, including past experiences that each brings to the situation.

contiguity disorder See under aphasia.

contingency management Manipulation of events that precedes and follows a response. In a therapy situation this may be the cue that precedes or evokes the target behavior, and may include the reinforcement (or the lack of reinforcement) that follows the target behavior. The target behavior, then, is not necessarily under the control of the cue provided by the therapist, but can be said to be under control of the event that follows (which may in some cases be a token reward).

contingent (kən-tin′jənt) Stimulus dependent on a response if the occurrence of the response causes the occurrence of the stimulus; this relationship of causation may be prearranged by an experimenter or clinician; *e.g.*, clinician's response of "good" after five minutes of fluent speech by the client should stimulate an additional five more minutes of fluent speech.

continuant (kon-tin′yu-ənt) **1.** See under consonant, manner of formation. **2.** See under distinctive features.

continuous reinforcement schedule See under reinforcement schedule.

contralateral (kon-trə-lat′ėr-əl) [L. *contra*, against, opposite + *latus*, side] **1.** Denoting association with an occurrence on the opposite side of the body. *Cf.* ipsilateral. **2.** In audiology, an effect that occurs in one ear when masking presented to that ear is intense enough to exert an effect on the other ear.

contralateral routing of signals (CROS) See under hearing aid.

contrastive distribution Parallel *distribution*.

contrastive linguistics See under linguistics.

control group In an experiment or study, those participants who do not experience the independent variable; used to verify the results by comparison with participants experiencing the variable.

controlled bite See under mature *bite*.

convergence circuit See under neuronal circuit.

conversational postulates See under pragmatic structures.

conversation board Communication board.

conversion (kən-vėr′shən) [con- + L. *versio*, turning] Change in character, form, or function.

conversion aphonia See under aphonia.

conversion deafness Psychogenic *deafness*.

conversion hysteria See under hysteria.

conversion reaction See under reaction.

convolution (kon-və-lu′shən) [L. *convolution*] Gyrus.

convulsion (kon-vəl′shən) [L. *convulsio*, to tear up] Violent involuntary contrac-

tion or series of contractions of voluntary muscles.

cooing (ku′iŋ) Early infantile sounds produced in comfortable states, usually in response to smiling or talking by the mother; the sounds are described as primarily vocalic, but some consonantal elements may appear; occurs between 6 and 8 weeks of age.

coordination (kō-ôr-di-nā′shən) [co- + L. *ordinatus*, arranged] Harmonious working together, especially of several muscles or muscle groups in the execution of complicated movements.

coprolalia (kop-rə-lā′lē-ə) [G. *kopros*, dung + *lalia*, talking] Obscene language uttered without provocation or reason.

copula (kop′yu-lə) Any form of *be* used to link a subject noun with a predicate noun or adjective; *e.g.*, she *is* my friend; we *are* late.

copy Imitation or reproduction of an object or act; usually noticeable in a child's imitation of an adult's language.

COR Conditioned orientation reflex audiometry.

cordectomy (kôr-dek′tə-mē) [G. *chordē*, cord + *ektomē*, excision] Surgical removal of one of the vocal folds.

core vocabulary See under vocabulary.

corniculate (kôr-nik′yə-lāt, -lit) [L. *corniculatus*, horned] Resembling a horn, or having hornlike appendages or prominences.

corniculate cartilages See under cartilage.

coronal (kə-rō′nəl) See under distinctive features.

coronal plane Frontal *plane*.

corpus, pl. **corpora** (kôr′pəs, kôr-pôr′ă) [L. body] **1.** In anatomy, the main portion of an organ, bone, or other structure. **2.** In linguistics, a sample of recorded utterances used as the basis of a descriptive analysis of a language or dialect. See also language sample.

corpus callosum (kôr′pus kə-lō′səm) Arched commissure of white matter beneath the longitudinal fissure of the cerebrum; connects the cerebral hemispheres.

corrective feedback See under feedback.

correlation (kôr-ə-lā′shən) **1.** Mutual or reciprocal relation of two or more items or parts. **2.** In acoustics, a measurement of similarity of two time series or waveforms; a function of the tone displacement between the two. **3.** In statistics, the relationship between two sets of scores or measures; the tendency of one set to vary with the other. The existence of a strong relationship, *i.e.*, a high degree of correlation between two variables, does not necessarily indicate that one has any causal influence on the other. See also coefficient of correlation.

   negative c. Inverse relationship of the values of two sets of measures; *e.g.*, children with good arithmetic skills and poor reading skills, and children with poor arithmetic skills and good reading skills.

   positive c. Direct relationship of the values of two sets of measures; *e.g.*, children with good arithmetic skills and good reading skills, and children with poor arithmetic skills and poor reading skills.

cortex, pl. cortices (kôr′teks, -tə-sēz) [L. bark] Outer portion of an organ, as distinguished from the inner (medullary) portion. See also cerebrum, under brain.

cortical (kôr′tə-kəl) Relating to a cortex.

cortical deafness Central *deafness* (1).

cortical lateralization Cerebral *dominance*.

cortical respiration See under respiration.

cortices (kôr′tə-sēz) Plural of cortex.

cosine wave See under wave.

Costen's syndrome [J. B. Costen, U.S. laryngologist, 1895–1962] Temporomandibular joint syndrome.

coulomb (Q) (ku-lom′) [C. de Coulomb, Fr. physicist, 1736–1806] Unit quantity of electricity or charge transferred by a current of 1 ampere in 1 second.

counter conditioning See under conditioning.

coup de glotte Glottal catch. See under voice disorders of phonation.

coupler (kup′lėr) In acoustics: **1.** Any device by which one portion of an acoustical system is joined to another; *e.g.*, earmold coupler; hearing aid. **2.** Cavity of predetermined shape and size used in measuring the acoustic output of earphones or receivers. **3.** Arrangement to transfer sound waves from their source to an amplifying system without first converting the sound waves to another form.

coupling (kəp′liŋ) Two or more resonators which are linked together and respond as one.

covert (kō′vėrt) **1.** Concealed, disguised, or kept secret, as opposed to overt. **2.** In stuttering, these tendencies may include such psychoemotional factors as fear, anxiety, negative emotion, guilt, and frustration. See also under stuttering, interiorized.

covert response See under response.

CPR Cochleopalpebral reflex.

CPS Cycles per second.

cranial (krā′nē-əl) [L. fr. G. *kranion*, skull] **1.** Relating to the cranium or skull. **2.** Toward the head.

cranial nerve Any one of twelve pairs of bundles or trunks of neurons emerging from the brainstem at points above the first cervical vertebra. Directly significant in speech and hearing are the trigeminal, facial, acoustic or vestibulocochlear, glossopharyngeal, spinal accessory, and hypoglossal nerves (cranial nerves V, VII, VIII, IX, XI, and XII). See *Cranial Nerves* table and figure.

craniofacial (krā′nē-ō-fā′shəl) Pertaining to or involving both the cranium (skull) and the face.

craniofacial anomalies Malformations of the cranium (skull) and face.

cretinism (krē′tə-niz-əm) [F. *crétin*, a cretin] Congenital condition caused by deficient thyroid secretion and charac-

CRANIAL NERVES

Nerve	Function	General Speech or Hearing Involvement Resulting From a Lesion
I Olfactory (sensory)	Sense of smell	
II Optic (sensory)	Vision	
III Oculomotor (motor)	Eye movement	
IV Trochlear (motor)	Sensory endings of muscles of the eye	
V Trigeminal (mixed)	Innervation of the mandible; chewing movements; primary sensory nerve to face and tongue	Articulation disorders which may be the result of a partial paralysis of the face or faulty control of mandibular movement
VI Abducens (motor)	Sensory endings in muscles of eye	
VII Facial (mixed)	Facial expressions; secretions of saliva; taste; extrinsic muscles of tongue	Dysarthria resulting from facial paralysis or faulty control of jaw and lip movements
VIII Acoustic or vestibulo-cochlear (sensory) Vestibular branch Cochlear branch	Balance or equilibrium Hearing	Impairment of hearing
IX Glossopharyngeal (mixed)	Taste buds of posterior third of tongue; mucous membranes of posterior third of tongue, pharynx, soft palate, and tonsils; carotid sinus	Palsy of palate, pharynx, and layrnx, depending on nature and extent of the injury
X Vagus (mixed)	Sensory and motor components to larynx, lungs, esophagus, heart, abdominal viscera, and stomach; has two principal branches; superior and inferior laryngeal nerves	In superior laryngeal paralysis there is inability of the vocal folds to tense; low and unsteady voice and anesthesia of the upper larynx and epiglottis may occur; in recurrent nerve parlaysis there is loss of adduction or abduction, and perhaps defects in tensing or relaxing, or loss of sphincteric action
XI Spinal accessory (motor)	Joins vagus nerve; motor to larynx and pharynx; shoulder movements; turning movements of head; movements of viscera	Impairment of action of muscles, depending on nature and extent of injury; faulty articulation and difficulty with guttural sounds
XII Hypoglossal (motor)	Muscles of tongue (proprioceptive); muscles of tongue and those connecting tongue with mandible and hyoid bone (movements)	Tongue deviates and may become atrophied; palatine paresis; many speech sounds are slurred

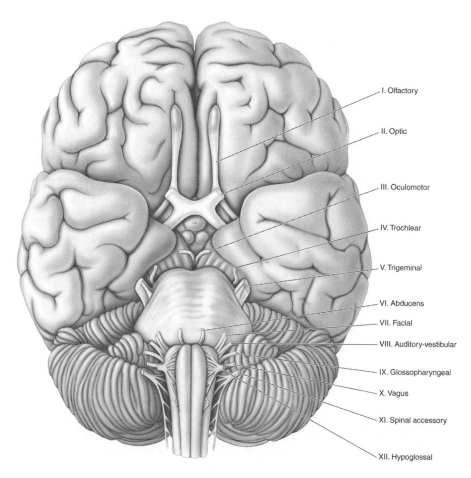

Cranial Nerves
From Bear MF, Connors BW, Paradiso MA. *Neuroscience: Exploring the Brain,* 2nd Ed. Baltimore: Lippincott Williams & Wilkins, 2001.

terized by physical and mental retardation.

crib-o-gram See under audiometer.

cricoarytenoid (krī′kō-ār-i-tē′noid, -ə-rit′ə-noid) Relating to the cricoid and the arytenoid cartilages.

cricoarytenoid ankylosis See under ankylosis.

cricoarytenoid joint Articulation between the base of each arytenoid cartilage and the upper border of the cricoid cartilage.

cricoarytenoid muscle See *Muscles of the Larynx* table, under larynx.

cricoid (krī′koid) [G. *krikos,* ring + *edios,* form] Ring-shaped, denoting the cricoid cartilage.

cricoid cartilage See under cartilage.

cricothyroid (krī-kō-thī′roid) Relating to the cricoid and thyroid cartilages.

cricothyroid muscle See *Muscles of the Larynx* table, under larynx.

cricothyroid paralysis See under laryngeal motor *paralysis.*

cri du chat syndrome (krē-du-shä′) [Fr. cry of the cat] Severe mental and physical retardation associated with varying craniofacial anomalies; a peculiar catlike cry is characteristic from birth to 5 months or more. Syn: cat cry syndrome.

cris-CROS Binaural CROS. See contralateral routing of signals (CROS), under hearing aid.

criteria, sing. **criterion** (krī-tēr′ē-ə, -ē-on) [G. *kritērion*, standard] Explicit standards for defining a category; in speech therapy, criteria for improvement are usually expressed as the number of consecutive responses or as percentages of correct responses. See also the specific term.

criterion-referenced test Assessment of an individual's development of certain skills in terms of absolute levels of mastery. The test items are objective and arranged in a hierarchical order of sequential skills; ratio scores are obtained.

criterion-related validity See under validity.

critical band 1. Restricted band of frequencies surrounding a pure tone; often used in audiological masking. See also critical band concept, under masking. **2.** Range of frequencies beyond which noise will not further decrease the audibility of a particular sinusoidal wave.

critical band concept See under masking.

CROS Contralateral routing of signals.

cross-bite See under teeth malpositions.

cross-consonant injection method See injection method, under esophageal speech, under alaryngeal *speech.*

crossed laterality See under laterality.

cross hearing Effect which occurs when sound pressure waves presented to one ear are heard in the other; the waves travel either around or through the head.

cross-modality perception See under perception.

cross-talk In auditory training units, extraneous speech heard on one loop-induction trainer system as a result of interference from another system

when the two systems are too close to one another.

croup (krup) Condition caused by obstruction of the larynx, especially in children, and characterized by a harsh cough and noisy difficult respiration; may result from an infection, allergy, growth, or foreign body.

> **inflammatory c.** Croup characterized by a breaking cough, inspiratory stridor, and swelling in the subglottic area; because of the swelling, the condition usually requires immediate medical attention.

> **spasmodic c.** Croup characterized by a hoarse ringing cough and sharp inspiratory stridor; largely confined to children, it appears suddenly (usually at night), lasts for about an hour, and then subsides.

crus, pl. **crura** (krus, kru′rə) [L. leg, shank] Limblike anatomical process, such as the short and the long crus of the incus, and the anterior and the posterior crus of the stapes.

CT Corrective therapy; computed tomography.

cue (kyu) An aid (visual, auditory, etc.) which promotes a correct response. For types of cues, see specific term.

cued speech See under sign systems.

cul-de-sac (kəl-də-sak′) [F. bottom of a sack] **1.** Blind pouch or tubular cavity closed at one end. **2.** See under voice disorders of resonation.

cultural norm Behavior which a society considers important in terms of group characteristics; behavior is judged by such a model, as opposed to real or theoretical standards, and individual personal idiosyncrasies are disregarded.

Culture Fair Intelligence Test See *Psychological Measures and Tests* in appendices.

cuneiform (kyu′nē-ə-form) [L. *cuneus,* wedge] Wedge shaped.

cuneiform cartilages See under cartilage.

current (kėr′ənt) **1.** Rate of electron flow through an electrical circuit; voltage divided by the resistance. Unit of measure is the ampere. **2.** Flow of electrons through a conductor.

alternating c. (AC) Electric current which periodically changes its value or direction of flow.

direct c. (DC) Electric current which flows continuously in one direction and does not change its value.

curve [L. *curvo*, to bend] Nonangular continuous bend, as in a graphic representation of a continuous line of shifting direction.

articulation c. In speech discrimination testing, a graphic configuration demonstrating the percentage of a specified list of words that the listener can identify as the words are spoken with increasing loudness to him. Syn: discrimination curve. See also speech discrimination, under speech *audiometry*.

Bell-shaped c. Normal *distribution*.

dipper c. Saddle curve. See under audiogram configurations.

discrimination c. Articulation *curve*.

frequency-response c. Graphic depiction for each frequency of the amount by which the instrument amplifies the incoming signal.

gaussian c. Normal *distribution*.

gradual falling or **gradual rising c.** See under audiogram configurations.

marked falling c. Sharply falling curve. See under audiogram configurations.

normal, normal probability, or **probability c.** Normal *distribution*.

saddle c. See under audiogram configurations.

saucer c. See under audiogram configurations.

shadow c. In audiometry, a false audiogram, usually the result of cross hearing, which indicates a threshold of hearing sensitivity in the poorer ear that parallels that of the better ear; may assume any configuration

and usually occurs when masking is not used.

sharply falling c. See under audiogram configurations.

ski slope c. See under audiogram configurations.

steep or **sudden drop c.** Ski slope curve. See under audiogram configurations.

trough or **"U"-shaped c.** Saddle curve. See under audiogram configurations.

waterfall c. Ski slope curve. See under audiogram configurations.

cusp [L. *cuspis*, point] On teeth, a conical elevation on the chewing surface of the crown.

cuspid teeth Canine *teeth*.

CV Consonant-vowel.

CVA Cerebral vascular accident.

CVC Consonant-vowel-consonant.

cyanosis (sī-ə-nō'sis) [G. *kyanos*, blue substance + *-ōsis*, condition] Dark bluish or purplish coloration of the skin and mucous membranes due to deficient oxygenation of the blood.

cybernetics (sī-bėr-net'iks) [G. *kybernētica*, things relating to control or piloting] **1.** Study of regulatory mechanisms, such as governors, thermostats, feedback systems, and reverberating circuits. **2.** Science based on the principles of control and communications as they apply to the operation of sophisticated electronic calculators and the function of the human nervous system, with the intent of the former explaining the latter.

cybernetic theory of stuttering See under stuttering theories.

cycle (sī'kəl) [G. *kyklos*, circle] **1.** Complete set of recurrent values of an alternating current or voltage, consisting of a positive rise and fall (alternation) and a negative rise and fall; a complete sinusoidal wave. **2.** One successive compression and rarefaction of a sound wave.

cycles per second (CPS) Former unit of measurement for the number of successive compressions and rarefactions of a sound wave within one second of time; now replaced by hertz (Hz).

cytomegalovirus (CMV) A viral disease which is passed from the mother to the fetus via the bloodstream; considered to be the most common viral disease to cause hearing loss. The loss is usually late in onset and may range from mild to profound.

dactyl (dak′təl) [G. *daktylos*, finger] **1.** A finger or, less commonly, a toe. **2.** Relating to a finger.

dactylology (dak-tə-lol′ə-jē) [G. *daktylos*, finger + *logos*, discourse] Fingerspelling.

dactyl speech Fingerspelling.

DAF Delayed auditory feedback.

damped wave See under wave.

damping Decrease in the amplitude of a vibrating body; systems are said to be *heavily damped* when the amplitude decays rapidly, *lightly damped* when the amplitude decays slowly over time, and *critically damped* if all vibration ceases before completion of one cycle.

dark lateral See lateral, under consonant, manner of formation.

dative See under parts of speech.

dB Decibel.

DBA dB scale used to measure environmental sounds.

DC Direct current.

de- [L. *de*, from, away] Prefix with a privative or negative sense, denoting away from, cessation.

dead room Anechoic chamber.

deaf (def) Denoting one in whom the sense of hearing is nonfunctional, with or without amplification, for the ordinary purposes of life. Such an individual may (a) have been born either totally deaf or sufficiently deaf to prevent the establishment of speech and natural language; (b) have become deaf in childhood before language and speech were completely established (prelingual deafness); or (c) have become deaf after having acquired speech and language skills (postlingual deafness), thus significantly impairing communication skills.

deaffrication See under substitution, under phonological processes.

deaf mute Old term for an individual who can neither hear nor speak, usually one born with a severe hearing loss.

deafness (def′nes) Loss of the ability to hear, without designation of the degree of loss or the cause. See also hearing impairment degrees.

   adventitious d. Loss of hearing sensitivity occurring after birth and due to injury or disease.

   catarrhal d. Hearing loss resulting from inflammation of the mucous membrane of the air passages in the head and throat, with congestion of the eustachian tube.

   central d. 1. Loss of hearing sensitivity as a result of damage to auditory nerve pathways in the brainstem or in the hearing centers in the cortex of the brain; acuity for pure tones is unimpaired, but phonemic regression prevails; sounds may be heard but not understood. **2.** Condition occurring during psychoneurotic disorders. Syn: cortical deafness. See also Wernicke's *aphasia*.

   conductive d. Impairment of hearing due to the failure of sound pressure waves to reach the cochlea through the normal air-conduction channels (outer or middle ear); the inner ear is usually normal.

   congenital d. Loss of hearing sensitivity existing at or dating from birth.

   conversion d. Psychogenic *deafness*.

   cortical d. Central *deafness* (1).

   functional d. Auditory impairment for which no organic basis can be determined or inferred. Syn: nonorganic deafness.

   high-frequency d. Loss of hearing acuity for high frequencies; may be associated with sensorineural damage.

   hysterical d. Psychogenic *deafness*.

   industrial d. Loss of hearing sensitivity as a result of relatively long exposure to industrial noise.

low-tone d. Low-frequency hearing loss; inability to hear low notes or frequencies.

mixed d. Combination of conductive and sensorineural hearing losses.

nerve d. See sensorineural *deafness*.

noise-induced d. Hearing impairment which develops gradually from continuous exposure to noise that is above acceptable levels. Syn: occupational deafness.

nonorganic d. Functional *deafness*.

occupational d. Noise-induced *deafness*.

postlingual d. Hearing impairment occurring after the development of speech and language.

prelingual d. Loss of hearing sensitivity occurring before the development of speech and language skills; may be congenital or adventitious.

prevocational d. Hearing impairment occurring prior to age nineteen.

psychogenic d. Auditory impairment which may result from emotional stress as an unconscious means of escape from an intolerable situation. Syn: conversion or hysterical deafness.

pure word d. See under pure *aphasias.*

retrocochlear d. Hearing loss resulting from a lesion behind the cochlea.

sensorineural d. Hearing impairment resulting from a pathologic condition in the inner ear or along

ETIOLOGIES OF SUDDEN AND PROGRESSIVE HEARING LOSS

Autoimmune Disorders	Vascular Disorders	Neurologic and Neoplastic Lesions	Trauma Insults	Infectious Disease
Autoimmune inner ear disease (AIED)	Cardiopulmonary bypass	Acoustic neuroma	Large vestibular aqueduct syndrome	Cryptococcal meningitis
Cogan's syndrome	Red blood cell deformability	Contralateral deafness after acoustic neuroma surgery	Inner ear concussion	Cytomegalovirus
Lupus erythematosus	Sickle cell disease	Focal pontine ischemia	Inner ear decompression sickness (caisson's disease)	Herpes
Ménière's disease	Vascular disease/ alteration of microcirculation	Leukemia	Otologic surgery (stapedectomy)	Human immunodeficiency virus
Polyarteritis nodosa	Vascular disease associated with mitochondrial myopathy	Meningeal carcinomatosis	Ototoxicity	Lassa fever
Relapsing polychondritis	Vertebrobasilar insufficiency	Metastasis to internal auditory canal	Perilymph fistula	Meningococcal meningitis
Ulcerative colitis		Migraine	Surgical complications	Mumps
Wegener's granulomatosis		Multiple sclerosis Myeloma	Temporal bone fracture	Mycoplasma Rubeola Rubella Syphilis Toxoplasmosis

From Muller, C. *Sudden sensorineural hearing loss.* Paper presented at Grand Rounds in the Department of Otolaryngology/Head and Neck Surgery, University of Texas Medical Branch, Galveston, TX, June 2001. Available at www.utmb.edu/otoret/grnds/suddenhearingloss-010613/ssnhl.htm

the nerve pathway from the inner ear to the brainstem; may be cochlear or retrocochlear, depending on the site of the lesion.

sudden and progressive hearing loss A sudden progressive sensorineural hearing loss whose prognosis depends on the underlying etiology which may vary from individual to individual. See table.

tone d. Inability to distinguish between two sounds of different frequencies within the normal hearing range when there is not any apparent loss of acuity in these frequencies, as in being unable to tell whether oneself or another is singing "off key" or "on key."

toxic d. Hearing loss resulting from the effect of drugs on the sensory mechanism, due to sensitivity to a drug or to an excessive dosage.

word d. See auditory *aphasia;* See also under pure *aphasias.*

deaf speech See under speech.

decay period or **rate** Speed with which a sound vibration fades at a specific place and time; usually expressed in decibels per second.

decentration (dē-sen-trā'shǝn) [de- + L. *centrum,* center] Ability to simultaneously attend to more than one dimension of an object; realization that shape and space do not necessarily change the size of an object. See also Period III, under cognitive development.

decibel (dB) (des'i-bel) One-tenth of a bel; a quantitative unit of sound intensity with a logarithmic relationship to the amplitude of the sound; *e.g.,* in audiology, sound intensity is measured in terms of the ratio between the intensity of the sound being measured and a standard reference intensity (0.0002 dyne/cm^2).

deciduous teeth See teeth.

declarative sentence See under sentence types.

decoder (dē-kōd'ėr) In electric computers, a network in which a combination of inputs produces a single output.

decoding (dē-kōd'iŋ) Receptive *language.*

deconditioning (dē-kǝn-di'shǝn-iŋ) Counter *conditioning.*

decruitment (de-krut'mǝnt) Failure of the sense of loudness to increase as intensity increases, a condition found in individuals exhibiting retrocochlear

DECIBEL LEVELS	
dB	*Sound Source*
20	Watch ticking
30	Whispering, library
40	Leaves rustling, refrigerator
50	Average home, neighborhood street
60	Normal conversation, dishwasher, microwave
70	Car, alarm clock, city traffic
80	Garbage disposal, noisy restaurant, vacuum cleaner, outboard motor
85	Factory, electric shaver, screaming child
90	Passing motorcycle, lawn mower, convertible ride on a freeway
100	Blow dryer, diesel truck, subway train, helicopter, chain saw
110	Car horn, snow blower
120	Rock concert, prop plane
130	Jet engine 100 feet away, air raid siren
140	Shotgun blast

The federal government advises wearing earplugs, earmuffs, or other hearing protection whenever exposed to 85 dB for a period of more than a few hours. Federal regulations require a hearing conservation program at any workplace where employees are exposed to 85 dB during their entire eight-hour workday. (From Better Hearing Institute Self-Help for Hard of Hearing People.)

lesions; demonstrated with loudness-balance tests and usually confined to one or two audiometric frequencies. See also recruitment.

decussation (de-kə-sā′shən) [L. *decussatio*] Intercrossing of similar nerve bundles as each crosses over to the opposite side of the brain in the course of ascending or descending through the brainstem or spinal cord.

deduction (dē-dək′shən) [L. a leading away from] Synthetic method of study moving from the general to the specific; *e.g.*, progression from a class to a component within the class.

deep articulation test See under articulation test.

deep structure See under structure.

Deep Test of Articulation See *Articulation Tests and Phonological Analysis Procedures* in appendices.

degeneration (dē-jen-ėr-ā′shən) [L. *degeneratio*] Retrogressive pathologic inhibition or destruction of a tissue or organ's ability to function; if the process cannot be reversed, necrosis will result.

deglutition (dē-glu-ti′shən) [L. *deglutio*, to swallow] Act of swallowing. See swallow.

deictic (dīk′tik) Denoting or characteristic of deixis.

deixis (dīk′sis) **1.** Linguistic device that anchors the utterance to the communicative setting in which it occurs. **2.** Purposeful exchange of information; requires a maintenance of interaction.
　person Linguistic device to indicate who is the speaker and who is the listener.
　place Linguistic device to indicate where the speaker and listener are at the time of the utterance.
　time Linguistic device to indicate when the utterance is taking place.

déjà vu (dā-zhä′vu) [Fr. already seen] Illusion that things perceived have occurred before, even though no memory trace of the previous experience(s) can be found; a normal experience for most people, but is often associated with aphasic individuals or may suggest a temporal lobe disorder.

Déjérine syndrome [J. J. Déjérine, Fr. neurologist, 1849–1917] Bulbar paralysis resulting from lesions in the medulla oblongata: (a) those in the upper part produce paralysis of the hypoglossal nerve (cranial nerve XII) on the side of the lesion and hemiplegia on the opposite side; (b) those in the lower part produce paralysis of the larynx and soft palate.

delayed auditory feedback (DAF) See under feedback.

delayed echolalia See under echolalia.

delayed feedback audiometry (DFA) See under audiometry.

delayed language See under language.

delayed reinforcer See under reinforcer.

delayed response See under response.

delayed speech See under speech.

deletion of final consonant See under syllabic structure, under phonological processes.

deletion of initial consonant See under syllabic structure, under phonological processes.

deletion of unstressed syllables See under syllabic structure, under phonological processes.

Del Rio Language Screening Test, English/Spanish See *Language Tests and Procedures* in appendices.

delta (del′tə) [G. letter d, Δ (capital) or δ (lower case)] **1.** In anatomy, a triangular surface. **2.** Denoting the fourth in a series, usually δ.

delta rhythm or **waves** See under electroencephalogram.

dementia (də-men′shē-ə) [L. fr. *de-* priv. + *mens*, mind] General mental deterioration due to organic or psychological factors, characterized by disorientation, impaired memory, judgment, and intellect, and a shallow labile affect.

demonstrative (də-mon′strə-tiv) In grammar, designating the one referred to and distinguishing it from others of the same class; *e.g.*, *that* ball.

demonstrative-entity See semantic relations.

denasal (dē-nā′zəl) Quality of the voice in hyponasality (denasality).

denasality (dē-nā-zal′i-tē) Hyponasality. See under voice disorders of resonance.

denasalization See under substitution, under phonological processes.

dendrite (den′drīt) [G. *dendritēs*, relating to a tree] See neuron.

denotation (dē-nō-tā′shən) [de- + L. *notatus*, designating] Relation of a symbol to its object, as defined in a dictionary; the literal definition of a word. *Cf.* connotation.

density (den′si-tē) [L. *densitas*, thickness] 1. Extent to which entries of a correlation plot are grouped closely together. 2. In acoustics, a measure of mass per unit volume.

dental (den′təl) [L. *dens*, tooth] 1. Pertaining to the teeth. 2. Denoting a speech sound made by tongue or lip contact with the teeth. See also consonant, place of articulation.

dental arch Curved structure formed by the teeth in their normal position.

dental lisp See under lisp.

dentition (den-ti′shən) [L. *dentitio*, to teethe] Natural teeth, considered collectively, in the dental arch.

Denver Articulation Screening Examination (DASE) See *Articulation Tests and Phonological Analysis Procedures* in appendices.

depalatization (dē′pal-ə-ti-zā′shən) Pal-

atal fronting. See under substitution, under phonological processes.

dependent clause Subordinate *clause.*

depressors (də-pres′ėrs) [L. *depressus*, pressed down] Infrahyoid muscles. See muscles of the larynx, under larynx.

derivation (dår-ə-vā′shən) [L. *derivatus*, drawn off (as from a stream)] 1. In grammar, a word or sentence made from another word or sentence; *e.g.*, manly from man. 2. In linguistics, steps leading from an initial string to a terminal string; the strings resulting from the application of branching rules.

derivation of a sentence Process of producing a sentence from phrase-structure rules, utilizing the initial string through the intermediate string(s) to the terminal string.

    initial string Beginning line in a derivation, represented by the symbol S for the complete sentence to be derived or explained.

    intermediate string Line that follows the initial string and explains in more detail the rest of a given sentence by using such symbols as S (sentence), NP (noun phrase), VP (verb phrase), MV (main verb), Aux (auxiliary), etc. Each string may indicate one explanation of the sentence's derivation at a time.

    terminal string Last line of the derivation of a sentence; consists wholly of symbols which cannot be developed further by phrase-structure rules, and may or may not then indi-

---

DERIVATION OF A SENTENCE

S → The girls are drinking water.	—*initial string*
S → NP + VP	
NP → Det + N	*intermediate string*
VP → Aux + MV + NP	
S → Det + NP + Aux + MV + NP	—*terminal string*
S → The girls are drinking water.	

cate the actual order and structure of the sentence.

derived adjective Adjective constructed from other parts of speech by additions or transformations; *e.g.*, *homely* boy, *drunken* man.

derived sentence See under sentence classification, transformational grammar.

descending pitch break See pitch break, under voice disorders of phonation.

descending technique In audiometry, a method of establishing threshold of hearing by going from an audible to an inaudible stimulus; opposite of ascending technique.

descriptive linguistics See under linguistics.

descriptive phonetics See under phonetics.

desensitization (dē-sen′si-ti-zā′shən) Therapy technique used to enable an individual to become comfortable in a situation that previously evoked fear or anxiety; usually based on a tolerance hierarchy of fear- or anxiety-producing situations.

desk-type auditory trainer See under auditory training units.

detectability threshold Absolute *threshold.*

detection (dē-tek′shən) Ability to react to the presence or absence of either auditory or visual stimuli; a prerequisite to, but not a guarantee of, perception.

detection threshold Absolute *threshold.*

determiner (dē-tėr′min-ėr) In transformational grammar, a name used for a word class which encompasses parts of speech known in traditional grammar as articles (regular determiners), demonstratives (predeterminers), and indefinite adjectives (postdeterminers).

development (də-vel′əp-mənt) Act or process of natural progression from a previous, lower, or embryonic stage to a later, more complex, or adult stage.

developmental ages Various ages at

which children acquire specific skills. See also appendices.

developmental aphasia See under aphasia.

developmental articulatory apraxia See under apraxia.

developmental disability A severe, chronic disability of a person which (a) is attributable to a mental or physical impairment or combination of mental and physical impairments; (b) is manifested before the person attains age 22; (c) is likely to continue indefinitely; (d) results in substantial functional limitations in three or more of the following areas of major life activity: (1) self-care, (2) receptive and expressive language, (3) learning, (4) mobility, (5) self-direction, (6) capacity for independent living, and (7) economic self-sufficiency; (e) reflects the person's need for combination and sequence of special, interdisciplinary, or generic care, treatment, or other services which are of lifelong or extended duration and are individually planned and coordinated [Public Law 95–602].

developmental hesitations Normal repetitions, prolongations, or stumblings in the speech of a child learning to talk.

developmental imbalance Discrepancy in the natural progressive patterns of intellectual skills. See also learning disability.

developmental period In humans, the period of time between birth and the eighteenth year.

developmental phonological processes See under phonological processes.

developmental scale Test or inventory for estimating stages of development attained by an individual.

deviant (dē′vē-ənt) Denoting a deviation.

deviant articulation See articulation disorder.

deviant language Language disorder.

deviant speech Speech disorder (1).

deviant swallowing Tongue thrust.

deviated septum Irregularity or separation of the nasal septum.

deviation (dē-vē-ā′shən) [L. *deviatus,*

turned from the straight road] **1.** Deflection; abnormality. **2.** In statistics, the amount by which a measure differs from a point of reference, generally from the mean.

    standard d. Statistic used to express the amount of the deviations of a score from the mean for the distribution; obtained by taking the square root of the mean of the square of the deviations from the mean of a distribution. If the group measured is a normal population, their scores, if plotted graphically, would yield a normal distribution curve; approximately two thirds (68.3%) of the scores would lie within the limits of one standard deviation above and one standard deviation below the mean. See also normal distribution.

devoicing of final consonants See under assimilatory phonological processes.

dexterity (deks-tăr′ə-tē) [L. *dexter*, right] Smooth and skillful movements, usually of the hands and fingers.

dextral (deks′trəl) [L. *dextra*, right] Pertaining to the right side; opposite of sinistral.

dextrality (deks-tral′ə-tē) Preferential use of organs or members of the right side of the body. See also laterality (1).

DFA Delayed feedback audiometry.

di- [G. *dis*, two] Prefix denoting two or twice.

diachronic linguistics See comparative *linguistics*.

diacritic (dī-ə-krit′ik) Mark added to an orthographic or phonetic character to indicate a phonetic or semantic difference; *e.g.*, affect (af′ekt, afekt′). See also transcription.

diadochokinesis (dī′ə-dō-kō-ki-nē′sis) [G. *diadochos*, working in turn + *kinēsis*, movement] In speech, the ability to execute rapid repetitive movements of the articulators; opposite of adiadochokinesis.

diadochokinetic rate The speed with which one can perform contrasting (or

repetitive) movements, as in saying the following syllables: puh-tuh-kuh.

diagnosis (dī-ag-nō′sis) [G. *diagnosis*, a deciding] Identification of a disease, abnormality, or disorder by analysis of the symptoms presented; may include a study of the origin and development of the symptoms. See also evaluation.

    differential d. Process of distinguishing between two similar-appearing conditions by discovering a significant symptom or attribute present in one condition but not the other.

diagnosogenic theory (dī′ag-nō-sō-jen′ik) See under anticipatory and struggle behavior theory, under stuttering theories.

diagnostic (dī-ag-nos′tik) Relating to or assisting in diagnosis.

diagnostic articulation test See under articulation test.

diagnostic audiometry See under audiometry.

diagnostic teaching Informal method of assessing abilities when formal diagnostic measures are ineffective; involves observation and teaching to determine whether the subject possesses the skills being assessed or whether remediation is necessary. Syn: diagnostic therapy.

diagnostic test Evaluation made to identify specific problems and to provide clues concerning the remedial measures to be applied.

diagnostic therapy (Dx) Diagnostic teaching.

dialect (dī′ə-lekt) Specific form of a language spoken in a given geographic area, differing sufficiently from the official standard of the larger language community (pronunciation, vocabulary, and idiomatic use of words) to be regarded as a distinct entity, yet not sufficiently different from other dialects of the language to be regarded as a separate language; *e.g.*, Pennsylvania Dutch, Cajun. See also basilect.

dialect speech community See under speech community.

diaphragm (dī′ə-fram) [G. *diaphragma*, partition wall] Muscular and tendonous partition separating the thorax from the abdominal cavities; the primary muscle of inhalation. See also *Muscles of Respiration* table, under respiration.

diaphragmatic-abdominal respiration See abdominal-diaphragmatic *respiration*.

diathesis (dī-ath′ə-sis) [G. arrangement, condition] Inherited tendency or predisposition toward certain diseases or disorders, such as otosclerosis and diabetes.

dichotic, dichotomic, dichotomous (dī-ko′tik, -ko′tə-mik, -ko′tə-məs) Denoting or characteristic of dichotomy.

Dichotic Consonant-Vowel Test See *Audiometric Tests and Procedures* in appendices.

Dichotic Digits See *Audiometric Tests and Procedures* in appendices.

dichotic listening Stimulation of both ears at the same time with different sounds; stimulation may be with tones of different frequencies or with different speech messages. Syn: competing or dichotic messages.

dichotic messages Dichotic listening.

dichotomy (dī-ko′tə-mē) [G. *dichotomia*, a cutting in two] Division of a group into two categories on the basis of the presence or absence of a certain characteristic.

diction (dik′shən) [L. rhetorical delivery] Ability to pronounce connected sounds clearly.

dielectric (dī-ə-lek′trik) Insulating material between two electrodes or plates in a capacitor.

diencephalon See under brainstem, under brain.

difference limen (DL) See under threshold.

difference tone See under tone.

differential diagnosis See under diagnosis.

differential function Parallel *distribution*.

differential reinforcement See under reinforcement.

differential relaxation Conscious tensing and releasing of a muscle group to learn to sense the specific action of various muscles, and to be able to voluntarily release tensed muscles; used as a form of voice therapy.

differential response See under response.

differential threshold Difference limen. See under threshold.

differentiation (di′fèr-en-shē-ā′shən) **1.** In phonetics, a phonetic change resulting in a sharpening of the difference between two phonemes if the two are in contact. *Cf.* dissimilation (2). **2.** Ability to discriminate between correct and incorrect responses. **3.** Functional separation of a finer movement from a larger one with which it formerly occurred.

auditory d. Auditory figure-ground *discrimination*.

Differentiation of Auditory Perception Skills (DAPS) See *Auditory Tests and Procedures* in appendices.

diffracted wave See under wave.

diffuse phoneme See under phoneme.

digastric muscle See *Muscles of the Larynx* table, under larynx.

digital (di′ji-təl) [L. *digitus*, finger or toe] **1.** Technology that allows sound waves to be converted into a binary system and transmitted by electronic or electromagnetic signals. **2.** Relating to or resembling a finger.

digital hearing aid See under hearing aid.

digital manipulation Voice therapy technique in which the clinician places external pressure with his fingers on the client's thyroid cartilage and helps the client learn to feel the movement of the larynx associated with different pitches; through this awareness technique, the client can learn to position his larynx and change his pitch.

diglossia (dī-glo′sē-ə) [di- + G. *glossa*,

tongue] Developmental abnormality of the tongue in which the two anterior portions fail to fuse. Syn: bifid or forked tongue; glossoschisis.

digraph (dī′graf) [di- + G. *graphō*, to write] Two letters written successively to represent one single sound. There are four English digraphs representing five different consonant sounds: sh = /ʃ/, ch = /tʃ/, wh = /hw/, th = /θ/, th = /ð/. Successively written vowels may also be digraphs; *e.g.*, *ea*ch = /i/.

diminutive (di-min′yə-tiv) Addition of /i/ on the end of nouns in children's speech. See also under phonological processes.

diode (dī′ōd) [di- + G. *hodos*, way (road, path)] Vacuum tube with two elements (anode and cathode), or a semiconductor manufactured to allow current to flow in one direction.

diotic (dī-ot′ik) [di- + G. *otikos*, fr. *ous*, ear] Pertaining to both ears.

diotic listening or **messages** Simultaneous stimulation of both ears with the same sound.

diphasic spike See under electroencephalogram.

diphthongs See under vowel.

diplacusis (di-plə-ku′sis) [G. *diplous*, double + *akousis*, hearing] Auditory condition in which one sound is heard as two.

   d. binauralis A condition in which a listener perceives a single pure tone as having a different pitch in each ear.

   d. monauralis A condition in which a pure tone in one ear sounds like two or more tones.

diplegia (dī-plē′jē-ə) [di- + G. *plēgē*, stroke] Bilateral paralysis affecting like parts on both sides of the body. *Cf.* hemiplegia; monoplegia; paraplegia; quadriplegia; triplegia.

diplophonia See under voice disorders of phonation.

dipper curve Saddle curve. See under audiogram configurations.

direct current (DC) See under current.

directionality (di-rek-shən-al′i-tē) Ability to discriminate left and right, up and down, and above and below in external space.

directional microphone See under microphone.

directivity (di-rek-tiv′ə-tē) In acoustics, the tendency of most sound sources to radiate sound more efficiently in some directions than in others.

direct laryngoscopy See under laryngoscopy.

direct motor system Pyramidal system.

direct object In grammar, any word or group of words acting as a noun that answers the question *what* or *whom*, and in some way is affected by the action of the verb in a particular sentence; traditionally stated, the direct object receives the action of the transitive verb; *e.g.*, He shoveled *snow*. He knows *what we need*.

direct selection communication board See under communication board.

dis- [L.] Prefix denoting separation, taking apart. *Cf.* dys-.

disability (dis-ə-bil′i-tē) Loss or impairment of a function, usually as a result of some injury to the structure.

disassimilation (dis′ə-sim-i-lā′shən) Alternative spelling for dissimilation.

disassociation (dis′ə-sō-sē-ā′shən) Alternative spelling for dissociation.

discomfort threshold See *threshold* of discomfort.

discourse (dis′kôrs) Connected communication of thought sequences; continuous expression or exchange of ideas.

discrimination (dis-krim-i-nā′shən) [L. *discriminatus*, separated] Process of distinguishing among stimuli and responding appropriately.

   auditory d. Ability to sort and sift sounds from each other; involves a comparison of heard sounds with other competing sounds, and may include differentiation of speech sounds as well as sounds of varying frequencies, intensities, and pressure-pattern components. See also *Auditory Processes* table; *Auditory Tests and Procedures* in appendices.

auditory figure-ground d. Selection of the relevant from the irrelevant auditory stimuli in an environment; *e.g.*, teacher talking while children whispering. Syn: auditory differentiation; auditory selective listening; competing messages integration.

oral sensory d. Oral *stereognosis.*

speech d. (SD) 1. In speech, the degree to which one is able to hear and recognize acoustic differences among all the phonemes in speech segments. *Cf.* auditory *discrimination.* **2.** See under speech *audiometry.*

speech sound d. Differentiation of speech sounds. See auditory *discrimination.*

visual d. Process of detecting differences in objects, forms, letters, or words.

visual figure-ground d. Ability to attend to one aspect of the visual field while perceiving it in relation to the rest of the world; *e.g.*, ability to pick out one object from the rest of a picture.

discrimination curve Articulation *curve.*

discrimination loss See speech discrimination, under speech *audiometry.*

discrimination score Percentage of words correctly repeated by a listener during an auditory differentiation or discrimination test.

discriminatory training Teaching of comparisons between pairs of syllables or words.

disfluency (dis-flu'ən-sē) Alternative spelling for dysfluency.

diskinesia (dis-ki-nē'zē-ə) Alternative spelling for dyskinesia.

displaced speech See under speech.

dissimilation (di-sim-i-lā'shən) [dis- + L. *assimilatus*, made alike] **1.** Phoneme changes which occur when one of two reoccurring phonemes is altered to become less like its neighbor; usually one

of the two repeated sounds is dropped or is changed into a different sound; *e.g.*, library/libary; surprise/suprise. **2.** Phonetic change which results in a sharpening of the difference between two phonemes if the phonemes are separated by others. *Cf.* differentiation (1).

dissociation (di-sō-sē-ā'shən) [dis- + L. *associatus*, joined to] Inability to synthesize separate elements into integrated meaningful wholes.

dissociative reaction See under reaction.

dissonance (di'sə-nəns) [L. *dissonus*, discordant] Inharmonious combination of musical sounds; sounds that do not complement each other. *Cf.* consonance (2).

distal (dis'təl) [L. *distalis*] Furthest from the center or point of origin; opposite of proximal.

distinctive (di-stiŋk'tiv) [L. *distinctus*, distinct] **1.** Distinguishing or differentiating among meanings. **2.** Making a speech item a phoneme rather than an allophone.

distinctive feature analysis See under phonological analysis.

distinctive features 1. Those indispensable attributes of a phoneme that are required to differentiate one phoneme from another in a language; based on a binary principle. In English, these elements include the presence or absence of voicing and contrasts in the various manners of articulation. See also binary principle; consonant; phoneme; vowel. **2.** Theory that the phonemic systems of all languages can be described by the use of 15 to 20 features, 13 of which apply distinctively to English; includes a plus or minus system, where plus indicates distinctive possession of a given feature and minus denotes a distinctive nonpossession of a feature. See *Distinctive Features of English Phonemes* table.

   Anterior is present when a sound is produced in the front region of the

DISTINCTIVE FEATURES OF ENGLISH PHONEMES

PHONEME	Anterior	Back	Consonantal	Continuant	Coronal	High	Low	Nasal	Round	Strident	Tense	Vocalic	Voice	LETTERS
j				+		+							+	y
w		+		+		+			+				+	w
ɔ		+		+			+		+			+	+	a
æ				+			+					+	+	ā
o		+		+					+		+	+	+	ō
ʌ		+		+								+	+	ù
ɛ				+								+	+	è
ʊ		+		+		+			+			+	+	o͞o
I				+		+						+	+	I
ɔI		+		+			+		+		+	+	+	oy
aI		+		+			+				+	+	+	ī
ou		+		+					+		+	+	+	ow
eI				+							+	+	+	ā
u		+		+		+			+		+	+	+	u
i				+		+					+	+	+	ee
h				+			+							h
ŋ		+	+			+		+					+	ng
g		+	+			+							+	g
k		+	+			+								k
ʒ			+	+	+	+				+			+	zh
ʃ			+	+	+	+				+				sh
dʒ			+		+	+				+			+	j
tʃ			+		+	+				+				ch
z	+		+	+	+					+			+	z
s	+		+	+	+					+				s
n	+		+		+			+					+	n
ð	+		+	+	+								+	ŧħ
θ	+		+	+	+									th
d	+		+		+								+	d
t	+		+		+									t
m	+		+					+					+	m
v	+		+	+						+			+	v
f	+		+	+						+				f
b	+		+										+	b
p	+		+											p
l	+		+	+	+							+	+	l
r			+	+	+							+	+	r

mouth, at the alveolar ridge or forward (negative: nonanterior).

Back is concerned with placement; the body of the tongue is retracted from the neutral position /ɛ/ (negative: nonback).

Consonantal is sound formed with a narrow constriction, as in the fricative consonants; all liquids, nasal consonants, and nonnasal consonants have this feature (negative: nonconsonantal).

Continuant requires a partial obstruction to the airflow in the vocal tract (negative: noncontinuant). Syn: interrupted.

Coronal is concerned with placement; the blade of the tongue is raised from the neutral position /ɛ/ (negative: noncoronal).

High is concerned with placement; the body of the tongue is raised above the neutral position /ɛ/ (negative: nonhigh).

Low is concerned with placement; the body of the tongue is lowered below the neutral position /ɛ/ (negative: nonlow).

Nasal is characterized by a lowering of the velum to allow the air to be directed through the nose; the nasal feature is present (negative: nonnasal).

Round is characterized by a narrowing of the lip orifice (negative: nonround).

Strident is characterized by noisiness resulting from a fast rate of airflow directed against the hard surface of the teeth (negative: nonstrident).

Tense is produced with considerable effort by supraglottal musculature as the articulatory organs maintain their configurations over a relatively long period of time (negative: nontense).

Vocalic requires the presence of two conditions: (a) the constriction in the oral cavity cannot be greater than that required for the /i/ and /ʊ/; and (b) the vocal folds must be positioned to allow spontaneous voicing (negative: nonvocalic).

Voiced requires the vocal folds to vibrate (negative—nonstrident).

distoclusion See under teeth malocclusion.

distortion (di-stôr′shən) **1.** In speech, a sound readily identified but not accurate enough to be considered correct. See also under articulation disorder. **2.** In cleft palate, a sound correctly articulated but obscured by nasal emission. See also nasal emission. **3.** In acoustics, an inexact reproduction of a sound wave pattern which is present when the output signal of the amplifying system differs in waveform from the original signal; reflects an undesired change in the relative intensity of the frequency components of the complex sound wave. See also articulation error.

amplitude d. Harmonic *distortion.*

figure-ground d. Inability to focus on an object or sound without having the background or setting interfere with perception.

harmonic d. In acoustics, new frequencies resulting from the addition of amplitude distortions (harmonic vibrations) not present in the input sound wave but harmonically related to the original frequency. Syn: amplitude or nonlinear distortion.

intermodulary d. In acoustics, new frequencies resulting when two pure tones occurring simultaneously produce an effect perceived as a warble or beat phenomenon; the new frequencies created by the distortion have no harmonic relationship.

nonlinear d. Harmonic *distortion.*

transient d. In acoustics, an inexact reproduction of a sound wave pattern resulting from sudden changes of voltage or load; occurs in the amplifier if the electrical and mechanical components are not adequately damped.

waveform d. Undesirable change in a waveform.

distortional bone conduction Compression bone *conduction.*

distortion product otoacoustic emissions (DPOAE) See under otoacoustic emissions.

distoversion See under teeth malpositions.

distractibility (dis-trak-tə-bil′ə-tē) Disorder of attention in which the mind is easily diverted by inconsequential occurrences.

distraction (dis-trak′shən) [L. *distractus,* pulling in different directions] In stuttering, filling the mind with other thoughts so that the expectancy of stuttering is avoided; keeping the anticipation of stuttering from conscious thought, thus temporarily effecting release from fear of stuttering and the performance of stuttering reactions.

distribution (dis-trə-byu′shən) [L. *distributus,* distributed] **1.** Systematic grouping of data into classes or categories. **2.** In linguistics, the occurrence of linguistic items in terms of context or geography; the total of the contexts of environments in which an element may occur; *e.g.,* The *boy* (subject) is playing; Bobby is playing with the *boy* (object of preposition); Bobby is a *boy* (predicate nominative). **3.** In statistics, the representation, tabular or graphic, of the frequency of occurrence of scores or measurements.

complementary d. In linguistics: **1.** Sounds that cannot be interchanged; the allophones together cover all possible positional occurrences but do not appear in the same linguistic environment. **2.** One of 12 methods by which sounds are combined into a phoneme; there may be several sounds, but each is used in a specific context; *e.g.,* aspirated /t/ of *top* appears initially versus the unaspi-

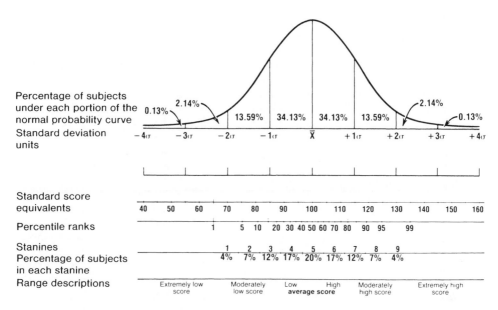

Normal Distribution

rated /t/ of *stop;* /n/ is generally produced with the tongue on the alveolar ridge, but when it occurs before a /th/ (as in *tenth*) the tongue moves forward to a position touching, or nearly touching, the front teeth. Syn: noncontrastive distribution.

contrastive d. Parallel *distribution.*

gaussian d. Normal *distribution.*

noncontrastive d. Complementary *distribution.*

normal d. In statistics, a specific bell-shaped frequency curve commonly assumed by statisticians to represent the infinite population of measurements from which a sample has been drawn; characterized by the mean and standard deviation. Syn: bell-shaped, gaussian, normal, normal probability, or probability curve; gaussian distribution.

parallel d. In linguistics, linguistic units that can be substituted for each other in the same linguistic environment; *e.g.*, in *fan*, /f/ and *an* occur; almost all of the consonants of En-

glish can be substituted for the /f/ of *fan* to form a standard word, such as *ban, can, man, pan, ran, tan.* Syn: contrastive distribution; differential function.

disyllable (dĭ′sil-ə-bəl) Bisyllable.

divergence circuit See under neuronal circuit.

DL Difference limen.

Doerfler-Stewart Test See *Audiometric Tests and Procedures* in appendices.

dominance (dom′ə-nəns) [L. *dominor,* to rule] Relation of being more prominent or important, of taking precedence, or of being more pressing. See also cerebral *dominance;* laterality.

  cerebral d. 1. Theory that in the brain one cerebral hemisphere is considered dominant over the other for particular tasks such as perception, ideation, memory, language, and other sensorimotor activities. **2.** Tendency for one cerebral hemisphere, usually the left, to be more fully developed in certain functions, especially speech and handedness.

Syn: cortical lateralization. See also laterality (1).

lateral d. Laterality (1).

dominant language See under language.

donkey breathing Technique used to obtain the use of the true vocal folds by prefacing the expiratory phonation with voiced inhalation; helps lessen hard glottal attacks and aids in the elimination of false vocal fold phonation.

Doppler effect, phenomenon, or **shift** [C. J. Doppler, Austrian mathematician and physicist in U.S., 1803–1853] Pitch which seems to change when a listener and a sound move rapidly away from or toward each other; *e.g.,* sound of a train whistle as the train approaches and passes by.

dorsal (dôr′səl) [L. *dorsum,* back] Toward the backbone; away from the front of the body; opposite of ventral.

dorsum, pl. **dorsa** (dôr′səm, -sə) [L. back] Upper or posterior surface, or the back, of any structure. See also under tongue.

Dos Amigos Verbal Language Scales See *Language Tests and Procedures* in appendices.

double assimilation See under assimilation.

double consonant See under consonant.

doubling (dəb′liŋ) Reduplication. See under syllabic structure, under phonological processes.

Down's syndrome [J. L. H. Down, Eng. physician, 1828–1896] Syndrome of mental retardation, ranging from mild to severe, associated with a variety of abnormalities caused by representation of chromosome 21 three times (instead of twice) in some or all cells. Characteristic abnormalities include retarded growth, flat hypoplastic face with short, prominent epicanthic skin folds, protruding lower lips, small rounded ears with prominent anthelix, fissured and thickened tongue, broad hands and feet, stubby fingers, and transverse palmar crease; varying degrees of hearing loss and speech im-pairment are associated. Syn: chromosome 21-trisomy syndrome; mongolism.

DPOAE Distortion product otoacoustic emissions.

drive Any compelling force toward or away from an intended goal.

drumhead Tympanic membrane. See under external *ear.*

drum membrane Tympanic membrane. See under external *ear.*

dry hoarseness See hoarseness, under voice disorders of phonation.

duration (du-rā′shən) **1.** Length of an audible sound. **2.** Length of (a) sounds or syllables, (b) pauses between phrases or sentences, or (c) overall rate of speech. **3.** Length of time taken by a moment of stuttering. See also speech sound flow.

duty cycle Interval of time that an instrument is actually *on;* usually refers to instruments and machines that work on an intermittent basis, such as pulse generators and electronic switches.

Dx Diagnostic therapy.

dynamic aphasia See under aphasia.

dynamic range 1. In speech, the difference in dB between the threshold of discomfort and the absolute threshold. **2.** In audiology, the difference in dB between the overload (distortion level) in a transducer or hearing aid and the minimum acceptable level.

dynamometer (dī-nə-mom′ə-tėr) [G. *dynamis,* force + *metron,* measure] **1.** In audiometry, an instrument used by the client during hearing testing to express judgment of sound loudness by squeezing a bulb. **2.** Instrument used to test muscular strength and motor function. Syn: ergometer.

dyne (dīn) [G. *dynamis,* force] Measure of energy or force; the amount of power necessary to accelerate a weight of one gram a distance of one centimeter per second; *e.g.,* in measuring sound pressure, the reference level is a pressure of 0.0002 dyne/cm^2, the force exerted against a field of one square centimeter.

dyplophonia (dip-lə-fō′nē-ə) Alternative spelling for diplophonia. See under voice disorders of phonation.

dys- [G]. Prefix denoting difficult. *Cf.* dis-

dysacusis (dis-ə-ku′sis) [dys- + G. *akousis*, hearing] Auditory *agnosia*.

dysarthria (dis-är′thrē-ə) [dys- + G. *arthroō*, to articulate] Term for a collection of motor speech disorders due to impairment originating in the central or peripheral nervous system. Respiration, articulation, phonation, resonation, or prosody may be affected; volitional and automatic actions, such as chewing and swallowing, and movements of the jaw and tongue may also be deviant. It excludes apraxia and functional or central language disorders. See also *Diagnostic Differences* in appendices.

  ataxic d. Dysarthria associated with damage to the cerebellar system and characterized by speech errors relating primarily to timing, giving equal stress to each syllable; articulation problems are typically characterized by intermittent errors ranging from mild to severe; vocal quality is harsh, with monotonous pitch and volume; prosody may range from reduced to unnatural stress.

  flaccid d. Dysarthria associated with disorders of the lower motor neurons; speech is characterized by mild to marked hypernasality coupled with nasal emission; continuous breathiness may be present during phonation, with audible inspiration of air; consonant production is imprecise.

  hyperkinetic d. Dysarthria in which involuntary movements are present, as a result of dysfunction of the extrapyramidal system; muscle tone is abnormal, ranging from hypotonic to hypertonic, and, in some cases, fluctuating between the two. It includes various subclassifications, all of which are marked by disorders of loudness, rate, and inappropriate interruption of phonation.

  hypokinetic d. Dysarthria associated with disorders of the extrapyramidal system and characterized by monotonous pitch and loudness, reduced stress, and imprecise consonants; when occurring in Parkinson's disease, speech is characterized by short rushes of speech, rapid rate increasing in contextual situations, and a reduced range of movements.

  parkinsonian d. [J. Parkinson, Eng. physician, 1755–1824] Condition characterized by rigid, mumbling, nonprosodic speech. See also hypokinetic *dysarthria*.

  peripheral d. Dysarthria resulting from dysfunction of brainstem nuclei or motor cranial nerves.

  somesthetic d. Disturbance of articulation as a tactile alteration of the oral region.

  spastic d. Dysarthria associated with a bilateral upper motor lesion and characterized by imprecise articulation, monotonous pitch and loudness, and poor prosody; muscles are stiff and move sluggishly through a limited range; speech is labored and words may be prolonged; it is often accompanied by facial distortions and short phrasing.

dysaudia (dis-ô′dē-ə) [dys- + L. *audio*, to hear] Defective articulation associated with auditory feedback difficulties; may occur as a result of hearing loss.

dyscalculia (dis-kal-kyu′lē-ə) [dys- + L. *calculo*, to add] See acalculia.

dysdiadochokinesia Impaired ability to undertake rapidly alternating movements.

dysfluency (dis-flu′ən-sē) [dys- + L. *fluēns*, flowing] Any type of speech which is marked with repetitions, prolongations, and hesitations; an interruption in the flow of speech sounds. It may (a) describe developmental hesitations of a child, or (b) refer to the dysrhythmic speech of a stutterer. Syn: nonfluency. See also stuttering.

dysglossia (dis-glo′sē-ə) [dys- + G. *glōssa*, tongue] See aglossia.

dysgraphia (dis-gra′fē-ə) [dys- + G. *graphō*, to write] See agraphia.

dyskinesia (dis-ki-nē′zē-ə) [dys- + G. *kinesis*, movement] Impairment of the capacity for voluntary movements, resulting in abnormal movement. See also athetosis, under cerebral palsy symptomatology.

dyslalia (dis-lā′lē-ə) [dys- + G. *lalia*, talking] **1.** Articulatory disorder for which no physiologic cause can be determined. **2.** Functional articulatory disorders. See articulation disorder.

dyslexia (dis-lek′sē-ə) [dys- + G. *lexis*, word or phrase] See alexia.

dyslexic (dis-lek′sik) Denoting dyslexia, a less severe form of alexia.

dyslogia (dis-lō′jē-ə) [dys- + G. *logos*, speech] See alogia.

dyslogomathia or **dysmathia** (dis-lō-gō-mā′thē-ə, dis-mā′thē-ə) [dys- + G. *logos*, speech + *ma(n)thano*, to learn] Term used to refer to a difficulty in learning, especially in learning language. See also aphasia.

dysnomia (dis-nō′mē-ə) [dys- + G. *ōnoma*, name] See anomia.

dysphagia (dis-fā′jē-ə) [dys- + G. *phagein*, to eat] **1.** Difficulty in swallowing; may include inflammation, compression, paralysis, weakness, or hypertonicity of the esophagus. **2.** Difficulty moving food from the mouth to the stomach. See also swallowing. *Cf.* Feeding.

dysphasia (dis-fā′zē-ə,-fā′zhə) [dys- + G. *aphasia*, speechlessness] See aphasia.

dysphemia (dis-fē′mē-ə) [dys- + G. *phēmē*, speech] Disorder of phonation, articulation, or hearing due to emotional or intellectual deficits.

dysphemia and biochemical theory See under breakdown theory, under stuttering theories.

dysphonia (dis-fō′nē-ə) [dys- + G. *phone*, voice] See aphonia, under voice disorders of phonation.

  hyperkinetic d. See under voice disorders of phonation.

  spastic d. See under voice disorders of phonation.

  ventricular d. See under voice disorders of phonation.

dysphrasia (dis-frā′zē-ə, -frā′zhə) [dys- + G. *phrasis*, speaking] See aphrasia.

dysplasia (dis-plā′zē-ə, -plā′zhə) [dys- + G. *plasis*, a molding] Abnormal tissue or organ development. See also aplasia; hypoplasia.

dyspnea (disp-nē′ə) [G. *dyspnoia*] Difficult or labored breathing; a shortness of breath. *Cf.* apnea.

dyspraxia (dis-prak′sē-ə) [dys- + G. *apraxia*, lack of action] See apraxia (3).

dysprosody (dis-pros′ə-dē) [dys- + G. *prosōdia*, voice modulation] See aprosody.

dysrhythmia (dis-riTH′mē-ə) [dys- + G. *rhythmos*, rhythm] **1.** In speech, prolongations, hesitations, and repetitions that disrupt the articulatory and syllabic flow of speech. See also stuttering. **2.** In acoustics, an abnormal wave function in an encephalogram.

dystomia (dis-tō′mē-ə) [dys- + G. *stoma*, mouth] Abnormally small mouth. *Cf.* astomia.

dystonia (dis-tō′nē-ə) [dys- + G. *tonos*, tension) Involuntary rhythmic twisting distortions of the trunk.

dystrophy (dis′trə-fē) [dys- + G. *trophē*, nourishment] Weakness of a tissue, especially of muscle, as may occur in a neuromuscular disorder; may result in atrophy.

  muscular d. Disease of unknown origin characterized by progressive deterioration of muscle function, with weakness and withering of the muscles.

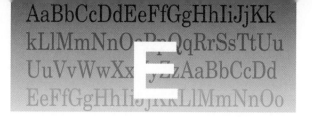

EA Educational age.

ear **1.** Organ of hearing, consisting of the external, middle, and inner ear. **2.** Commonly used to refer to the auricle or pinna.

external e. Concave funnel-like structure for receiving sound. It is composed of three main parts: (a) auricle or pinna, (b) external auditory meatus, and (c) outer surface of the tympanic membrane.

Auricle or **pinna,** the most visible part of the ear, is the concave cartilaginous structure which collects sound from the atmosphere and funnels it into the external auditory meatus. Although not prominent in function, the following parts are used as anatomical landmarks: anthelix (antihelix), antitragus, concha, helix, lobule, and tragus.

External auditory meatus is the passageway or tube extending from the auricle to the tympanic membrane through which sound waves travel. It is composed of an outer cartilaginous portion and an inner bony portion. Syn: auditory or ear canal.

Tympanic membrane is the thin, concave, parchment-like membrane, the edges of which are held in place by a bony ring, which closes the inner end of the external auditory meatus; the deepest or central part of the membrane is called the **umbo,** where the **manubrium** ends its attachment on the medial surface. Like the diaphragm of a microphone, it vibrates and transmits all audible sound frequencies at the same frequency as those of the sounding body. Syn: eardrum; drumhead; drum membrane; myrinx.

inner e. **1.** That part of the ear in which mechanical energy becomes electrical energy through vibrations which stimulate this end organ of hearing. It is composed of (a) the cochlea, (b) the internal auditory meatus, (c) the organ of Corti, (d) the semicircular canals, and (e) the vestibule. **2.** Sensory organ for balance.

Cochlea is the hearing part of the inner ear which resembles a snail shell and consists of three areas: (a) **scala media** or **cochlear duct,** which contains the sensory end organs of the organ of Corti; (b) **scala tympani,** which communicates with the round window and is on the bottom of the cochlear curve; it helps transmit sounds back into the middle ear to help restore equilibrium to the middle ear; and (c) **scala vestibuli** or **vestibular canal,** which communicates with the oval window to transmit the vibrations of the footplate of the stapes to the vestibule and to the organ of Corti.

Internal auditory meatus or **canal** is an opening in the petrous portion of the temporal bone through which pass the auditory and facial nerves.

Organ of Corti is a sensory part of the cochlea resting on the basilar membrane and containing hair cells, the sensory receptors whose function is to convert sound pressure waves into nerve impulses which are transmitted to the brain by cranial nerve VIII. Syn: end organ of hearing.

Semicircular canals are three looped bony tubes, the **anterior vertical, posterior vertical,** and **horizontal** or **lateral canals,** located in planes at right angles to each other and opening into the vestibule. They help an individual to maintain his sense of balance.

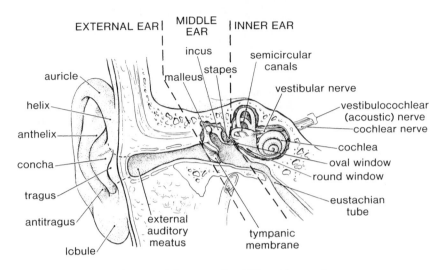

Diagram of the External, Middle, and Inner Ear
Section through the petrous portion of the temporal bone.

Vestibule is the bony cavity of the inner ear communicating between the cochlea and the semicircular canals, and with the tympanum through the oval window. Included in the vestibule are two membranous sacs: (a) **saccule,** the smaller of the two vestibular sacs, is globular in form and lies near the opening of the scala vestibuli of the cochlea; located within it are the saccular filaments of the acoustic nerve; (b) **utricle,** the larger of the two vestibular sacs, occupies the superior and posterior part of the vestibule; part of the structure is pouchlike and receives the utricular filaments of the acoustic nerve.

middle e. That part of the ear which directs sound energy via the ossicular chain (incus, malleus, and stapes) to the oval window to match the impedance of the air to the inner ear, and to protect the inner ear from intense sound; includes the inner surface of the tympanic membrane, the ossicular chain, the eustachian tube, and the outer surfaces of the oval and round windows. Syn: tympanic cavity.

Eustachian tube is an air duct from the nasopharynx which enters the anterior wall of the middle ear at its lowest point. It is usually closed at one end but opens with yawning and swallowing, thus ventilating the middle ear cavity and equalizing the pressure of the middle ear.

Incus or **anvil** is the middle of the three bones comprising the ossicular chain and serves to join the malleus and stapes. The body of the bone is moved by the malleus, while the longer process moves the head of the stapes.

Malleus or **hammer** is the first and largest bone in the ossicular chain. The handle (manubrium) is attached to the eardrum and serves to activate the saddle-shaped surface on the body of the incus to transmit sound waves.

Stapes or **stirrup** is the third and smallest bone in the ossicular chain, and articulates with the incus and moves its footplate into the oval window to transmit sound waves from the middle ear into the inner ear. It controls the loudness of sounds by being able to rotate on its transverse axis and dissipate some of the sound energy. Most conditions of conductive hypacusis (primarily otosclerosis) involve this bone.

Windows are the oval and round windows, portions of which are located in the inner ear but which function primarily in the middle ear. The **oval** or **vestibular window** is the resting place for the footplate of the stapes; its membrane pulsates from its location in the middle ear into the inner ear, allowing the mechanical action of the ossicular chain to be translated into fluid waves in the perilymph of the cochlea. Syn: fenestra ovalis or vestibuli. The **round** or **cochlear window** is located in the bony casing of the cochlea; its membrane works in opposition to that of the oval window by pulsating into the middle ear to allow movement of the fluid waves to compensate for the movement caused by the stapes at the oval window, and to restore equilibrium to the middle ear. Syn: fenestra cochlea or rotunda.

ear canal External auditory meatus. See under external *ear*.

eardrum Tympanic membrane. See under external *ear*.

Early Language Milestone Scale—Second Edition See *Language Tests and Procedures* in appendices.

earmold Fitting, usually made of plastic and fitting in the auricle of the ear, designed to conduct amplified sound waves into the ear from a receiver (earphone) of a hearing aid. See also coupler (1).

   nonoccluding e. Open *earmold*.

   open e. Earmold in which the vent is greatly enlarged and all of the canal portion is eliminated except for a small part used to retain the tubing; designed for maximum reduction of low-frequency gain; often used with CROS hearing aid. Syn: nonoccluding earmold.

   perimeter e. Skeleton *earmold*.

   shell e. Standard earmold with all possible bulk removed for maximum comfort; retains the same acoustic properties as those of the standard earmold; used with ear level hearing aid.

   skeleton e. Standard earmold in which the bowl has been cut out, leaving an outer concha rim; retains the acoustic characteristics of the standard earmold but is generally more comfortable and less conspicuous; used with behind-the-ear and eyeglass hearing aids. Syn: perimeter earmold.

   standard e. Oldest type of earmold, with a bowl completely filling the concha; may be fitted with any type of receiver but is mainly used with body hearing aids.

   vented e. Earmold with a hole bored through the bowl into the canal to relieve pressure or alter the acoustic response; allows passage of low-frequency energy out of the vent, resulting in a high-pass filtering effect.

earmuffs See under hearing protection device.

earphone See receiver.

earplugs See under hearing protection device.

ear training Technique used in articulation therapy which stresses self-hearing of speech deviations and standard utterance; the individual is taught to listen selectively and to differentiate internally or externally between sounds or tones, to associate the desired sound or tone, to match it, and to incorporate it into language or vocal production. See also auditory training.

earwax Colloquialism for cerumen.

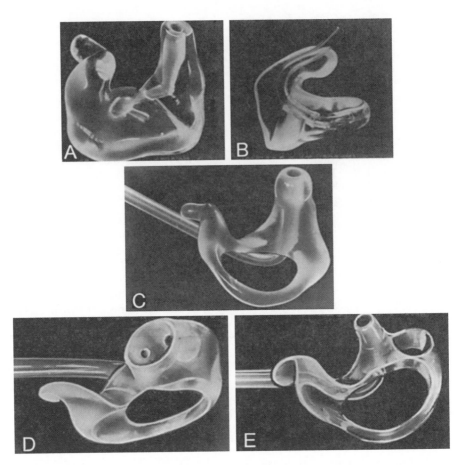

Earmolds
A, standard; B, shell style; C, perimeter or skeleton; D, vented; E, open. Courtesy of Westone Laboratories, Inc.

easy onset In stuttering, starting the voicing of a sound, syllable, or word at an extremely slow, smooth rate. The start is relaxed and produced without effort. Syn: gentle onset.

ebonics (ē-bon′iks) [L. *hebeninus*, fr. G. *ebeninos*, ebony] Linguistic continuation of Africa in African-American language; not genetically the same as European-American English because it is phonologically, morphophonemically, and morphosyntactically different. Syn: Black English.

echo (ek′ō) [L. fr. G. *ēchē*, sound] A reverberating sound.

echo chamber Reverberation room.

echoic operant See under operant, verbal.

echolalia (ek′ō-lā′lē-ə) [echo + G. *lalia*, talking] Tendency for an individual to repeat without modification that which is spoken to him; normally occurs between 18 and 24 months of age and usually considered to be involuntary, but may include voluntary repetitions. Syn: echologia; echophasia; echophrasia; echo or mimic speech; shadowing. See also imitation.

    delayed e. Repetition of an original utterance at some later time, with an intervening different utterance.

immediate e. Instant repetition of the original utterance.

mitigated e. Repetition of the original utterance with slight modification. It is observed (a) among adult aphasics and (b) as reflecting developmental progress in receptive and expressive language; *e.g.*, stimulus: Where do you sleep? response: I sleep.

unmitigated e. Unchanged repetition; exact duplication of the original utterance.

echologia (ek′ō-lō′jē-ə) [echo + G. *logos*, speech] Echolalia.

echophasia (ek′ō-fā′zē-ə) [echo + G. *aphasia*, speechlessness] Echolalia.

echophrasia (ek′ō-frā′zē-ə) [echo + G. *phrasis*, speaking] Echolalia.

echo speech Echolalia.

eclecticism (ek-lek′ti-si-zəm) [G. *eklekitos*, selective] **1.** System of finding, selecting, and ordering features from seemingly diverse sources; the resulting system is open to constant revision, even in its major outlines. **2.** Derivation of a method from several theories rather than from a single theory. Syn: syncretism.

ECoG, ECochG Electrocochleography.

-ectomy [G. *ektomē*, excision] Suffix denoting excision or removal.

EDA Electrodermal audiometry.

edema (e-dē′mə) [G. *oidēma*, a swelling] Accumulation of an excessive amount of fluid in cells, tissues, or serous cavities; usually results in a swelling of the tissues and may be associated with various inflammatory conditions.

EDRA Electrodermal response test audiometry.

educational age (EA) Grade level of an individual as measured by standardized achievement tests scored in age units.

educational audiology See under audiology.

educational quotient (EQ) Ratio of the educational age, expressed in months, to the chronological age, also ex-

pressed in months, multiplied by 100, *i.e.*,

$$EQ = \frac{EA}{CA} \times 100;$$

interpreted as an index of grade achievement.

Education for All Handicapped Children (Public law 94–142) A federal law passed in 1975 that mandates that states provide special education ("a free appropriate public education in the least restrictive environment") to meet the needs of children with disabilities from ages 5 to 21 years.

Education of the Handicapped Amendments of 1986 (Public law 99–457) A federal law passed in 1986 that amends and becomes a part of PL 99–457, which mandates that states provide preschool education for children with special needs (beginning at age 3 years). Part H focuses on the development of services to at-risk and handicapped infants and toddlers.

EEA Electroencephalic audiometry.

EEG Electroencephalogram.

effect For types of effect, see specific term.

effective amplitude See under amplitude.

effective masking See under masking.

effector (ə-fek′tėr) [L. producer] Peripheral tissue (muscle or gland) which receives nerve impulses and reacts by contraction (muscle) or secretion (gland).

effector operation System which controls and coordinates the individual output motor mechanisms of respiration, phonation, articulation, and resonance.

efferent (ef′ėr-ənt) [L. *efferens*, bringing out] Conducting outward from a given organ or part thereof, as of nerves leading out from the central nervous system. *Cf.* afferent.

efferent (kinetic) motor aphasia See under aphasia.

efferent nerve See under nerve.

effort level Term used by some to describe the degree of perceived labor in the production of phonation.

effusion (ə-fyu′zhən) [L. *effusio*, a pouring out] **1.** Escape of a fluid into a body cavity or tissue. **2.** The escaped fluid.

ego (ē′gō) [L. I] The self, particularly one's conception of oneself.

egocentric (ē-gō-sen′trik) Self-centered; denoting egocentrism.

egocentric language See under language.

egocentric speech Egocentric *language.*

egocentrism (ē-gō-sen′tri-zəm) [L. *ego,* I + G. *kentron,* center] State in which one sees the external world only from his viewpoint, without awareness of other points of view.

eidetic (ī-de′tik) [G. *eidon,* saw] Relating to the ability to visualize an object previously seen or imagined.

eidetic imagery See under imagery.

eighth cranial nerve See *Cranial Nerves* table, under cranial nerves.

eighth nerve tumor Acoustic *neurilemoma.*

elasticity (ē-las-tis′i-tē) Property of some materials which causes them to resist deformation and to be able to recover their original shape and size when the deforming forces are removed.

elected mutism Mutism (2).

electrical artificial larynx See under artificial larynx.

electrical measurement of speech production Language may be monitored, from its conception at the level of the brain to its expression by the speaker and interpretation by the listener, by the following: (a) **electroencephalography,** measures the discharge patterns of electrochemical energy from the cortex of the brain; (b) **electromyography,** measures the coordination of contraction and relaxation of muscles for respiration, phonation, and articulation; (c) **cineradiography,** shows speech energy changing into the physical movements of the speech organs; (d) **spectrographs** and **oscilloscopes,** measure acoustic energy and help classify it into defined phonetic units; and (e) **response,** although not a formal measuring instrument, is measured in the ears of the listener.

electrical potential Electromotive *force.*

electric field Space or medium surrounding positive or negative charged bodies, and in which other positive or negative charged bodies are subject to forces of attraction or repulsion.

electric irritability See under irritability.

electricity (ē-lek-tris′i-tē) Physical agent consisting of elementary negative particles (electrons) and positive particles (protons); the comparative number of protons and electrons determines whether it is positive or negative.

electric response audiometry (ERA) Evoked response audiometry. See under electrophysiologic *audiometry.*

electroacoustic, electroacoustical (ē-lek-′trō-ə-ku′stik, -sti-kəl) Relating to electroacoustics.

electroacoustics (ē-lek′trō-ə-ku′stiks) Combination of electricity and sound; sound energy patterns are converted into electric energy patterns for recording, displaying, and analyzing; *e.g.,* a microphone converts acoustic energy into electrical energy, while a loudspeaker converts electrical energy into acoustic energy.

electrocochleography (ē-lek′trō-kōk-lē-og′rə-fē) See under electrophysiologic *audiometry.*

electrode (ē-lek′trōd) [G. *ēlektron,* amber (electricity) + *hodos,* way] Terminal of an electric source or device, such as a battery, electrolytic cell, or electron tube, by which current enters or leaves; an electrical terminal specialized for a particular electrochemical reaction.

electrodermal audiometry (EDA) See under electrophysiologic *audiometry.*

electrodermal response test audiometry (EDRA) Electrodermal audiometry. See under electrophysiologic *audiometry.*

electroencephalic audiometry (EEA) See under electrophysiologic *audiometry.*

electroencephalic response audiometry (ERA) See under electrophysiologic *audiometry.*

electroencephalogram (EEG) (ē-lek′-trō-en-sef′ə-lə-gram) [G. *ēlektron,* amber (electricity) + *enkephalon,* brain + *gramma,* a writing] Recording of the electrochemical potentials of the brain, usually of the cortex, produced by an electroencephalograph.

    alpha waves or **rhythm** One of the fundamental waves of the EEG; ranges in frequency from 8 to 13 Hz in adults, somewhat slower in children.

beta waves or **rhythm** Waves of 14 to 25 Hz in frequency on the EEG; considered abnormal when of very high amplitude.

delta waves or **rhythm** Slow wave pattern on the EEG at a frequency slower than 4 Hz; normal during sleep, but abnormal during a waking state and may suggest depressed brain function.

diphasic spike Pattern on the EEG characteristic of a sudden burst of electricity first in a negative and then in a positive direction.

fourteen-and-six-hertz positive spikes Pattern on the EEG, usually observed

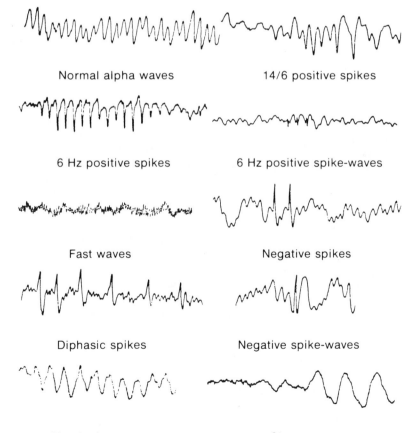

Normal alpha waves

14/6 positive spikes

6 Hz positive spikes

6 Hz positive spike-waves

Fast waves

Negative spikes

Diphasic spikes

Negative spike-waves

Notched waves

Slow waves

Electroencephalograms

in drowsiness and sleep, characteristic of sudden bursts of positive electricity and giving the appearance of a "spike" at a mixed frequency of 14 Hz and 6 Hz; thought to arise from deep structures within the brain.

negative spikes Pattern on the EEG characteristic of a sudden burst of negative electricity and appearing like a "spike"; thought to arise from the surface parts of the brain.

negative spike-waves Pattern on the EEG characteristic of a sudden burst of negative electricity and appearing like a "spike" followed by a slow wave.

notched waves Pattern on the EEG in which a slow wave, usually 6 Hz, has a depression or notch in it.

six-hertz positive spikes Pattern on the EEG, usually observed in drowsiness and sleep, characteristic of sudden bursts of positive electricity and giving the appearance of a "spike" arising at a frequency of 6 Hz; thought to arise from deep structures within the brain.

six-hertz positive spike-waves Pattern on the EEG, usually found in the waking state, characteristic of sudden bursts of positive electricity and appearing like a "spike" followed by a wave at a rhythm of 6 Hz; thought to arise from deep structures within the brain.

slow waves Waves on the EEG at a frequency of 7 Hz or slower; some are normal during sleep, but all are abnormal during a waking state. Waves 4 to 7 Hz are **theta waves;** waves slower than 4 Hz are **delta waves.**

theta waves or **rhythm** Slow wave pattern on the EEG at a frequency of 4 to 7 Hz; occur mainly in children but also in adults during periods of emotional stress.

electroencephalograph (ē-lek′trō-en-sef′-ə-lə-graf) Instrument used to record the electrochemical potentials of the brain; ten or more disc-shaped electrodes are pasted to various parts of the scalp and are connected to a high-fidelity amplifier, which in turn drives a series of pens on a strip of paper to produce an electroencephalogram. It is useful in localizing intracranial lesions and brain tumors, and in distinguishing between diffuse and focal brain lesions in epilepsy.

electroencephalography (ē-lek′trō-en-se-fə-log′rə-fē) [G. *elektron*, amber (electricity) + *enkephalon*, brain + *graphō*, to write] Measurement of the discharge patterns of electrochemical energy from the cortex of the brain by an electroencephalograph. See also electrical measurement of speech production.

electroglottograph (ē-lek′trō-glot′ə-graf) [G. *ēlectron*, amber (electricity) + glottis + *graphō*, to write] Instrument that measures the relative conductance or impedance between two small electrodes placed on either side of the larynx; indicates vocal fold contact for each vibratory cycle. Syn: laryngograph.

electrolarynx (ē-lek-trō-lăr′iŋks) Electrical or electronic *artificial larynx.*

electrolyte (ē-lek′trō-īt) [G. *ēlektron*, amber (electricity) + *lytos*, soluble] Any chemical compound (acid or alkaline) which when in solution conducts a current of electricity and is decomposed by it; *e.g.*, batteries; electrolytic capacitors.

electromagnetic wave See under wave.

electromotive force (EMF) See under force.

electromyography (EMG) (ē-lek′trō-mī-og′rəfē) [G. *ēlektron*, amber (electricity) + *mys*, muscle + *graphō*, to write] **1.** Recording the electrical potential accompanying muscle contraction by inserting an electrode into the fibers of a muscle or by applying an electrode to the surface of the skin. **2.** A visual recording of muscular electrical activity during spontaneous or voluntary movements.

electron (ē-lek′tron) [G. *ēlektron*, amber (electricity)]. One of the negatively charged subatomic particles that are distributed around a positively charged nucleus to form an atom.

electronic artificial larynx See under artificial larynx.

electronics [G. *ēlektron*, amber (electricity)] Field of science concerned primarily with the flow of electrons; important in audiology and speech science.

electronystagmography (**ENG**) (ē-lek′-trō-nī-stag-mog′rə-fē) See *Audiometric Tests and Procedures* in appendices.

electrophysiologic audiometry See under audiometry.

element For types of elements, see specific term.

elements of performance objective See performance objective.

elevators (el′ə-vā-tėrz) [L. *elevatus*, lifted up] Suprahyoid muscles. See *Muscles of the Larynx* table, under larynx.

eleventh cranial nerve See *Cranial Nerves* table, under cranial nerves.

elicit (ē-lis′it) [L. *elicitus*, drawn out] **1.** To draw forth or bring out. **2.** To derive by reason or argument.

elicited imitation See imitation (2).

elision (ē-li′zhən) **1.** Omission of phonemes or morphemes when speaking. **2.** Speech forms that lack final or initial phonemes of a variant speech form; *e.g.*, /′s/ instead of the full contraction *what's*.

ellipsis, pl. **ellipses** (e-lip′sis, -sēz) [G. *ek*, out + *leipsis*, leaving] **1.** Construction which is literally incomplete but in which the missing term is understood; derived from a specific sentence containing a complete predicate; *e.g.*, Mother: Eat your spinach. Child: I will (eat my spinach). Syn: predicate truncation. See also cohesive devices. **2.** In cluttering, a term used by some to describe such characteristics as omis-

sion of sounds, syllables, and whole words.

embed (em-bed′) To enclose in a surrounding mass.

embedded clause Subordinate *clause.*

embedded sentence Constituent sentence. See under sentence classification, transformational grammar.

embedded sound Any sound surrounded by other sounds; *e.g.*, /t/ in bottle.

embolism (em′bō-liz-əm) [G. *emboisma*, something thrust in] Obstruction of a blood vessel by a transported clot or other mass.

embryo (em′brē-ō) [G. *embryon*, fr. *en*, in + *bryō*, to be full, swell] In humans, the developing unborn organism during its period of most rapid growth, which extends from about two weeks after conception to the end of the seventh or eighth week of pregnancy. *Cf.* fetus.

embryonic (em-brē-on′ik) Denoting or characteristic of an embryo; rudimentary.

emergent (ē-mėr′jənt) Denoting anything arising as a natural or logical consequence.

emergent language See under language.

EMF Electromotive force.

EMG Electromyography.

EMH Educationally mentally handicapped.

emotion (ē-mō′shən) [L. *emotus*, agitating] Complex reaction, more intense than feelings, involving an aroused mental state or intense state of drive or unrest which is evidenced in both behavior and psychological changes, and directed toward a definite entity.

emotional disturbance Continuous anxiety, drive, and aroused mental state, with manifested difficulty in conforming to cultural norms.

empathy (em′pə-thē) [G. *en(em)*, in + *pathos*, feeling] Conscious or unconscious imitation or identification of one person with another, usually through participation in behaviors, feelings, or attitudes.

emphasis (em'fə-sis) Logical stress for expressing meaning; pertains primarily to words. See also stress.

empiric, empirical (em-pēr'ik, -i-kəl) [G. empeirikos, experience] Founded on practical experience but not proven scientifically.

empiricist theory See under language theories.

EMR Educationally mentally retarded.

encephalitis, pl. **encephalitides** (en-sef'ə-lī'tis, -lit'i-dēz) [G. enkephalos, brain + -itis, inflammation] Inflammation of the brain, usually of viral origin.

encoder (en-kō'dėr) Computer or network in which each separate input produces a combination of outputs.

encoding Expressive language.

encoding communication board See under communication board.

endentulous space (en-den'tyu-ləs) Area in the maxillary or mandibular arch devoid of teeth.

endocentric construction See under construction.

endocrine system (en'dō-krin) [G. endon, within + krinō, to separate] Any of the ductless glands, such as the adrenals, thyroid, and pituitary, whose products are transfused directly from the secreting cell of the gland through the gland tissue in the veins and throughout the vascular system; relates to speech functioning by affecting the tissues of the nerves that control speech muscles.

endogenous (en-doj'ə-nəs) [G. endon, within + -gen, production] Originating or developing from within an organism or one of its parts, as from congenital or hereditary factors. Cf. exogenous.

endolymph (en'dō-limf) [G. endon, within + L. lympha, clear fluid] Fluid contained within the membranous labyrinth of the ear.

endolymphatic hydrops (en'dō-lim-fat'ik hī'drops) Ménière's disease.

end organ Special structure in peripheral tissue which contains the terminal of a nerve fiber.

end organ of hearing Organ of Corti. See under inner ear.

endoscope (en'də-skōp) [G. endon, within + skopeō, to examined] Instrument for examination of the interior of a canal or hollow space.

endoscopy (en-dos'kə-pē) [See endoscope] Examination of the interior of a canal or hollow space.

energy (en'ėr-jē) [G. energeia] Capacity for doing work; measurements are usually expressed in foot-pounds, ergs, or joules. All forms of energy are convertible into one another and are measured by the quantity of work done in the process of transfer from one form to another.

　acoustic e. Vibration of a particle in a medium.

　kinetic e. Energy of a mass that results from its motion.

　potential e. Power possessed in a body at rest by virtue of its position.

ENG Electronystagmography.

engram [G. en, in + gramma, mark] Memory trace or pattern supposedly left in the brain cells following a mental stimulus.

ENT Ear, nose, and throat.

entity (en'ti-tē) **1.** An independent thing; that which contains in itself all the conditions essential to individuality or which forms of itself a complete whole. **2.** In linguistics, a semantic term referring to nominals; any word used as a noun.

entity-locative See semantic relations.

enunciate (ē-nən'sē-āt) [L. enuntiatus] To articulate; to pronounce; to articulate sounds.

envelope (en'və-lōp) Overall output signal of an acoustic or electroacoustic device; the total distribution of frequencies contained in a sound signal.

environment (en-vī'ron-ment) [Fr. environ, around] **1.** Totality or any aspect of the physical and social phenomena which surround or affect an organism or any of its parts. **2.** In linguistics, the circumstances or surroundings in which a phoneme or morpheme is found; *e.g.*, /s/ preceding /p/ in *spin* causes the /p/ to lose the aspiration it would have if it came initially.

Environmental Language Inventory (ELI) See *Language Tests and Procedures* in appendices.

Environmental Prelanguage Battery See *Language Tests and Procedures* in appendices.

epenthesis (e-pen-thē′sis) [G. *epi-*, following + *en*, in + *thesis*, placing] Insertion of an additional phoneme in a word or in a group of sounds; *e.g.*, tree = tʌri, film = fɪləm. See also phonological processes.

epiglottis (e-pi-glot′is) [G. *epiglōttis*] Cartilaginous structure of the larynx above the glottis, forming the anterior wall of the passage from the glottis to the pharynx; closes over the upper part of the larynx during swallowing to prevent foreign particles from entering.

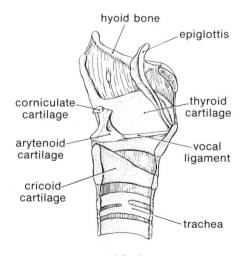

Epiglottis
Sagittal section of the larynx, showing the epiglottis and adjacent structures.

epilepsy (ep′i-lep-sē) [G. *epilēpsia*, seizure] Chronic disorder characterized by attacks of brain dysfunction usually associated with some alternation of consciousness; attacks or seizures may be confined to elementary or complex impairment of behavior (petit mal) or may progress to a generalized convulsion (grand mal). See also petit mal; grand mal.

episodic variation In stuttering, the tendency for young children to fluctuate cycles or periods of developmental nonfluency, followed by a return to more normal fluency, and then back to nonfluency again.

epithelium, pl. **epithelia** (ep-ə-thē′lē-ēm, -lē-ə) [G. *epi*, upon + *thēlē*, nipple (originally applied to thin skin covering the nipples and border of the lips)] A vascular cellular outer layer of the skin and mucous membrane. See also tissue.

EQ Educational quotient.

equal loudness contours Sound pressures necessary at each frequency to produce sensations of equal loudness for normal hearing. For input sounds of a sound pressure level of 50 dB and above, the sensitivity of the ear is essentially flat across the frequency range from 300 to 4000 Hz. At normal conversational intensity, the normal ear favors the middle frequencies in the speech range more than others.

equilibrium (ē-kwə-lib′rē-əm) [L. *aequilibirium*, horizontal position] **1.** Static or dynamic state of balance between two opposing forces; *e.g.*, in humans, the sense of balance is dependent on receptors in the semicircular canals in the inner ear. See also balance. **2.** State of adjustment between opposing or divergent influences; *e.g.*, in cognitive development stages, the balance between assimilation and accommodation is referred to as equilibrium.

equivalent speech reception threshold See under threshold.

ERA Electric response audiometry. Electroencephalic response audiometry. Evoked response audiometry.

erg [G. *ergon*, work] Unit of work in the decimal system which equals the amount of work done (energy) by a force of one dyne acting through a distance of one centimeter.

ergometer (ėr-gom′ə-tėr) [erg + meter] Dynamometer (2).

ERV Expiratory reserve volume.

escape (es-kāp′) Act of avoiding or evading something undesirable.

escape learning Situation in which the regulating drive is punishment; the desired response brings relief from punishment.

escape reaction See under reaction.

esophageal (ē-sof-ə-jē′əl) Relating to the esophagus.

esophageal speech See under alaryngeal *speech.*

esophageal voice Esophageal speech. See under alaryngeal *speech.*

esophagitis Inflammation of the esophagus.

    reflux e. Inflammation of the esophagus caused by a reflux of acid and pepsin from the stomach. Syn: Peptic esophagus.

esophagostomy See under nonoral *feeding.*

esophagram See barium swallow.

esophagus (ē-so′fə-gəs) [G. *osiophagos*, gullet] That portion of the digestive canal between the pharynx and stomach; extends from the lower border of the cricoid cartilage to the cardiac orifice, and is supplied by the vagus nerve (cranial nerve X).

ethmoid bone See under skull.

etiology (ē-tē-ol′ə-jē) [G. *aitia*, cause + *logos*, discourse] Study of the causes of a disease or condition, including (a) **perpetuating factors,** variables which are currently continuing the disease or condition; (b) **precipitating factors,** agents which are considered to have brought the disease or condition to its present state; and (c) **pre-**

disposing factors, agents that incline the patient toward a specific disease or condition.

etymology (et-i-mo′lə-jē) [G. *etymologia*, studying words] Study of the derivation of words.

eugnathia (yu-nā′thē-ə, yu-na′-) [G. *eu-*, good + *gnathos*, jaw] Abnormalities that are limited to the teeth and their immediate alveolar supports.

eunuchoid voice See under voice disorders of phonation.

euphemism (yu′fə-miz-əm) [G. *euphēmismos*, use of words of good omen] Word or phrase used as a substitute for an expression which is felt to be crude, improper, or vulgar.

eupnea (yup-nē′ə) [G. *eupnoia*] Quiet, normal respiration.

eustachian tube (yu-stā′shē-ən) [B. E. Eustachio, It. anatomist, 1520–1574] Air duct from the nasopharynx which enters the anterior wall of the middle ear at its lowest point. Syn: auditory tube. See under middle *ear.*

Evaluating Acquired Skills in Communication (EASIC) See *Language Tests and Procedures* in appendices.

Evaluating Communicative Competence See *Language Tests and Procedures* in appendices.

evaluation (ē-val-yu-ā′shən) Global appraisal of the significance and implications of a diagnostic assessment; includes formal and informal procedures. Syn: assessment. See also diagnosis. For types of evaluation, see specific term.

evoked Elicited, stimulated, or activated.

evoked response audiometry (ERA) See under electrophysiologic *audiometry.*

evolution (ev-ə-lu′shən) [L. *evolutus*, rolling out] Continuing process of change from one state, condition, or form to another; *e.g.*, in linguistics, the lack of strong differentiation in the usage of *will* and *shall* in spoken English.

evolutionary phonetics See under phonetics.

Examining for Aphasia See *Language Tests and Procedures* in appendices.

excessive nasality See hypernasality, under voice disorders of resonance.

exclamatory sentence See under sentence types.

excrescence (eks-kre′səns) [L. *excresco*, to grow forth] **1.** Unconscious insertion of /p/ or /b/, found in the phonological and morphological structures of various persons, formed as the articulators move from the position of one sound to that of another. **2.** Evolutionary changes in spellings which may reflect the insertion of such sounds; *e.g.*, the often pronounced /p/ in Samson may be a result of the spelling Sampson. Syn: anaptyxis. See also assimilation; neutralization.

executive aphasia See under aphasia.

exhalation (eks-hə-lā′shən) [L. *exhalatus*, breathing out] Expiration.

exocentric construction See under construction.

exogenous (eks-oj′ə-nəs) [G. *exō*, outside + *-gen*, production] Resulting from other than congenital or hereditary factors, *i.e.*, factors external to the organism; *e.g.*, a language impairment resulting from cerebral trauma. *Cf.* endogenous.

exophoric (ek-sə-fôr′ik) [G. *exō*, outside + *phoros*, bringing (back)] In grammar, relating to a preceding word or group of words. Syn: anaphoric.

exophoric pronoun See pronoun, under parts of speech.

exostosis, pl. **exostoses** (eks-os-tō′sis, -sēz) [G. *exo-*, outside + *osteon*, bone + *-osis*, condition] Of the ear: rounded hard bony nodule, usually bilateral and multiple, protruding from the external auditory meatus near the tympanic sulcus, often on opposing walls; ear function is normal unless obstruction or infection occurs. *Cf.* osteoma.

expansion (eks-pan′shən) [L. *expansus*, spreading out] **1.** Interpretation by an adult of a child's utterances, usually involving addition of words and indicating, through the adult's intonation, that what the child said was correct; most expansions are made in relation to the circumstances that prompted the child's utterance, thus helping the adult to correctly interpret the child's utterance and to expand it; *e.g.*, child: John candy. adult: Yes, John is eating candy. **2.** Building on or adding to an expression.

experimental audiology See under audiology.

experimentally delayed auditory feedback Delayed auditory *feedback*.

experimental phonetics See under phonetics.

experimental psychology See under psychology.

expiration (eks-pi-rā′shən) [L. *expiratus*, breathing out] Air flow from the lungs. Syn: exhalation. See also respiration.

expiratory reserve volume (ERV) See under respiratory volume.

expletive (eks′plə-tiv) [L. *expletus*, filled up] **1.** Extra word, phrase, or syllable which does not serve a grammatical function; often a profane interjection. **2.** Special type of absolute construction; *it* and *there* are commonly accepted as expletives; *e.g.*, It is hard to see if *there* are two books. See also absolute *construction*.

explosion (eks-plō′zhən) See plosive, under consonant, manner of formation.

expressive aphasia See under aphasia.

expressive language See under language.

Expressive Language Test See *Language Tests and Procedures* in appendices.

Expressive One-Word Picture Vocabulary Test—2000 See *Language Tests and Procedures* in appendices.

Expressive Vocabulary Test (EVT) See *Language Tests and Procedures* in appendices.

expressive-receptive aphasia See under aphasia.

extended jargon paraphasia See under paraphasia.

extension semantics See under seman-tics.

extensor (eks-ten′sėr) [L. one who stretches] A muscle, the contraction of which tends to straighten a limb; the antagonist of a flexor.

exteriorized stuttering See under stut-tering.

external auditory meatus See under ex-ternal *ear.*

external ear See under *ear.*

exteroceptor (eks′tėr-ō-sep′tėr) [L. *ex-terus*, outside + *receptor*, receiver] One of the sense organs of afferent nerves in the skin or mucous mem-brane which receives sensations of touch, pressure, pain, and tempera-ture.

extinction See under reinforcement schedule.

extraneous movement Any irrelevant movement, such as unnecessary tap-ping of the fingers or feet.

extraneous noise Ambient *noise.*

extrapolation (eks-trap-ə-lā′shən) [L. *extra-*, additional + *politus*, refine-ment] In statistics, a process of esti-mating values of a variable beyond the range of available data.

extrapyramidal system or **tract** (eks′-trə-pir-ə-mid′əl) Functional, rather than anatomical, unit comprising nuclei and nerve fibers (other than those of the pyramidal system) chiefly involved in subconscious, automatic aspects of motor coordination, but which also helps regulate postural and locomotor movements. Syn: indirect motor sys-tem.

extreme hearing loss See profound, in *Hearing Impairment Degrees* table.

extrinsic (eks-trin′sik) [L. *extrinsecus*, from without] Originating or acting from outside of the part where located or acting. *Cf.* intrinsic.

extrinsic muscles of the larynx See *Mus-cles of the Larynx* table, under larynx.

extrinsic muscles of the tongue See *Mus-cles of the Tongue* table, under tongue.

extroversion (eks-trō-vėr′zhən) [L. *extra*, outside + *versus*, turned] Gregarious-ness, with an emphasis on social inter-course and involvement with the ex-ternal world. *Cf.* introversion.

extrovert (eks′trō-vėrt) Person manifest-ing extroversion.

eye contact "Looking him in the eye" while talking to the listener; generally a natural, although not a constant, in-teraction of the speaker's eyes with those of the listener.

eye teeth Canine *teeth.*

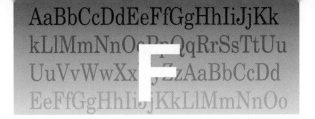

F Fahrenheit.

face validity See under validity.

facial nerve See *Cranial Nerves* table, under cranial nerves.

facial paralysis See under paralysis.

facies, pl. **facies** (fā′shēz) [L. face, countenance] The face, the countenance as revealing a mood, emotion, disease, or physical anomaly.

facilitated communication A method of assisting persons who are unable to speak or who are unable to speak clearly to communicate with others. A "facilitator," using some form of physical contact, assists the individual in using various augmentative communication systems; *e.g.*, communication boards, computers, and typewriters.

facilitation (fə-sil-i-tā′shən) [L. *facilitas* fr. *facilis*, easy] **1.** Promotion or acceleration of any natural process. **2.** Effect produced in nerve tissue by the passage of an impulse; the resistance of the nerve is diminished so that a second application of the stimulus evokes the reaction more easily.

facilitation of resonance Vibration of any sound-producing structure which is supported by the reaction of the resonance chamber.

facioversion See under teeth malpositions.

factitive See under parts of speech.

faking In stuttering, simulating stuttering behaviors or emotional reactions, and pretending to have difficulty talking when the person would otherwise be able to talk without difficulty. See also malinger.

falling curve See gradual, marked, and sharply falling curve, under audiogram configurations.

false fluency See under fluency.

false-negative response See under response.

false paracusis *Paracusis* willisi.

false-positive response See under response.

false role disorder Stuttering viewed as consisting largely of all the tricks, crutches, and false behaviors used by an individual to conceal his difficulty from a listener. See stuttering phases; stuttering stages.

false threshold See under threshold.

falsetto (fôl-set′ō) [It.] Highest voice register. See also under disorders of phonation.

false vocal folds Ventricular folds. See under vocal folds.

familial (fə-mil′ē-əl) [L. *familia*, family] Occurring in members of the same family; said of certain diseases or disorders.

farad (făr′əd) [M. Faraday, Eng. physicist and chemist, 1791–1867] Unit of electrical capacity; the capacity of a condenser which, charged with 1 coulomb, gives a difference of potential of 1 volt.

fascia, pl. **fasciae** (fä′shə, -shē-ə; -shē-ē) [L. band or fillet] Sheet of fibrous tissue which envelops the body beneath the skin and also encloses muscles and groups of muscles, and separates their several layers or groupings.

fasciculation (fə-sik′-yu-lā′shən) Small local involuntary contractions, or twitchings, of groups of muscles; may be visible through the skin. It represents a spontaneous discharge of muscle fibers innervated from a single motor unit.

fasciculus, pl. **fasciculi** (fə-sik′-yu-ləs,-lī) [L. dim. *fascis*, bundle] Band or bundle of fibers, usually of muscles or nerve fibers.

fatigue (fə-tēg′) [Fr. fr. L. *fatigo*, to tire] **1.** Exhaustion of strength, weariness from exertion, or diminished ability to do work, either physical or mental. **2.** Condition of cells or organs in which, through overactivity, the power or capacity to respond to stimulation is diminished or lost. **3.** Normal temporary loss of sensation, such as hearing or smell, following a period of stimulation.

auditory f. Temporary *threshold shift.*

voice f. See under voice disorders of phonation.

fauces (fä′sēz) [L. throat] Narrow passage between the cavity of the mouth and the pharynx, bounded laterally by two curved folds (pillars): the anterior being the glossopalatine arch, and the posterior being the pharyngopalatine arch. Syn: isthmus of fauces.

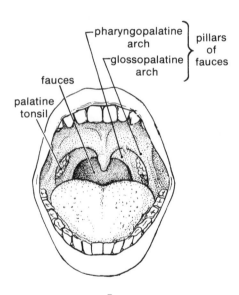

Fauces

fear [A.S. *faer*] Apprehension, dread, or alarm; it has an identifiable, actual or anticipated, stimulus, and thus is differentiated from anxiety which has no easily identifiable stimulus; one of the major characteristics of stuttering.

feared words See Jonah words.

feature (fē′chėr) **1.** Prominent part or characteristic. **2.** In speech, articulatory, auditory, linguistic, and phona-tory aspects of speech. For types of features, see specific term.

feature contrasts processes Substitution. See under phonological processes.

feedback 1. Process of monitoring and modifying one's own responses, as in a cybernetic system; it includes both an internal form, where part of the response pattern is fed back into the system prior to effecting the response, and an external form, where the overt response is monitored. **2.** Returning of a fraction of the output of a transmission system to its input in a self-regulating system.

acoustic f. Squealing sound produced by an amplification system when the microphone and receiver (speaker) are placed in close proximity, allowing recirculation and reamplification of sound waves.

afferent f. Proprioceptive *feedback.*

auditory f. Return of one's own speech; hearing oneself talk; part of the control system of the speaking act in which output is fed back to the ear to produce a self-monitoring regulation of speech. Syn: simultaneous auditory feedback.

biofeedback Use of modern electronic devices to train individuals to control certain unconscious body functions, such as blood pressure.

corrective f. Response to error signals and the effort to revise or adjust output to more closely approximate the intended output signal.

delayed auditory or **experimentally delayed auditory f. 1.** Time lapse, usually experimentally produced, in returning one's speech output to auditory input; used in voice and stuttering therapy. **2.** System by which the speaker's words are returned (feedback) through earphones after a time delay of a few milliseconds; used in voice and stuttering therapy.

haptic f. Collective term denoting the return of information through kinesthetic and tactile feedback.

inverse f. Negative *feedback.*

kinesthetic f. Return of movement patterns; in speech, the awareness of the location of the articulators during the production of phonemes.

negative f. 1. In speech, self-rejection of incorrect performance; when signals (acoustic and sensation) do not match the intended output, this information is fed back and future output is corrected until desired performance is achieved. **2.** In acoustics, out-of-phase return from the output circuit to the input circuit of an amplifier, resulting in a decrease of amplification, distortion, noise, and hum. Syn: inverse feedback.

proprioceptive f. Return of information from muscles, tendons, and joints; in speech, important in awareness of the location of the articulators. Syn: afferent feedback.

simultaneous auditory f. Auditory *feedback.*

tactile f. Return of information received through the sense of touch; in speech, the response to articulatory contacts.

feedforward In the perceptual and expressive processes of oral language, a neurobiological control system that increases neural activity, accelerates conductance, and heightens the electrical potential in strategic cortical areas mediating the response.

feeding 1. Placement, manipulation, and mastication of food in the oral cavity prior to initiation of the swallow. **2.** The giving or taking of food; administration of nourishment.

nonoral f. Procedures used to feed patients who are unable to take nutrition by mouth. Syn: forced feeding.

nasogastric (NG tube) f. This technique utilizes a tube placed through the nose, pharynx, and esophagus into the stomach.

pharyngostomy f. A hole or stoma is created from the skin into the pharynx through which a tube is placed into the esophagus and the stomach.

esophagostomy f. A creation of a hole from the skin into the cervical esophagus through which a feeding tube is passed which extends into the esophagus and stomach.

gastrostomy (G tube) f. A surgical procedure that creates an external opening in the abdomen leading into the stomach; may be performed as a general surgical procedure or percutaneously under a local anesthetic with an endoscope. Food is passed through the tube directly into the stomach. The patient can take puréed table food through the tube.

jejunostomy (J tube) f. A surgical procedure that may be performed under a general anesthetic or with a local anesthetic and a percutaneous approach. Both procedures create an opening into the abdominal wall that leads to the jejunum. This method requires prepared feedings.

feeding, normal development See *Normal Development of Feeding* in appendices.

feeling 1. Any kind of conscious experience of sensation. **2.** Mental perception of a sensory stimulus. **3.** A quality of any mental state, whereby it is recognized as being pleasurable or the reverse.

feeling-of-knowing Tip-of-the-tongue phenomenon.

feeling threshold See *threshold* of feeling.

FEES Fiberoptic endoscopic evaluation of swallowing.

fenestra, pl. **fenestrae** (fə-nes′trə, -trē) [L. window] Small opening or window in a bony structure, usually closed by a membrane. See windows, under middle *ear.*

f. cochleae Cochlear window. See windows, under middle *ear.*

f. ovalis Oval window. See windows, under middle *ear.*

f. rotunda Round window. See windows, under middle *ear.*

f. vestibuli Vestibular window. See windows, under middle *ear.*

fenestration (fen-ə-strā′shən) [See fenestra] Surgical procedure in which an artificial opening is made into the labyrinth of the inner ear; performed when otosclerotic conditions are present.

fetal (fē′təl) Denoting or characteristic of a fetus.

fetal alcohol syndrome (FAS) A cluster of severe congenital abnormalities caused by maternal drinking during pregnancy. Characteristics may include mental retardation, attention deficit/hyperactivity disorder, and motor delays. Facial anomalies may also be present. These may include small eyes, epicanthal folds (a vertical skin fold at the inner corner of the eyes), small jaw, flat midface, indistinct or long philtrum, thin upper lip, short nose, ear anomalies, and short palpebral fissures (the opening between the upper and lower eyelids). A diagnosis of FAS involves both the head and face, and the central nervous system.

fetus (fē′təs) [L. offspring] In man, the developing unborn organism from the end of the seventh or eighth week of pregnancy until birth. *Cf.* embryo.

FEV Forced expiratory volume.

fiber [L. *fibra*] **1.** An elongated, threadlike or filamentous structure. **2.** A single nerve fiber. See also neuron.

    nerve f. Axon of a neuron.

fiberscope (fī′bėr-skōp) Endoscope with a slender flexible tube containing bundles of thin glass fibers, some of which convey light for illumination while others transmit back the illuminated image for viewing; the tube is passed through the nasal meatus to the velopharyngeal area and can be attached to either a still or motion picture camera for recorded observation, or can be used for direct viewing, even by the subject. It is used to assess muscle activity in velopharyngeal closure and as a source of visual feedback in therapy.

fiberoptic endoscopic evaluation of swallowing (FEES) This procedure allows for a comprehensive assessment of the functions of the swallowing mechanism at the velopharyngeal, oropharyngeal, pharyngeal, and laryngeal levels of swallowing.

field [A.S. *feld*] In acoustics, the area over which a sound wave may be distributed.

    free f. Area over which a sound wave may be distributed in which the boundaries have little effect on sound pressure waves; *e.g.,* an anechoic chamber.

    sound f. 1. Area over which a sound wave may be distributed; limited by reflections and boundaries. **2.** Area in which an auditory stimulus is presented to subjects through a loudspeaker, as opposed to presentation through earphones.

fifth cranial nerve See *Cranial Nerves* table, under cranial nerves.

figure-ground 1. That aspect of perception wherein the perceived is separated into at least two parts, each with different attributes but influencing one another. Figure is the most distinct; ground, the least formed; *e.g.,* a bird (figure) seen against the sky (ground). **2.** Tendency of one part of a perceptual configuration to stand out clearly while the rest forms a background. See also perception.

    auditory f-g. Relevant acoustic stimuli in the presence of complex and competing background stimuli. See auditory figure-ground *discrimination.* See also *Auditory Processes* table.

    visual f-g. Relevant visual stimuli in the presence of complex and competing background stimuli. See visual figure-ground *discrimination.*

figure-ground distortion See under distortion.

figure of speech **1.** Manner of expressing a thought by referring to one thing in terms of another which it actually or symbolically resembles. **2.** Unusual use of words to produce a desired effect.

    allusion (ə-lu'zhən) [L. *allusus*, played with] Real imagery suggestive of a similarity between people, places, or events; *e.g.*, The Babe Ruth of football, Joe Namath.

    apostrophe (ə-pos'trə-fē) [G. a turning away] Addressing an inanimate object or abstract idea as if it were capable of understanding; *e.g.*, "You stupid machine. . . . "

    hyperbole (hī-pèr'bə-lē) [G. *hyperbolē*, exaggeration] Overstatement (see below).

    idiom (i'dē-əm) Utterance whose meaning cannot be predicted from the individual morphemes within the utterance; *e.g.*, kick the bucket; bury the hatchet; a red herring.

    irony (ī'èr-nē) [L. *ironia*] Statement which says one thing but means the opposite; *e.g.*, " . . . Brutus is an honorable man."

    litotes (līt'ə-tēz) [G. *litotēs*, simple, plain] Understatement (see below).

    metaphor (met'ə-fôr) [L. *metaphora*] Implied comparison of two or more objects, which in most respects are totally unlike, omitting the word *like* or *as*; *e.g.*, "Taxes are a walking shadow ever hanging over us." Syn: transferred meaning.

    metonymy (mə-ton'ə-mē) [G. *metonymia*, fr. *meta-*, subsequent + *onoma*, name] Figure of speech that consists of using the name of one thing for something else with which it is associated; *e.g.*, "the deep" for "the sea."

    overstatement Deliberate exaggeration for effect; *e.g.*, I'm so happy I could burst. Syn: hyperbole.

    personification (pèr-son'i-fə-kā'shən) Giving of human characteristics and qualities to animals and inanimate objects; *e.g.*, The breeze kissed her hair.

    simile (sim'ə-lē) [L. likeness] Comparison of two or more objects, which in most respects are totally unlike, using *like* or *as* to introduce the comparison; *e.g.*, He walks *like* an elephant. She is lovely *as* a rose.

    synechdoche (si-nek'də-kē) [G. *synekdochē*, receiving same from one another] Figure of speech by which a part is used for the whole and the whole for the part; *e.g.*, "fifty-two" for "fifty-two people"; "dead of the year" for "winter."

    understatement Deliberate minimizing of a fact; *e.g.*, That four-karat ring is a pretty trinket. Syn: litotes.

filler Any interruption of oral discourse during which the speaker emits sounds such as "er," "um," "ah," etc. to initiate or maintain an utterance. Syn: vocalized pause.

filter [L. *filtro*, to strain through felt (filtrum)] In acoustics: **1.** Device used for separating components of sound waves on the basis of their frequency; allows components in one or more frequency bands to pass relatively unattenuated, and attenuates components in other frequency bands. **2.** Device used to control the frequencies allowed to pass through an amplifying system.

    active f. Amplifier that is part of the filter circuit and whose response is dependent on the gain of the amplifier.

    band-pass or **pass-band f.** Electrical device which allows a fixed or predetermined band of frequencies to be transmitted; acoustic signals or frequencies above or below the band pass are not effectively transmitted or amplified.

    High-pass filter is a band-pass filter which transmits all sound wave components whose frequencies are

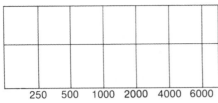

Frequencies in Hz

No filter: sound wave extends from 250 Hz to 6000 Hz with no interruptions.

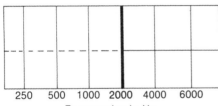

Frequencies in Hz

Band pass: only frequencies within the band of 1000 Hz and 2000 Hz will be heard; those higher and lower than the band pass will be weakened or cut out.

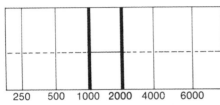

Frequencies in Hz

High pass: frequencies above the filter point of 2000 Hz are heard; those below that point are weakened or cut out.

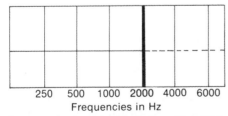

Frequencies in Hz

Low pass: frequencies below the filter point of 2000 Hz are heard; those above that point are weakened or cut out.

Filters

above a certain cutoff frequency; *e.g.*, 800 Hz, the cutoff frequency, transmits all components whose frequencies are higher than 800 Hz but weakens those below 800 Hz.

Low-pass filter is a band-pass filter which transmits all sound wave components whose frequencies are below a certain cutoff frequency; *e.g.*, 1000 Hz, the cutoff frequency, transmits all components of the input wave whose frequencies are lower than 1000 Hz but weakens components above 1000 Hz.

Octave-band filter is a band-pass filter which allows the measurement of the sound pressure level of each octave band of a complex noise.

pass-band f. See band-pass *filter.*

third-octave f. Band-pass filter that is one-third octave wide and transmits all sound wave components within that range, while attenuating all frequencies above and below the band.

wave f. Instrument which separates waveforms on the basis of their frequencies.

filtered speech Speech that has been passed through filters to alter its characteristics, *i.e.*, altered by removal of a portion of the frequency spectrum; this type of distorted speech is often used in research on auditory perception; *e.g.*, words from which frequencies above 800 Hz have been eliminated.

final consonant position See under consonant position.

fine motor See under motor.

finger agnosia See under agnosia.

fingerspelling Art of communicating ideas by movements made with the fingers, as with the manual alphabet of the deaf; uses the conventional language system with its vocabulary, spelling, and grammar. Syn: dactylology; dactyl speech. See also manual method, under aural rehabilitation; American

Manual *Alphabet;* unaided *augmentative communication.*

finite (fī'nīt) [L. *finitus*, limited] Having measurable limits.

finite grammar See under grammar.

first cranial nerve See *Cranial Nerves* table, under cranial nerves.

first deciduous molar or **first premolar teeth** Bicuspid *teeth.*

first sentences Earliest use of combinations of two or more words, one of which is either a verb form or implies a verb form; *e.g.*, Baby hit; Daddy go.

first words Earliest utterances which are recognizable words or approximations of words; may be the result of vocal play or meaningless imitation of adult syllables, but will eventually signify meaningful needs or appropriate responses to a given situation.

Fisher-Logemann Test of Articulation Competence See *Articulation Tests and Phonological Analysis Procedures* in appendices.

fissure (fish'ėr) [L. *fissura*] A deep furrow, cleft, or slit.

  f. of Rolando [L. Rolando, It. anatomist, 1773–1831] Central *sulcus.*

  f. of Sylvius [J. Sylvius, Fr. anatomist, 1614–1672] Lateral *sulcus.*

  longitudinal cerebral f. Deep midline cleft separating the right and left cerebral hemispheres.

fistula (fis'tyu-lə) [L. pipe or tube] **1.** Abnormal passage leading from an abscess or hollow organ to the body surface or from one abscess or hollow organ to another. **2.** In cleft palate surgery, a minute opening left after surgery.

Fitzgerald Key [Edith Fitzgerald, 1937] In aural rehabilitation, a method of teaching grammar and syntax to the deaf which provides visible sentence patterns so the individual can generate his own sentences and recognize and correct his mistakes; various symbols are used to identify the various parts of speech. See also grammatic method, under aural rehabilitation.

Five Slate System See Barry Five Slate System.

fixation (fik-sā'shən) [L. *fixus* fr. *figo*, to fix or fasten] In stuttering, the prolongation or maintenance of an articulatory or phonatory posture for an abnormal duration.

fixed interval reinforcement schedule See under reinforcement schedule.

fixed ratio reinforcement schedule See under reinforcement schedule.

flaccid dysarthria See under dysarthria.

flaccidity (flə-sid'ə-tē) [L. *flaccidus*, flaccid] Inability of a muscle to contract volitionally when it can do so reflexively and is not atrophied. See under cerebral palsy symptomatology.

flaccid paralysis See under paralysis.

flap consonant See under consonant.

flat See under audiogram configurations.

flexion (flek'shən) [L. *flectus*, bent] **1.** Bending of a joint so as to approximate the parts it connects. **2.** Act of bending or condition of being bent.

flexion reflex See under reflex.

flexor (fleks'ėr) A muscle the action of which is to move a joint; the agonist of an extensor.

Flowers Auditory Screening Test (FAST) See *Auditory Tests and Procedures* in appendices.

Flowers-Costello Test of Central Auditory Abilities See *Auditory Tests and Procedures* in appendices.

Flowers Test of Auditory Selective Attention (FTASA) See *Auditory Tests and Procedures* in appendices.

fluency (flu'ən-sē) [L. *fluens*, flowing] Smoothness with which sounds, syllables, words, and phrases are joined together during oral language; lack of hesitations or repetitions in speaking. See also speech sound flow; stuttering.

  basal f. In stuttering: **1.** Length of time a stutterer can speak continuously with no stuttering. **2.** Removal of all pressures and the facilitation of fluency which result in a period of speaking free from stuttering. See also desensitization.

false f. In stuttering: **1.** Period of almost complete freedom from stuttering, usually occurring early in a treatment program and attributed to attitudinal changes; referred to as a "flight into health." **2.** Fluent speech achieved by the stutterer by the use of tricks, devices, verbal asides, or by assuming the role of someone else (such as a clown or boor) in an attempt to deny the problem.

verbal f. 1. Production of utterances in connected sequences without any extraneous pauses, hesitations, or repetitions. **2.** Superior speaking skill.

fluency disorder 1. Term used to describe any interruption in the flow of oral language; not restricted to stuttering. **2.** Deviations from acceptable rhythm of speech noticeable enough to cause concern.

fluency-initiating gestures Fluency-enhancing techniques such as slow speech, loudness control, smooth speech, syllable stress, and easy onsets.

fluent (flu′ənt) [see fluency] Denoting facility, smoothness, flowing.

fluent aphasia See under aphasia.

Fluharty Speech and Language Screening Test See *Articulation Tests and Phonological Analysis Procedures* in appendices.

fluoroscopy (flu-ros′kə-pē) [fluorescence + G. *skopeō*, to examine] Radiologic procedure in which the physiologic and pathologic speech activities are momentarily displayed on a fluorescent screen by x-rays transmitted through tissue densities in the body area under study; permanent records of these findings can be made during the studies by cinefluoroscopy or videofluoroscopy. See also cinefluoroscopy, videofluoroscopy, x-ray. *Cf.* radiography; tomography.

FM Frequency modulation.

FOCALCROS See under contralateral routing of signals (CROS), under hearing aid.

fold Ridge or margin formed by the doubling back of a thin layer of tissue. For types of fold, see specific term.

footplate Base of the stapes that rests in the oval window. See also stapes, under middle *ear*.

foot-pound Unit of energy, or work, being equal to the work done in raising one pound of weight against the force of gravity to the height of one foot.

foramen, pl. **foramina** (fôr-ā′men, -am′i-nə) [L. aperture] Passage or opening; cavity of an organ or an aperture in a bone for passage of blood vessels or nerves.

incisive f. Funnel-shaped aperture centrally located in the hard palate just behind the central incisors and opening into paired incisive canals, which transmit the descending palatine artery and the nasopalatine nerve; considered by some to be the reference point for the classification of clefts (lip and palate).

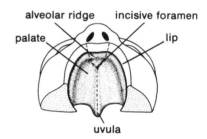

Incisive Foramen
From Sadler, TW. *Langman's Medical Embryology*, 5th ed. Baltimore: Williams & Wilkins, 1985.

force 1. Energy or power which starts or stops motion. **2.** Condition that produces a change in behavior or experience.

electromotive f. (EMF) Pressure or potential difference required to produce a flow of electrical current; the capacity to do work. The practical unit of electromotive force is the volt. Syn: electrical potential.

forced expiratory volume (FEV) See under respiratory volume.

forced feeding See under nonoral *feeding*.

forced vibration See under vibration.

fore-glide On-glide.

forked tongue Diglossia.

form [L. *forma*] **1.** Distinguishing property of a figure; the shape or outline of an object. **2.** In linguistics, one of the different aspects a word may take as a result of inflection, change of spelling, or change of pronunciation. See also morpheme; word.

formal method Analytic method. See aural rehabilitation.

formal operations period See Period IV under cognitive development stages.

formal universals See under linguistic universals.

formant or **formant frequency 1.** Frequency region, for vowels and resonant consonants, in which a relatively high degree of acoustic energy is concentrated. **2.** Natural mode of air vibration in the vocal tract characterized on a spectrogram by a dark area indicating a relatively high intensity of a group of frequency components. **3.** Concentrations of vowels; the primary resonances of vowels are usually studied in terms of three formants.

   singer's f. Resonant frequency around 3000 Hz considered to give the voice a musical quality.

formulation (fôr-myu-lā′shən) **1.** Organization of relevant elements of a specific project into a clear and concise pattern. **2.** In language, selection of words and grammatical structures in the construction of meaningful verbal expressions, utilizing knowledge of the syntactic and semantic components of language.

form word Content *word*.

fortis consonant See under consonant.

forward coarticulation See under coarticulation.

forward masking See under masking.

fossa, pl. **fossae** (fos′ə, fos′ē) [L. trench, ditch] Depression, usually more or less longitudinal in shape, below the level of the surface of a part.

Fourier analysis or **Fourier's law** [J. B. J. Fourier, Fr. mathematician and physicist, 1768–1830] Mathematical principle that any complex wave, such as a sound wave or light wave, may be analyzed into simple sine waves; discloses the frequencies and amplitudes of the constituent simple waves which make up the complex periodic wave.

fourteen-and-six-hertz positive spikes See under electroencephalogram.

fourth cranial nerve See *Cranial Nerves* table, under cranial nerves.

fragile X syndrome (FXS) An inherited abnormality of the X chromosome which causes disabilities ranging from varying degrees of learning problems to mental retardation. Features commonly associated with the syndrome are: severe language delays, behavior problems, autism or autistic-like behaviors (including poor eye contact and hand-flapping), enlarged testicles, large or prominent ears, hyperactivity, delayed motor development, and poor sensory skills.

fragment Any utterance that does not express a complete thought; may consist of a single word, a phrase, or a subordinate clause. Some are acceptable in conversation because of the previous information given; *e.g.,* "What do you want to eat?" "Lasagna."

Franceschetti's syndrome [A. Franceschetti, Swiss ophthalmologist, 1896–1968] Mandibulofacial dysostosis.

FRC Functional residual capacity.

free field See under field.

free field room Anechoic chamber.

free form Free *morpheme*. See also content *word*.

free morpheme See under morpheme.

free variation In linguistics: **1.** Use in the same environment, by the same or different speakers, of forms perceptually different but semantically the same and idiomatically normal; *e.g.*, *grease* pronounced /grēs/ or /grēz/; *with* pronounced /wɪð/ or /wɪθ/. **2.** Term indicating any of several possible versions of a phoneme which can occur, with no change in meaning.

free vibration See under vibration.

French method [after C.-M. de l'Epee, a Frenchman, 1712–1789] First method of instruction for the deaf in the United States; used signs to denote objects and ideas. See also manual communication, under aural rehabilitation.

frenulum, pl. **frenula** (fren′yu-ləm, -lə) [L. dim. *frenum*] A small frenum.

frenum, pl. **frena, frenums** (frē′nəm, -nə, -nəmz) [L. bridle] Fold of skin or mucous membrane which checks or limits the movement of an organ.

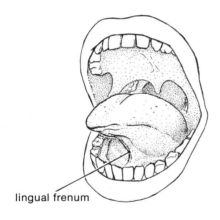

Lingual Frenum

lingual f. Small, white cord of tissue extending from the floor of the mouth to the midline of the inferior surface of the tongue blade; important in speech because if too short it may restrict the elevation and extension of the tongue.

frequency (frē′kwen-sē) [L. *frequens*, repeated, often, constant] **1.** In acoustics, number of repetitions of compressions and rarefactions of a sound wave that occur at the same rate over a period of time, expressed in hertz (Hz);

e.g., if 15 cycles occur in 1 second, the vibration has a frequency of 15 Hz. **2.** In acoustics, number of hertz of a wave. See also wave. **3.** In speech, the rate of glottal vibration (opening and closing of the glottal space between the vocal folds in a given time period); the main determinant of what is heard as pitch. **4.** In measurement, the number of times a score or phenomenon occurs.

band f. Range of frequencies extending between specified limits either controlled or natural, as by an audiometer or the human ear.

formant f. Formant.

fundamental f. 1. Lowest component frequency of a periodic wave; the principal component of a sound wave; the component having the greatest wavelength. **2.** Lowest partial in a complex sound wave. **3.** Tone produced by the vibration of the vocal folds before the air reaches any cavities.

high f. (HF) Sound at 2000 Hz or higher; the range of pitch for sibilants [s-z], [ʃ-ʒ] and fricatives [f-v], [θ-ð].

infrasonic f. Frequency below the range of 20 Hz. Sounds in this frequency are not perceived by the human ear.

low f. (LF) Indefinite term which refers to a frequency of 1000 Hz and below.

modal f. Habitual *pitch*.

natural or **resonant f. 1.** In electricity, the rate of oscillation; approximately equal to that frequency at which the inductive reactance is equal to the capacitive reactance. **2.** Inherent power of a vibrating body to go into free oscillation with regard to frequency. **3.** Frequency at which a mass vibrates with the least amount of external force.

respiratory f. Number of breaths per minute.

speech f.'s Frequencies at which the majority of speech sounds occur;

considered to be 500, 1000, and 2000 Hz on a pure-tone audiometer.

ultrasonic f. Frequency above the range of 20,000 Hz. Sounds in this frequency are not perceived by the human ear.

frequency jitter Jitter (3).

frequency-modulation (FM) Modification of the frequency of the carrier wave in accordance with speech or signal.

frequency-modulation auditory trainer See under auditory training units.

frequency range See band *frequency*.

frequency response See under response.

frequency response curve See under curve.

frequency theory See under hearing theories.

fricative See under consonant, manner of formation.

frictionless Glide. See under consonant, manner of formation.

frog in the throat Colloquialism for syllabic aphonia. See under voice disorders of phonation.

frontal (frən′təl) [L. *frontalis*] Relating to the anterior part of a structure or organ.

frontal bone See under skull.

frontal gyri See under gyrus.

frontal lisp See under lisp.

frontal lobe See under lobe.

frontal plane See under plane.

frontal sulci See under sulcus.

frontolateral laryngectomy See under laryngectomy.

front phoneme See under phoneme.

front routing of signals (FROS) See under contralateral routing of signals (CROS), under hearing aid.

front vowel See under vowel.

FROS Front routing of signals.

frustration (frəs-trā′shən) [L. *frustratus*, deceived] Increased emotional tension resulting from failure to achieve sought gratification or satisfaction, ordinarily as a result of external forces.

frustration tolerance In stuttering, the capacity of the stutterer to resist feelings of frustration because of an inability to speak without difficulty.

Fullerton Language Test for Adolescents See *Language Tests and Procedures* in appendices.

function (fəŋk′shən) [L. *functio*, to perform] Physiologic activity of an organ or structure. For types of function, see specific term.

function word Functor. See under word.

functional aphonia Conversion *aphonia*.

functional articulation disorder See under articulation disorder.

Functional Communication Profile See *Language Tests and Procedures* in appendices.

functional deafness See under deafness.

functional disorder Condition in which one or more of the normal activities of the organism cannot be properly performed, although there is no known pathologic change in organic structure which can be related to the disorder.

functional residual capacity (FRC) See under respiratory capacity.

functor (fəŋk′tėr) See under word.

fundamental frequency See under frequency.

fusion (fyu′zhən) [L. *fusio*, a pouring] **1.** Blending, uniting, or joining together of two entities into one. **2.** Phonetic changes that occur in a language; the unifying process by which the speech measure becomes a single configuration. For types of fusion, see specific term. See also assimilation.

future perfect progressive tense See progressive *tense*.

future perfect tense See under tense.

G

g Gram.

GA Gestational age

gag 1. To retch. **2.** To forcibly restrain from talking.

gag reflex Pharyngeal *reflex.*

gain Ratio of the output power, voltage, or current to the input power, voltage, or current measured in decibels; *i.e.*, output – input = gain.

> **acoustic g.** In hearing aids, the output of the instrument minus the input; *e.g.*, if at 1000 Hz the output is 100 dB and the input is 60 dB sound pressure level, the gain would be 40 dB.
>
> **HAIC g.** Formula presented by the Hearing Aid Industry Conference for arriving at an expression of acoustic gain; achieved by averaging the actual acoustic gain at 500, 1000, and 2000 Hz; *e.g.*,

Frequency (Hz)	Acoustic Gain (dB)
500	35
1000	50
2000	65
	150

150 dB ÷ 3 = 50 dB HAIC gain

Now replaced by high-frequency average full-on gain.

> **high-frequency (HF) average full-on g.** Average of the 1000, 1600, and 2500 Hz values of full-on gain; current ANSI standard for determining average gain, replacing HAIC gain.
>
> **peak acoustic g.** Maximum gain provided by an amplification system at any single frequency.
>
> **real-ear g.** The output of a hearing aid as measured in the individual's ear in a sound-field setting.

gain control Volume control.

> **automatic g. c.** Automatic *volume control.*

galvanic [L. Galvani, It. physician and anatomist, 1737–1798] Pertaining to galvanism, a unidirectional electric current derived from a chemical battery or from a physiochemical phenomenon, as in galvanic skin response.

galvanic skin resistance Galvanic skin *response.*

galvanic skin response (GSR) See under response.

galvanic skin response audiometry (GSRA) Electrodermal audiometry. See under electrophysiologic *audiometry.*

galvanometer (gal-və-nom′ə-tėr) Instrument for measuring the strength of an electric current.

ganglion, pl. **ganglia, ganglions** (gaŋ′ lēon, -lē-ə, -lē-onz) [G. swelling or knot] Currently, an aggregation of nerve cell bodies in the peripheral nervous system. Originally, any group of nerve cell bodies whether in the central or peripheral nervous system.

Garliner's Classification See under tongue thrust classifications.

gastroesophageal reflux (GER) The spontaneous return of gastric contents into the esophagus. Aspiration of this material may result in respiratory disease.

gastrostomy (G tube) See under feeding, nonoral.

gaussian curve or **distribution** [J. K. F. Gauss, Ger. physicist, 1777–1855] Normal *distribution.*

gaussian noise [J. K. F. Gauss, Ger. physicist, 1777–1855] White *noise.*

gender (jen′dėr) **1.** Grammatical classification of nouns. **2.** Anatomical sex of an individual.

general intellectual functioning Results obtained by assessment with one or more of the individually administered general intelligence tests developed for that purpose.

generalization (jen′ėr-ə-li-zā′shən) **1.** Reasoning by which a basic conclusion is

135

reached which applies to different items, each having some common factor. **2.** In conditioning, the eliciting of a conditioned response by stimuli similar to a particular conditioned stimulus. See also generalization, under response. **3.** Transfer of learning from one environment to a similar environment; the more similar the environments or situations, the more transfer takes place. See also carryover.

generalized intellectual impairment Reduction of cognitive functioning, with the primary deficit being in the area of memory for abstract material.

generalized reinforcer See under reinforcer.

general linguistics See under linguistics.

general oral inaccuracy See under articulation disorder.

general phonetics See under phonetics.

general semantics See under semantics.

generative grammar See under grammar.

generative semantics See under semantics.

generative transformational grammar See under grammar.

generator (jen′ə-rā-tèr) [L. *generatus*, begotten] **1.** Device for converting mechanical energy into electrical energy. **2.** Force which sends a body into oscillation.

genetics (jə-ne′tiks) [G. *genesis*, origin or production] **1.** Branch of science concerned with heredity, *i.e.*, the origin, history, and development of an organism. **2.** Study of the resemblances and differences between all organisms related to one another. **3.** In psychology, the study of the influence of heredity on behavior.

genioglossus muscle (jē′ni-ō-glos′əs) See *Muscles of the Tongue* table, under tongue.

geniohyoid muscle (jē′ni-ō-hī′oyd) See *Muscles of the Larynx* table, under larynx.

genitive case See case.

gentle onset Easy onset.

gentle onsets Precision fluency shaping.

geriatric (jăr-ē-a′trik) Of or relating to geriatrics, old age, and the aging process.

geriatric audiology See under audiology.

geriatrics (jăr-ē-a′triks) [G. *gēras*, old age + *iatrikos*, healing] Branch of medicine devoted to the study and treatment of physiologic and pathologic aspects of old age. Syn: gerontology (2).

German measles (mē′zəlz) Rubella.

German method Oral-aural method. See under aural rehabilitation.

gerontological (jăr′ən-tō-loj′i-kəl) Of or relating to gerontology.

gerontology (jăr-ən-tol′ə-jē) [G. *gēras*, old age + *logos*, discourse] **1.** Specialized study of the phenomenon of aging and of the problems of the aged. **2.** Geriatrics.

Gerstmann syndrome [J. Gerstmann, Austrian neurologist, *1887] Collection of disorders characterized by finger agnosia, agraphia, confusion of laterality of body, and acalculia; caused by lesions between the occipital lobe and the angular gyrus.

gerund See verbal, under parts of speech.

gestalt (gə-stôlt′) [Ger. shape] **1.** Structure or configuration of physical, biological, or psychological phenomena so integrated as to constitute a functional unit which is greater than the sums of its parts. **2.** Pattern involving relationships with a whole rather than isolated actions.

gestalt psychology See under psychology.

gestational age (GA) The duration of pregnancy measured from the first day of the last normal menstrual period.

gesture (jes′chèr) Movement of any part of the body to express or emphasize an idea, emotion, or function; not intended to include formalized symbolic methods of communication, such as fingerspelling, signed English, etc.

gesture language See under language.

gibberish (jib′èr-ish) Unintelligible and incoherent language.

Gilles de la Tourette syndrome [G. E. A. B. Gilles de la Tourette, Fr. physician, 1857–1904] Facial and vocal tics beginning in early childhood, usually in boys, and progressing to generalized jerking of other parts of the body; initial inarticulate expiratory laryngeal noises progress to loud exclamations and coprolalia; echolalia and palilalia may also develop.

Glasgow Coma Scale Widely used intensive care clinical scale that measures the depth and duration of unconsciousness. Three components (eye opening, verbal ability, and motor ability) are scored and then combined into a composite score from 3 to 15. A patient with an initial score of 8 or lower is usually admitted to an intensive care unit.

glide 1. See under consonant, manner of formation. **2.** Diphthong. See under vowel.

gliding of fricatives See under substitution, under phonological processes.

gliding of liquids See under substitution, under phonological processes.

global (glō'bəl) Denoting the complete, generalized, overall, or total aspect.

global aphasia See under aphasia.

gloss 1. Brief explanation of a difficult or obscure word or expression (as in the margin or between the lines of a text). **2.** Immediate parental or adult interpretation of a child's telegraphic utterances, often used to seek confirmation that the interpretation made was what the child intended to say; *e.g.*, child: "Baby eat." mother: "Baby wants to eat?" See also expansion (1). **3.** Identification of meaningful units in a language by exploring their likenesses and differences; often used by linguists when studying an unknown language. **4.** A false interpretation.

gloss-, glosso- [G. *glossa*, tongue] Combining forms relating to the tongue.

glossal (glos'əl) Pertaining to the tongue.

glossectomy (glo-sek'tə-mē) [gloss- + G. *ektomē*, excision] Surgical removal of all or part of the tongue.

glossitis (glo-sī'tis) [gloss- + G. *-itis*, inflammation] Inflammation of the tongue.

glossograph (glos'ō-graf) [glosso- + G. *graphō*, to write] Instrument for recording the movements of the tongue during speech.

glossolalia (glo-sə-lā'lē-ə) [glosso- + G. *lalia*, talking] Unintelligible jargon which has meaning to the originator but has no meaning for the listener.

glossopalatine (glo-sō-pal'ə-tīn) Relating to the tongue and palate.

glossopalatine arch See fauces.

glossopalatine muscle See *Muscles of the Palate* table, under palate.

glossopharyngeal (glos'ō-fə-rin'jē-əl) Relating to the tongue and pharynx.

glossopharyngeal nerve See *Cranial Nerves* table, under cranial nerves.

glossopharyngeal press See injection method, under speech, methods of esophageal speech.

glossoptosis (glos-op-tō'sis) [glosso- + G. *ptōsis*, a falling] Downward displacement of the tongue.

glossoschisis (glos-ō-skē'sis) [glosso- + G. *schistos*, split + -*osis*, condition] Diglossia.

glottal (glot'əl) Pertaining to the glottis.

glottal area See under consonant, place of articulation.

glottal attack Glottal catch. See under voice disorders of phonation.

glottal catch See under voice disorders of phonation.

glottal chink Space between the vocal folds when they are not adducted.

glottal click Glottal catch. See under voice disorders of phonation.

glottal cycle Vibratory cycle.

glottal fry See under voice disorders of phonation.

glottal pulse See under pulse.

glottal replacement See under syllabic structure, under phonological processes.

glottal seizure Glottal catch. See under voice disorders of phonation.

glottal stop 1. Approximation of plosive sound made by stopping and releasing the breath stream at the level of the glottis; may be a compensatory behavior in the presence of inadequate velopharyngeal closure. **2.** Plosive sound produced by the sudden release of subglottic air pressure; represented phonetically as /[IL]/. Syn: ubiquitous glottal stop. **3.** Glottal catch. See under voice disorders of phonation.

glottal stroke Glottal catch. See under voice disorders of phonation.

glottal tone See under tone.

glottal vibration Opening and closing of the glottis when the vocal folds are adducted for phonation.

glottic (glot′ik) **1.** Pertaining to the glottis. **2.** One of the three divisions of the larynx, *q.v.*

glottis (glot′is) [G. *glōttis*, aperture of the larynx] Vocal apparatus of the larynx, consisting of the true vocal folds and the opening between them. Syn: rima glottidis.

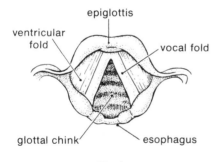

epiglottis

ventricular fold

vocal fold

glottal chink

esophagus

Glottis

glottograph (glot′ə-graf) [glottis + G. *graphō*, to write] Instrument used to measure the relative amount of light that shines through the glottis; indicates the extent of the glottal opening but not the shape.

glue ear Mucoid *otitis* media.

Glycerol Test See *Audiometric Tests and Procedures* in appendices.

gm Former abbreviation for gram, now g.

gnathic (na′thik) [G *gnathos*, jaw] Pertaining to the jaw.

goal 1. End result toward which action, muscular or mental, is directed. **2.** Any object or objective that an organism seeks to attain or achieve.

Goldman-Fristoe Test of Articulation—Second Edition See *Articulation Tests and Phonological Analysis Procedures* in appendices.

Goldman-Fristoe-Woodcock Auditory Skills Battery See *Auditory Tests and Procedures* in appendices.

Goldman-Fristoe-Woodcock Test of Auditory Discrimination See *Auditory Tests and Procedures* in appendices.

Goodenough "Draw-A-Man" See *Psychological Measures and Tests* in appendices.

gradual falling or **gradual rising curve** See under audiogram configurations.

gradual topic shift See under topic shift.

gram (g) Basic unit of weight and mass in the metric system; one gram is equal to slightly less than 1/30 of an ounce, and also equal to the weight of one cubic centimeter of water.

grammar (gram′ėr) [G. *gramma*, word] **1.** Principles or rules for speaking or writing according to the form and usage of a language. **2.** Rules that outline the way sequences of words can be combined to form acceptable sentences; a description of the intrinsic structure of a linguistic system.

    case g. 1. Semantic approach to grammar which attempts to provide underlying as well as superficial representations of sentences; syntactically significant semantic concepts called case relations constitute the deep structure and comprise a set of concepts which identify certain innate human judgments. **2.** Set of rules that define the relationship between a sentence structure and the semantic roles played by the constituent structures (noun phrase, verb phrase, etc.).

finite g. Grammar consisting of a limited number of options and producing a limited number of sentences; *e.g.*, computer language.

generative g. Any grammar which accounts for the derivation of meaningful language.

generative transformational g. 1. System which contains a list of symbols (English words) and a list of rules for combining these symbols in various ways to produce all the possible grammatical sentences in a language. It consists of: (a) a deep structure component which provides the semantic interpretation of a sentence; (b) a set of transformations which operate on the deep structures; and (c) a surface structure component which constitutes the terminal sentence string; it generates the surface structure of a sentence in more than one step, *e.g.*,

deep structure
  components
      $\rightarrow$ *transformations* $\rightarrow$
          surface structure
          components

2. System of rules that derives an infinite set of well-formed sentences and assigns them correct structural description. Syn: transformational or transformational generative grammar.

particular g. Study of the functions of universal features which are present in an individual language or features peculiar to a specific language. See also linguistic universals.

pedagogical g. Grammar utilized by an instructor in a classroom to teach students; it acts as the basis for an explanation of how individuals understand sentences.

phrase structure g. Grammar concerned with the identification of the

constituents of constructions and how they are related; structural regularity is a primary concern. It indicates which strings of words are sentences (those which can be produced by a specific procedure) and describes the surface structure of sentences, *e.g.*,

phrase structure
  grammar
        $\rightarrow$ surface structures

pivot g. Term used to describe the earliest stages of syntactic development, the early appearance of a small number of words (pivot) occurring frequently in a relatively fixed position in combination with a large number of other words (open) occurring less frequently; *e.g.*, baby tired, baby eat, baby play *(baby* is the pivot; *tired, eat,* and *play* are open).

prescriptive g. Set of rules which dictate precisely the usage to be followed by all speakers and writers.

scientific g. Grammar concerned with logical generalizations about the operation of a language; it attempts to provide a logical, complete, and self-consistent explanation for the manner in which any particular language operates.

traditional g. Set of rules derived from Greek and Latin grammars, and based on the assumption that the structure of various languages (especially Latin) contains universally valid laws of logic. The rules for English are based on Latin models and are almost always prescriptive.

transformational or **transformational generative g.** Generative transformational *grammar.*

universal g. 1. General principles basic to grammatical phenomena of all languages. **2.** Theory of grammar which maintains that the variations of particular grammars are but cultural instances of an underlying universal grammar with which all humans are endowed. See also linguistic universals.

grammatic, grammatical (grə-ma'tik, -ti-kəl) Of or pertaining to grammar, or conforming to standard usage.

grammatical analysis Determination of the categories and the functions of words in a sentence; *e.g.*, *Mary* ran home (Mary = noun = subject).

grammatical categories See parts of speech.

grammatical component See linguistic component.

grammatical equivalent Word whose meaning is so similar to another word that its substitution in a sentence does not change or affect the meaning of the sentence.

grammatical meaning Relationship of ideas, the meaning a word assumes in relation to the context in which it is formed; every word has a lexical (dictionary) and a grammatical meaning. See also connotation; denotation.

grammatical morpheme See under morpheme.

grammatical structure Structural relationship between the morphemes of a sentence.

grammatic closure See under closure.

grammatic method See under aural rehabilitation. See also under specific term.

grand mal (gran-môl') [Fr. large sickness] Type of epileptic seizure; may be characterized by loss of consciousness and possible muscular contractions followed by a convulsion.

granuloma (gran-yu-lō'mə) [L. *granulum*, granule + *-oma*, tumor] Localized nodular inflammatory lesion, usually small, firm, and granular. See also under laryngeal anomaly.

grapheme (gra'fēm) **1.** Smallest unit of writing or printing that distinguishes one meaning from another. **2.** Printed symbols.

gravel voice Glottal fry. See under voice disorders of phonation.

grave phoneme See under phoneme.

grimace (grim'əs, gri-mās') Distorted facial expression resulting from paralysis, muscular imbalance, or momentary emotional states.

grommet (grom'ət) Silicone tube that can be inserted into the tympanic membrane to equalize the air pressure on both sides; creates an artificial eustachian tube to ventilate the middle ear. Syn: tympanostomy tube, ventilation, pressure equalization tube (PE tube).

groove fricative See fricative, under consonant, manner of formation.

gross motor See under motor.

gross sound Sound originating from the environment.

group audiometer See under audiometry.

GSR Galvanic skin response.

GSRA Galvanic skin response audiometry.

G tube Gastrostomy tube. See under feeding

guilt Feeling of responsibility, regret, or remorse for an offense (real or imagined), about the difference between role expectation and role performance, or from not measuring up to self-expectations; considered by some to be a major factor in stuttering.

guttural (gət'ėr-əl) [L. *guttur*, gullet, throat] **1.** Pertaining to the throat. **2.** Denoting a low-pitched, raspy, throaty voice quality.

guttural voice See under voice.

gutturophonia See under voice disorders of phonation.

gyrus, pl. **gyri** (jī'rəs, -rī) [L. fr. G. *gyros*, circle] One of the many convolutions of the cerebral hemispheres which are separated by deep grooves (fissures) or shallow grooves (sulci). Syn: convolution.

  angular g. Cerebral convolution which together with the supramarginal gyrus forms the posterior portion of the parietal lobe, where impressions from the primary somes-

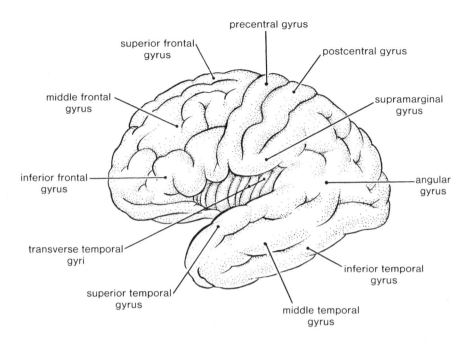

Gyri

Lateral view of the left cerebral hemisphere with the banks of the lateral sulcus drawn apart to expose the transverse temporal gyri.

thetic area are correlated and blended.

frontal gyri Three sets of cerebral convolutions comprising the majority of the frontal lobe. The **inferior f. g.** comprises the lower third of the lobe below the inferior frontal sulcus; the left one is usually more highly convoluted than the right, and its posterior portion is known as Broca's area. The **middle f. g.**, between the inferior and superior frontal sulci, contains the center for intelligence according to Brodmann's classification. The **superior f. g.**, above the superior frontal sulcus, contains in its posterior portion the premotor area, where the cortically originating portion of the extrapyramidal system is said to be located.

Heschl's gyri [R. L. Heschl, Aus. pathologist, 1824–1881] Transverse temporal *gyri*.

postcentral g. Cerebral convolution of the parietal lobe immediately posterior to the central sulcus; it constitutes the primary somesthetic area for all parts of the body.

precentral g. Cerebral convolution of the frontal lobe immediately anterior to the central sulcus (fissure of Rolando) which constitutes the primary motor area for all parts of the body.

supramarginal g. Cerebral convolution, which together with the angular gyrus forms the posterior portion of the parietal lobe, where impressions from the primary somesthetic area are correlated and blended.

temporal gyri Three sets of cerebral convolutions comprising the temporal lobe. The **inferior t. g.**, below the inferior temporal sulcus, the **middle t. g.**, between the inferior and superior temporal sulci, and the **superior t. g.,** between the superior sulcus and lateral sulcus (fissure of Sylvius), contain centers concerned with associative auditory functions in conjunction with the primary auditory area in the transverse temporal gyri (Heschl's gyri).

transverse temporal gyri Several short oblique convolutions on the inner bank of the lateral sulcus (fissure of Sylvius) adjacent to but concealed from lateral view by the temporal gyri; they comprise the primary auditory area of the temporal lobe. Syn: Heschl's gyri.

AaBbCcDdEeFfGgHhIiJjKk
kLlMmNnOoPpQqRrSsTtUu
UuVvWwXxYyZzAaBbCcDd
EeFfGgHhIiJjKkLlMmNnOo

habilitation (hə-bil-i-tā′shən) [L. *habili-tatus*, equipped] Act or process of developing a skill in order to be able to function within a given environment. *Cf.* rehabilitation.

habit [L. *habitus*, condition] Behavior that has become, by repeated performance, relatively fixed, consistent, and almost automatic; often performed unconsciously.

habitual pitch See under pitch.

habituation (hə-bich-yu-ā′shən) [See habit] **1.** Act or process of becoming natural. **2.** In audiology, becoming accustomed to a sound or a noise to the degree that it can be ignored. **3.** Carryover.

HAE Hearing aid evaluation.

HAIC Hearing Aid Industry Conference.

HAIC gain See under gain.

HAIC output See under output.

hair cells Sensory receptors in the organ of Corti. See also organ of Corti, under inner *ear.*

hallucination (hə-lu-si-nā′shən) [L. *hallucinatio*, a wandering of the mind] **1.** Acceptance of sensory imagination as real. **2.** False perception, auditory or visual.

halo effect (hā′lō) Inclination, when making an estimate or rating of one characteristic of a person, to be influenced by another characteristic or by a general impression of that person; *e.g.*, a bright-eyed, good-looking, verbal youngster: classified on the basis of these features as an intelligent child.

hammer Malleus (so called because of fancied resemblance). See under middle *ear.*

handedness Preferential use of either the right or left hand for activities such as writing, eating and drinking, and throwing.

handicapped (hand′i-kapt) Denotes one who is hindered in performing specific tasks because of limited physical or mental capabilities; when more than one disability occurs at the same time, the individual is said to be multiply handicapped.

handle of malleus See manubrium.

hapaxepy (hə-paks′ə-pē) Haplology.

haplology (hap-lol′ə-jē) [G. *haplous*, simple form + *logos*, discourse] **1.** Omission of syllables in producing words because of an excessive rate of utterance; *e.g.*, *probli* for *probably*. **2.** Group of phonemes articulated once when they should be articulated twice in succession; *e.g.*, *morphonology* for *morphophonology*. Syn: hapaxepy.

haptic [G. *haptō*, to grasp, touch] Denoting the combination of tactile and kinesthetic sensations. See also proprioception.

haptic feedback See under feedback.

haptic perception See under perception.

haptic system Neural processes by which an individual perceives his body in relation to objects and space; includes the sensations of touch and kinesthesis; the system by which speech is felt.

hard contacts In stuttering, hypertensed articulatory postures assumed by stutterers when attempting to produce feared words. See also glottal catch, under voice disorders of phonation.

hard glottal attack Forceful approximation of the vocal folds during the initiation of phonation. See also hypervalvular *phonation* (1).

hard-of-hearing 1. Denoting reduced acuity or sensitivity of the organs of hearing, although the ability to communicate orally is retained. **2.** Denoting one in whom the sense of hearing, although defective, does function with or without a hearing aid. See also deaf; deafness.

hard palate See under palate.

hard-wire auditory trainer See under auditory training units.

harelip (hār′lip) Cleft lip (so called because of fancied resemblance to that of a rabbit).

harmonic [G. *harmonikos*, musical, suitable] In acoustics, any whole number multiple of the fundamental frequency of a complex wave; the fundamental frequency equals the first harmonic and produces the fundamental tone. Integral multiples of the first harmonic produce higher frequency components called overtones; thus, the second harmonic evokes the sensation of the first overtone, and so forth. See also overtone.

harmonic distortion See under distortion.

harmony processes Assimilation *phonological processes.*

harshness See under voice disorders of phonation.

HAS High-amplitude sucking technique.

Haws Screening Test for Functional Articulation Disorders See *Articulation Tests and Phonological Analysis Procedures* in appendices.

head shadow effect In unilateral hearing impairment, the difference in reception at the good ear created by the degree of interposition of the head between the good ear and the sound source.

head turn technique See under behavioral *audiometry.*

hearing The sense, receptive in nature, through which spoken language is received by response to sound pressure waves. The ears, the auditory nerve, and the brain are involved in the process of hearing.

hearing aid Any electronic amplifying device whose function is to bring sound more effectively into the listener's ear; consists of a microphone, amplifier, and receiver; may be worn with the amplifier attached in a unit on the body, or all three parts may be at ear level (behind the ear, in the ear, or combinations of these). See also auditory training units.

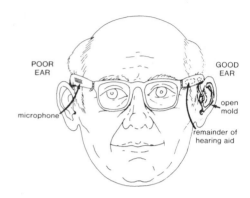

Hearing Aid (CROS)
Typical arrangement for contralateral routing of signals (CROS). From Hodgson, WR. *Hearing Aid Assessment and Use in Audiologic Habilitation,* 3rd ed. Baltimore: Williams & Wilkins, 1985.

air-conduction h. a. Aid designed to amplify sound pressure waves and transmit the signal to the external ear through the medium of air.

behind-the-ear h. a. An aid worn behind the ear and coupled to the ear by tubing attached to an earmold.

binaural h. a. Type of aid which allows sound to be directed to each ear via separate microphones, amplifiers, and receivers; attempts to duplicate "two ears." Some types incorporate a control that permits the relative output at each of the two phones to be varied; helps to localize and discriminate speech from conflicting noise stimuli.

body h. a. Aid designed to provide high levels of amplification and a wide frequency range for individuals with severe hearing impairments; amplification unit is usually strapped to the body with earmolds worn in the ear.

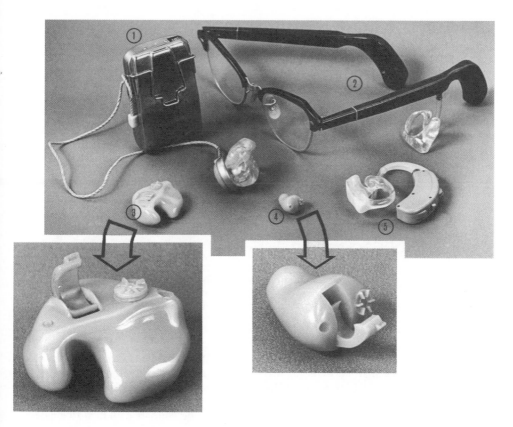

Hearing Aids
Different types of hearing aids: (1) body aid; (2) eyeglass; (3) in-the-ear aid; (4) in-the-canal aid; and (5) behind-the-ear aid. From Bess, FH, and Humes, LE. *Audiology: The Fundamentals,* 3rd ed. Baltimore: Lippincott Williams & Wilkins, 2003.

bone-conduction h. a. Aid designed to amplify sound pressure waves and transmit the signal to a bone-conduction vibrator placed behind the ear on the mastoid process; vibrations of the bone-conduction vibrator cause a signal to be presented directly to the inner ear by vibrating the bones of the skull. It is utilized when an air-conduction hearing aid cannot be worn or is not effective.

canal h. a. Hearing aid that fits mostly in the ear canal, with a small part extending into the concha.

contralateral routing of signals (CROS) Hearing aid in which sounds originating on the side of the impaired ear are picked up by a microphone mounted near that ear, amplified slightly, and routed electronically across the head to a receiver mounted near the good ear; traditionally utilized in unilateral hearing loss to avoid head shadow effect. Originally developed by Earl Hartford, with various modifications being subsequently developed.

Bilateral contralateral routing of signals (BICROS) is used with individuals who demonstrate a bilateral

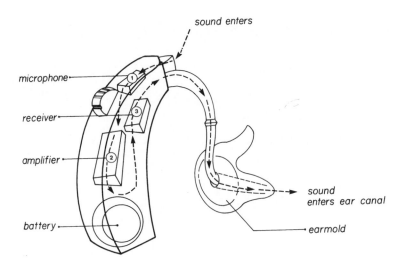

Conventional Hearing Aid

Components are (1) microphone; (2) amplifier; and (3) receiver. From Bess, FH, and Humes, LE. *Audiology: The Fundamentals,* 3rd ed. Baltimore: Lippincott Williams & Wilkins, 2003.

hearing loss but have only one ear with usable hearing; microphones are mounted on both sides of the head, and the amplified signal is transmitted to the better ear.

Binaural CROS or **criss-CROS** is utilized to separate the microphone from the receiver to provide more power by reducing the probability of feedback; microphones are mounted on both sides of the head, and amplified signals are routed across the head to the opposite ear.

FOCALCROS is a CROS or BICROS arrangement with a plastic tube to channel sound from the concha of the unaided ear into a microphone placed on that side.

Front routing of signals (FROS) or **ipsilateral frontal routing of signals (IFROS)** is used with individuals requiring little more amplification than that afforded by IROS; a microphone is placed on the eyeglasses near the midline of the head or near the front of the temple bar on the same side as the hearing aid,

thus providing some separation of microphone and earphone.

High-frequency CROS (HICROS) provides high-frequency emphasis for individuals with high-frequency hearing loss.

Ipsilateral routing of signals (IROS) is used only for mild hearing losses requiring little amplification; it utilizes a monaural hearing aid fitted with a high-frequency circuit and an open earmold connection to the ear.

MINICROS is a CROS system without an earmold and with only a short sound tube (or no tube) from the receiver part way to the good ear; in cases of unilateral hearing loss, it helps alleviate overamplification by disbursing some sound of contralateral origin in the direction of the good ear.

MULTICROS is a CROS system with an off-on switch on each microphone so the user can change at will the aid from a CROS to a BICROS or to a conventional hearing aid.

Power CROS is a monaural system designed to provide greater amplification without feedback by placement of the head between the microphone and receiver.

digital h. a. Instrument that converts electric signals from a microphone to digital values, modifies them according to the program stored in a microcomputer, and converts them back into an electric signal fed to the earphone.

in-the-ear h. a. Hearing aid that fits entirely in the concha, with a case molded to fit the user's ear and an overall shape like that of a standard (receiver) earmold.

monaural h. a. Aid worn in a case on the body, behind the ear, or in the ear, with the receiver and microphone near the same ear.

pseudobinaural h. a. Y-cord *hearing aid.*

vibrotactile h. a. Device that delivers amplified vibratory energy to the skin by means of special transducers; such instruments are designed for individuals whose hearing losses are so severe that assistance hearing cannot be obtained from traditional hearing aids.

Y-cord h. a. Body hearing aid with one microphone and one amplifier which are wired to both ears by a "Y"-shaped cord. Syn: pseudobinaural hearing aid.

hearing aid evaluation (HAE) Process by which an amplification system is selected for an individual to help him utilize his residual hearing. The traditional test battery, conducted in sound-field conditions, includes speech reception threshold testing, speech discrimination testing performed in quiet and noise at a normal conversational listening level (50 dB, HTL), and tolerance testing; comparisons are then made between aided and unaided conditions for several hearing aids, and the instrument which pro-

duces the best aided results, both objectively and subjectively, is recommended.

Hearing Aid Industry Conference (HAIC)- Organization, comprising hearing-aid manufacturers, that provides standardization of measurement and reports on hearing-aid performance data.

hearing conservation Programs designed for the preservation of auditory acuity, primarily through prevention of hearing loss; may be accomplished through dissemination of information and screening programs.

hearing impairment Hearing losses that may range from slight to deafness. See also deafness.

hearing impairment degrees Generally, six categories are used to identify the amount of auditory impairment: slight, mild, moderate, moderately severe, severe, and profound. Each category has its own characteristics and indicates the probable resulting handicap. See *Hearing Impairment Degrees* table.

hearing level (HL) Number of decibels above audiometric zero at which an individual receives sound.

hearing loss See deafness, hearing impairment degrees.

hearing protection device (HPD) Apparatus used to protect an individual's hearing from excessive environmental noise; may include items that block the ear canal, that are inserted into the external ear canal, and that cover the external ear.

    canal caps Semiaural *hearing protection device.*

    circumaural h. p. d. Earmuffs. See below.

    earmuffs Cups, attached to a tension headband, that fit over the pinna. The interior of the cup is lined with a material such as acoustic foam, the perimeter of the cup is fitted with a cushioned seal that rests against the head, and the clamping force of the headband presses the cushions against the head to form a seal

HEARING IMPAIRMENT DEGREES

Category	Handicap	Needs
15–25 dB (ANSI) (slight)	No significant delay in speech or language; may adversely affect auditory perceptual abilities	Condition should be monitored
26–40 dB (ANSI) (mild)	Faint or distant speech may be difficult	Preferential seating and lipreading may facilitate learning; speech and language are learned through auditory channel
41–55 dB (ANSI) (moderate)	Conversational speech can be understood at a distance of 3 to 5 feet; as much as 50% of class discussions may be missed if voices are faint or not in line of vision; vocabulary may be limited and misarticulations may be present; language skills are mildly affected; reading and writing skills may be delayed	Need early language and speech instruction; can attend regular classes if preferential seating given; vocabulary work needed; attention should be given to reading and writing skills; may profit from amplification
56–70 dB (ANSI) (moderately-severe)	Group discussion will be difficult to follow; language usage and comprehension may be deficient and confused; speech can be understood only if it is loud; speech and language are delayed; early speech is unintelligible	Speech and language can be learned through the ear with amplification; speech and language should be aided with cues through visual channel; child may benefit from regular class placement along with special assistance in special classes; may require speech and language training during preschool years; later may require tutorial assistance in academic subjects
71–90 dB (ANSI) (severe)	Voices are heard only from a distance of about one foot from the ear; environmental sounds and vowel sounds may be discriminated, but many consonants will be distorted; speech and language will be distorted and may not develop spontaneously if the loss is present before one year	Speech, language, and auditory training are necessary; auditory amplification is necessary; child is considered educationally deaf; enrollment in preschool program is necessary; needs speechreading; special education placement is necessary, with emphasis on speech and language
More than 91 dB (ANSI) (profound)	May hear some loud sounds, but is more aware of vibrations than tonal patterns; speech and language are defective and will not develop spontaneously if loss is present before one year of age	Requires special classes; may profit from hearing aids to monitor own voice and to discriminate loudness, inflection, and rhythm patterns of other talkers; enrollment in preschool program is necessary

around the pinna. Syn: circumaural hearing protection device.

earplugs Devices designed to be worn in the outer portion of the ear canal and to fit tightly against its cartilaginous walls to create an acoustic seal. Syn: insert hearing protection device.

insert h. p. d. Earplugs. See above.

semiaural h. p. d. Flexible caps, attached to a tension headband, which block the entrance to the ear canal but do not intrude into the canal. Syn: canal caps.

hearing science See speech and hearing science.

hearing theories Hypotheses concerning the displacement effect of a sound wave on the basilar membrane within the cochlea.

   frequency theory Generally discounted belief that pitch discrimination is dependent on the number of times per second that sound impulses pass over the auditory nerve [W. Rutherford, 1886].

   place theory Belief that pitch discrimination is dependent on the response to the stimulation of specific areas along the basilar membrane; sometimes extended to say that "places" in the brain are stimulated, depending on the pitch. Advocates of this hypothesis hold that tones of high frequency stimulate the area near the oval window, while tones of low frequency stimulate the apex of the cochlea [H. von Hemholtz, Ger. physician, 1821–1894].

   resonance-volley theory Combination of the place and frequency theories which states that pitch has a twofold representation: low tones are represented by frequency, high tones by place, and other tones by a combination of the two.

   telephone theory Volley theory (see below).

   traveling wave theory Hypothesis that the movement of the footplate of the stapes causes movement along the basilar membrane, with a rise and fall in amplitude; the point where the wave reaches its maximum amplitude is the point at which the frequency of the sound is detected [G. von Békésy, 1960].

   volley theory Theory that pitch discrimination in the lower frequencies is dependent on nerve impulses firing in series; for tones at higher frequencies, advocates of this theory accept

the place theory [E. G. Wever and C. W. Bray, 1949]. Syn: telephone theory.

hearing threshold level (HTL) Absolute *threshold.*

helix (hē′liks) [L. fr. G. *helix*, coil] Anatomical landmark of the auricle of the ear. See auricle, under external *ear.*

Help Test, The See *Language Tests and Procedures* in appendices.

helping verb Auxiliary verb.

hemilaryngectomy See under laryngectomy.

hemiplegia (hem-i-plē′jē-ə) [G. *hemi-*, half + *plēgē*, stroke] Paralysis of one side of the body. *Cf.* diplegia; monoplegia; paraplegia; quadriplegia; triplegia.

hemisphere (hem′is-fer) Half of a spherical structure; usually used in reference to brain structures.

hemorrhage 1. Discharging of blood from a ruptured artery. **2.** To bleed profusely.

hereditary (hə-red′i-tār-ē) Denoting genetic transmission from parent to offspring. *Cf.* congenital.

heredity (hə-red′i-tē) [L. *hereditas*, inheritance] Sum total of the abilities and potentialities genetically derived from one's ancestors.

herpes simplex virus (HSV) A sexually transmitted disease. The virus is passed on to the fetus in utero during the birth process; may result in a variety of complications including hearing loss.

hertz (Hz) [H. R. Hertz, Ger. physicist, 1857–1894] Unit of vibration adopted internationally to replace cycles per second (CPS), the number of successive compressions and rarefactions of a sound wave in a time period of one second; *e.g.,* 1 Hz = 1 CPS.

Heschl's gyri See under gyrus.

hesitation phenomena Any of several disruptions in speech production, such as false starts, repetitions, unusual pauses, and fillers.

heterogeneous (het′ĕr-ə-jē′nē-əs) [G. *heteros*, other + *genesis*, production]

Composed of parts having various or dissimilar characteristics.

heterogeneous word Syntagmatic *word*.

heterolalia (het′ėr-ə-lā′lē-ə) [G. *heteros*, other + *lalia*, talking] Heterophemy.

heterophemy (het′ėr-ə-fē′mē) [G. *heteros*, other + *phēmē*, a speech] Saying or writing something other than what is intended. Syn: heterolalia.

heterotopy (het-ə-rot′ə-pē) [G. *heteros*, other + *topos*, place] Sound displacement during speech; a characteristic of cluttering; *e.g.*, *silp* for *slip*.

HF High frequency.

HF average SSPL 90 High-frequency average saturation sound pressure level.

HICROS High-frequency CROS.

hierarchy (hī-är′kē) [G. *hierarchia*, power of the high priest] List of stimulus situations arranged by an individual in an order representing the degree of negative emotion with which he reacts to them; used in determining the order in which desensitization will take place; often used as a technique in stuttering therapy. See also response hierarchy.

high See under distinctive features.

high-amplitude sucking technique (HAS) See under behavioral *audiometry*.

high frequency (HF) See under frequency.

high-frequency audiometry See under audiometry.

high-frequency (HF) average full-on gain See under gain.

high-frequency average saturation sound pressure level (HF average SSPL 90) See under output.

high-frequency CROS (HICROS) See under contralateral routing of signals (CROS), under hearing aid.

high-frequency deafness See under deafness.

High Level SISI See *Audiometric Tests and Procedures* in appendices.

high-pass filter See under band-pass *filter*.

high-stimulus speech In stuttering, a technique in which an individual is trained to hear or feel his normal speech patterns and to contrast them with his dysfluent speech patterns.

high vowel See under vowel.

Hiskey-Nebraska Test of Learning Aptitude See *Psychological Measures and Tests* in appendices.

histogram (his′tō-gram) [G. *histos*, web (tissue) + *gramma*, writing] Graph of amplitude density distribution.

historical linguistics See under linguistics.

historical phonetics Evolutionary *phonetics*.

HL Hearing level.

hoarseness See under voice disorders of phonation.

holophrastic utterances (hō-lə-fra′stik) [G. *holos*, whole + *phrasis*, phrase of speech] Stage in the development of language where single-word verbalizations may express complete and complex ideas; *e.g.*, baby saying "ball" may mean "I want the ball," "Look at the ball," or "Where is the ball?" See also language.

home language See under language.

homeostasis (hō′mē-ə-stāsis) [G. *homoios*, like + *stasis*, a standing] In humans, a regulated equilibrium to maintain an internal steady state through a coordinated response of the psychophysiologic systems to any potential or actual disruption of normal conditions.

homogenous (hə-mäj′ə-nəs) [G. *homos*, same + *genos*, kind, family] Having a similarity, usually structural, because of descent from a common predecessor.

homogenous word Paradigmatic *word*.

homograph Ambiguous *word*.

homonym See under word.

homophene See under word.

homophone Homonym. See under word.

homorganics (hō-môr-gan′iks) Phonemes articulated in the same area of the speech mechanism but different in one or more features; *e.g.*, [t]-[d], [p]-[b]-[m].

Hood technique See under masking techniques.

horizontal canal See semicircular canals, under inner *ear*.

horizontal plane See transverse *plane*.

HPD Hearing protection device.

HSV Herpes simplex virus.

HTL Hearing threshold level.

hum **1.** Low continuous murmur. **2.** Electrical disturbance at the power supply frequency or its harmonic which is manifested in electronic equipment. *Cf.* sixty-cycle hum.

Hunt's syndrome Ramsay Hunt syndrome.

huskiness Hoarseness. See under voice disorders of phonation.

Hx History.

hydrocephalus (hī-drō-sef'ə-ləs) [G. *hydor*, water + *kephalē*, head] Condition, congenital or acquired, in which there is excessive accumulation of cerebrospinal fluid within the cranial cavity; marked by enlargement of the head, underdeveloped or atrophied brain, and mental deterioration.

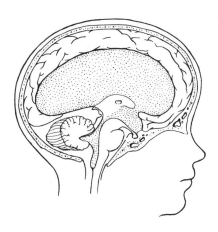

Hydrocephalus

hyoglossus muscle (hī-ō-glos'us) See *Muscles of the Tongue* table, under tongue.

hyoid bone (hī'oid) [G. *hyoeidēs*, shaped like the letter upsilon, υ] "U"-shaped bone situated at the base of the tongue and above the thyroid cartilage which acts as a support for the tongue root above and as a suspension for the larynx below; many laryngeal muscles are attached to this bone. It is considered a part of the laryngeal structure insofar as its function in speech and voice is concerned, and is the only bone in the body not directly connected to another bone.

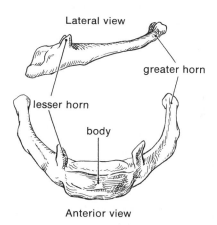

Hyoid Bone

hypacusis (hī-pə-ku'sis) [G. *hypo*, under + *akousis*, hearing] Auditory acuity impairments which may be conductive or sensorineural. Syn: hypoacusis. See also deafness.

hyper- [G. *hyper*, above, over] Prefix denoting excessive, above the normal; corresponds to Latin *super-*.

hyperactivity (hī'pėr-ak-tiv'ə-tē) Abnormal excess of physical action. In children, it is characterized by almost continuous action accompanied by restlessness, distractibility, and low tolerance for frustration, which usually abates during adolescence; may be a result of neurochemical imbalance, brain damage, or psychosis.

hyperacusis (hī'pėr-ə-ku'sis) [hyper- + G. *akousis*, hearing] Exceptionally acute sense of hearing.

hyperbole (hī-pėr′bə-lē) Overstatement. See under figure of speech.

hypercorrect language See under language.

hyperesthesia (hī′pėr-es-thē′zē-ə, -thē′-zhə) [hyper- + G. *aisthēsis*, sensation] Abnormal acuteness of sensitivity to sensory stimuli.

   laryngeal h. See under laryngeal sensory *paralysis.*

hyperfunction See under voice disorders of phonation.

hyperkeratosis (hī′pėr-kār-ə-tō′sis) [hyper- + G. *keras*, horn + *-osis*, condition] **1.** Hypertrophy of the horny layer of the skin. **2.** Oral disease characterized by grayish-white, flat, soft, and smooth patches whose margins fuse with surrounding tissues. See also under laryngeal anomaly.

hyperkinesia, hyperkinesis (hī′pėr-ki-nē′zē-ə, -nē′sis) [hyper- + G. *kinēsis*, motion] Incessant and excessive movement or motor activity. See also hyperactivity.

   h. of the false folds See under laryngeal anomaly.

hyperkinetic (hī′pėr-ki-net′ik) Pertaining to hyperkinesia.

hyperkinetic dysarthria See under dysarthria.

hyperkinetic dysphonia See under voice disorders of phonation.

hyperkinetic syndrome See attention deficit/hyperactive disorder.

hypernasality See under voice disorders of resonance.

hyperplasia (hī-pėr-plā′zē-ə, -plā′zhə) [hyper- + G. *plasis*, a molding] Excessive cell formation, excluding tumor formation, in a tissue or organ; abnormal or unusual increase in the elements composing tissue cells. *Cf.* hypertrophy.

hyperplastic (hī-pėr-plas′tik) Pertaining to hyperplasia.

hyperplastic laryngitis See under laryngitis.

hyperrecruitment See under recruitment.

hyperrhinolalia (hī′pėr-rī-nō-lā′lē-ə) [hyper- + G. *rhis*, nose + *lalia*, talking] Hypernasality. See under voice disorders of resonance.

hyperrhinophonia (hī′pėr-rī-nō-fō′nē-ə) [hyper- + G. *rhis*, nose + *phone*, voice] Hypernasality. See under voice disorders of resonance.

hypertonic (hī-pėr-ton′ik) [hyper- + G. *tonos*, tone] Denoting excessive tone or tension, as of a muscle.

hypertrophy (hī-pėr′trə-fē) [hyper- + G. *trophē*, nourishment] Enlargement of a part or an organ due to an increase in the bulk (but not number) of its elements, not due to tumor formation. *Cf.* hyperplasia.

hypervalvular phonation See under phonation.

hypnosis (hip-nō′sis) [G. *hypnos*, sleep + *-osis*, condition] Artificially induced trancelike state in which the subject is highly susceptible to suggestion, oblivious to all else, and responds readily to the suggestions of the hypnotist.

hypnotherapy (hip-nō-thėr′ə-pē) [G. *hypnos*, sleep + *therapia*, therapy] Use of hypnosis either as an aid or as the primary method of treating physical or mental disorders.

hypo- [G. *hypo*, under] Prefix, equivalent to sub-, denoting (a) location beneath something else; or (b) diminution or deficiency.

hypoactivity (hī′pō-ak-tiv′ə-tē) Diminished motor function.

hypoacusis (hīpō-ə-ku′sis) Hypacusis.

hypofunction See under voice disorders of phonation.

hypoglossal nerve See *Cranial Nerves* table, under cranial nerves.

hypoglottic (hī-pō-glot′ik) **1.** Denoting those parts of the larynx below the vocal folds. **2.** One of three divisions of the larynx, *q.v.*

hypokinesia, hypokinesis (hī′pō-ki-nē′zē-ə, -nē-sis) [hypo- + G. *kinēsis*, motion] Diminution of normal amounts of bodily movements or motor activity; listlessness. See also hypoactivity.

hypokinetic (hī′pō-ki-net′ik) Pertaining to hypokinesia.

hypokinetic dysarthria See under dysarthria.

hypologia (hī-pō-lō′jē-ə) [hypo- + G. *logos*, word] Lack of normal ability for speech resulting from either low intelligence or a cerebral disorder.

hyponasality See under voice disorders of resonance.

hypopharynx (hī′pō-fär′iŋks) [hypo- + G. *pharynx*, throat] Laryngopharynx.

hypophonia See under voice disorders of phonation.

hypophrasia (hī-pō-frāzē-ə, -frā′zhə) [hypo- + G. *phrasis*, phrase of speech] Lack of speech or the reduction of speech that characterizes the depressed phase of certain psychotic states.

hypoplasia (hī-pō-plā′zē-ə, -plā′zhə) [hypo- + G. *plasis*, a molding] Defective or incomplete development of any tissue. See also aplasia; dysplasia.

    lingual h. Incomplete development of the tongue.

    mandibular h. Micrognathia.

hypoprosody (hī-pō-pros′ə-dē) [hypo- + G. *prosōdia*, voice modulation] Aprosody.

hyporhinolalia (hī′pō-rī-nō-lā′lē-ə) [hypo- + G. *rhis*, nose + *lalia*, talking] Hyponasality. See under voice disorders of resonance.

hyporhinophonia (hī′pō-rī-nō-fō′nē-ə) [hypo- + G. *rhis*, nose + *phone*, voice] Hyponasality. See under voice disorders of resonance.

hypothesis (hī-poth′ə-sis) [L. fr. G. *hypotithenai*, to propose] Preliminary assumption usually based on enough observation to place it beyond the class of mere speculation but which requires further experiments for its verification.

hypotonic (hī-pō-ton′ik) [hypo- + G. *tonos*, tone] Denoting diminution or absence of tone or tension, as of a muscle.

hysteria (his-tār′ē-ə) [G. *hystera*, womb (formerly thought to be of uterine causation)] Emotional disorder characterized by anxiety, excitability, and lack of emotional control.

    conversion h. Substitution through psychic conversion of physical signs and symptoms for anxiety; fainting under emotional stress is a common example, but generally it is applied to major symptoms such as blindness, deafness, and paralysis resulting from psychogenic factors.

hysterical (his-tār′i-kəl) Denoting or pertaining to hysteria.

hysterical aphonia Conversion *aphonia.*

hysterical deafness Psychogenic *deafness.*

hysterical stuttering See under stuttering.

Hz Hertz.

-ia [G. suffix denoting action or abstraction] Suffix denoting condition, used in the formation of names of disorders and diseases.

iambic stress See under stress.

IC Inspiratory capacity.

icons (ī′konz) [G. *eikōn*, image] Signs that are related to the things they represent by virtue of some direct physical resemblance; *e.g.*, a hieroglyphic picture of a house.

idea (ī-dē′ə) [G. semblance] Any mental image or concept not directly sensory in nature.

ideation (ī-dē′ā-shən) Organization of concepts into meaningful relationships; the process of forming ideas.

identification (ī′den-tə-fi-kā′shən) [L. *idem*, same + *facio*, to make] **1.** In articulation, the methods used to recognize the essential features of a sound. **2.** Attributing to oneself (consciously or unconsciously) the feelings and characteristics of another person, with a resulting feeling of close emotional association.

identification audiometry Screening *audiometry.*

ideographs (i′dē-ō-grafs) Symbols representing ideas. See also Blissymbolics.

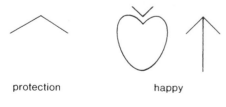

protection   happy

Ideographs

idioglossia (i-dē-ō-glo′sē-ə) [G. *idea*, semblance + *glossa*, tongue] **1.** Any unique speech code invented by an individual which differs markedly from normal language standards. Although the speaker may know what he is saying, the code is generally unintelligible to the listener; this linguistic form should be distinguished from artificial codes affected to achieve secrecy of communication. **2.** Omissions, substitutions, distortions, and transpositions of phonemes so numerous during speech that speech is unintelligible and appears to be an invented language; often associated with mental retardation. **3.** Type of jargon often used by twins for communication between each other to the exclusion of others. Syn: idiolalia.

idiolalia (i-dē-ō-lā′-lē-ə) [G. *idea*, semblance + *lalia*, talking] Idioglossia.

idiolect (i′dē-ō-lekt) Personal dialect of a speaker.

idiom See under figure of speech.

idiopathic (i-dē-ō-pa′thik) [G. *idea*, semblance + *pathos*, suffering] Denoting a disease or disorder of unknown etiology.

idiopathic language retardation Delayed language development for which no physiologic cause is known.

idiosyncratic meaning (i′dē-ō-sin-kra′-tik) [G. *idea*, semblance + *syn*, together, with + *krasis*, a blending] Meaning specific to one's limited experiences; a peculiar meaning.

IFROS Ipsilateral frontal routing of signals.

iliocostalis dorsi muscle See *Muscles of Respiration* table, under respiration.

iliocostalis lumborum muscle See *Muscles of Respiration* table, under respiration.

Illinois Test of Psycholinguistic Abilities (ITPA)—Third Edition See *Language Tests and Procedures* in appendices.

illocution (i-lō-kyu′shən) [L. *in-*, within + *locutus*, spoke] **1.** That which a speaker is performing when verbalizing, such as thanking, promising, requesting, describing, and reporting. *Cf.* locutions; perlocution. **2.** All that is entailed in an effort to communicate; the intent of the communication act. **3.** Meaning intended by the speaker.

illusion (i-lu'zhən) [L. *illusus*, mocked] False interpretation of a real sensation; a perception which misinterprets the object perceived.

image (im'ij) [L. *imago*, likeness] **1.** Accumulated, organized knowledge that one has about himself and his world. **2.** Mental or physical representation of an object.

imagery (im'ij-rē) [See image] Formation of mental images, especially by imagination.

  eidetic i. Vivid type of pretending, common in childhood, in which the individual seems to perceive an object which is not actually present; *e.g.*, a child's imaginary playmate.

imagination (i-ma-ji-nā'shən) [L. *imaginatus*, imagined] Act or ability of forming a mental image of something not present to the senses or never before wholly perceived in reality.

I marker Intention marker.

imitation (i-mi-tā'shən) [L. *imitatus*, copied] **1.** Behavior that copies, almost exactly, the behavior of another. **2.** In speech, repetition of a verbal stimulus; may be **elicited** (by request) or **spontaneous** (volitional).

immature (i-mə-chur') [L. *immaturus*, unripe (untimely)] **1.** Denoting an organism, or part or aspect of an organism, which has not achieved full development. **2.** Denoting behavior which would be more appropriate at an earlier age.

immediate echolalia See under echolalia.

immediate sentence constituents See sentence constituents.

immittance (i-mit'əns) [L. *immitto*, to send in] In audiology, an all-encompassing term to describe measurements made of eardrum membrane impedance, compliance, or admit-

tance. See also acoustic immittance measurement.

immittance tests See *Audiometric Tests and Procedures* in appendices.

immune Protected from a disease.

impacted cerumen Blockage of the ear canal with cerumen; a common cause of conductive hearing loss.

impairment (im-pãr'mənt) Deterioration, weakening, or partial loss of function; may be the result of injury or disease. For various impairments, see specific terms.

impedance (im-pē'dens) Resistance to a vibratory force which may be acoustic, mechanical, or electric, particularly when such resistance is selective as to frequency; *e.g.*, a hearing aid coupler may demonstrate resonance to some frequencies and impedance to others.

  static acoustic i. Point of maximum compliance, as compared with the point of least compliance; one of the three measurements used in acoustic immittance measurement. See also acoustic impedance.

impedance bridge An instrument designed to measure the resistance of the mechanism of the ear to acoustic stimuli.

impedance matching Impedance equalized in two connected parts of a circuit, such as using an 8-ohm earphone with the 8-ohm output of an amplifier.

impediment of speech An obsolete term. See speech defect.

imperative mood See under mood.

imperative sentence See under sentence types.

imperception (im-pér-sep'shən) [L. *in-*, neg. + *perceptio*, a receiving] Defective awareness of stimuli. See also perception.

  auditory i. Auditory *agnosia*.

implant Any device that is placed into a surgically or naturally formed cavity of the human body if it is intended to remain there for a period of 30 days or more (FDA).

implicit language Inner *language*.

implicit stuttering Interiorized *stuttering.*

implosive See under consonant, manner of formation.

impressionistic phonetics See under phonetics.

impulse [L. *impulsus*, pushed against] **1.** Sudden determination to act without deliberation or consideration of the consequences. **2.** Action potential of a nerve fiber. **3.** Momentary surge of voltage or current in an electrical circuit.

in- [L.] Prefix denoting (a) negation, without, not; equivalent of English *a-* and *un-*; (b) within, inside; or (c) intensive action. Appears as *im-* before b, p, or m.

inanimate (in-an′ə-mit) Not animate; said of a vegetable (lacking conscious life and deliberate movement) or a mineral (nonliving).

inarticulate (in-är-tik′yu-lit) [in- + L. *articulatus*, jointed (distinct)] Unable to satisfactorily express oneself with words; difficulty with verbal expression of thoughts, attitudes, feelings, etc.

incidence (in′si-dəns) [L. *incido*, to happen] Frequency of occurrence.

incident wave See under wave.

incipient stuttering Primary *stuttering stage.*

incisive foramen See under foramen.

incisor teeth See under teeth.

incoherence (in-kō-hēr′əns) [in- + *cohaereo*, to cling together] Lack of organization or integration especially in oral expression; confusion; disjointedness.

incompatible behavior See under behavior.

incomplete cleft palate See under cleft palate.

incomplete recruitment See under recruitment.

incoordination (in′kō-ôr-di-nā′shən) [in- + L. *co-*, together + *ordinatus*, arranged] Absence of the normal adjustment of muscular motions; failure of

organs to function harmoniously; in speech, often results in the imprecise production of speech sounds.

incus (in′kəs) [L. anvil] The middle bone of the ossicular chain in the middle ear. Syn: anvil. See under middle *ear.*

indefinite vowel Neutral *vowel.*

independent clause Main *clause.*

index See indices. For individual index, see specific term.

indicative mood See under mood.

indices, sing. **index** (in′də-sez, in′deks) [L. *index*, one that points out, an informer, fr. *indico*, to declare] Signs that relate to the entities which they represent because they participate in or are actually part of the event or object for which they stand; *e.g.*, smoke indicates the existence of fire by virtue of the fact that the two are part of the same phenomenon.

indirect laryngoscopy See under laryngoscopy.

indirect motor system Extrapyramidal system.

indirect object In grammar, any noun (or its equivalent) which is indirectly affected by the action of the verb and which states *to* or *for* whom something is done; *e.g.*, He gave *me* an apple.

Individuals with Disabilities Education Act (PL 101–476) A federal law passed in 1991 that reauthorizes and amends PL 94–142. Part H of PL 101–476 focuses on services to infants and toddlers who are at risk or have developmental disabilities.

inductance (in-dək′təns) [L. *inductio*, a leading in] In electricity: **1.** Property of a conductor, coil, or circuit to store energy in a magnetic field and to resist any change in the current flowing through that conductor, coil, or circuit. **2.** Electric circuit element that opposes a change in current by its electromagnetic field energy.

induction (in-dək′shən) [L. *inductio*, a leading in] **1.** In logic, reasoning from the specific to the general. **2.** In physiology, the arousal of an activity in one part as a result of the spread of activity from an adjoining area.

induction coil Device designed to transform electrical current into higher or lower voltages.

induction loop Continuous wire conducting electrical energy from an amplifier; the flux or magnetic field thus created when it surrounds a room makes possible auditory training systems which utilize a wearable hearing aid. See also loop-induction auditory trainer, under auditory training units.

inductive reactance See under reactance.

inductor Device, usually some form of a coil, used in electronic circuits to introduce the element of inductance.

industrial audiometry See under audiometry.

industrial deafness See under deafness.

inertia (in-èr′shə, -shē-ə) [L. want of skill, laziness] **1.** Tendency of a body to persist in its state of rest or motion; a resistance to a change in the state or position in space of a body. **2.** Time gap between the stimulus and the onset of activity in the particular organ. **3.** Inactivity or lack of force; absence of mental or physical vigor; sluggishness of thought or action.

inertial bone conduction See under conduction.

infantile (in′fən-tīl) Relating to or characteristic of infants or infancy.

infantile aphasia Developmental *aphasia.*

infantile autism See under autism.

infantile perseveration 1. Persistence of early developing speech and language characteristics beyond the age of normalcy; characterized primarily by inconsistent omissions and substitutions of sounds. **2.** Pattern of speech reflecting immaturity in the utterance of speech sounds. Syn: baby talk; infantile speech; pedolalia.

infantile psychosis See under psychosis.

infantile speech Infantile perseveration.

infantile swallowing Tongue thrust.

infection (in-fek′shən) [L. *infectus,* corrupted] Invasion of the body by pathogenic microorganisms and the reaction of the tissues to their presence.

inferior (in-fēr′ē-èr) [L. lower] Lower than or below in relation to another structure; opposite of superior.

inferior maxillary bone Mandible. See under skull.

inferior nasal concha See nasal conchae, under skull.

inferior pharyngeal constrictor See *Muscles of the Pharynx* table, under pharynx.

inferior turbinated bone Inferior nasal concha. See nasal conchae, under skull.

infinitive See verbal, under parts of speech.

inflammatory croup See under croup.

inflection (in-flek′shən) [L. *inflectus,* bent] **1.** Modulation of pitch during phonation; *e.g.,* rising, falling, circumflex (combination of rising-falling or falling-rising pattern). **2.** In linguistics, alteration in the forms of a word to express grammatical distinctions; the process of adding affixes (prefixes or suffixes) to a base word. **3.** A bending or change in the shape of a curve.

inflectional endings Small class of suffixes: /-s/, /-es/, /-'s/, /-ed/, /-ing/, /-er/, /-est/.

informal method Synthetic method. See aural rehabilitation.

infra- [L. below] Prefix denoting a position below the part indicated by the word to which it is joined.

infraglottic (in-frə-glot′ik) **1.** Denoting those parts of the larynx below the vocal folds. **2.** One of three divisions of the larynx, *q.v.*

infrahyoid muscles See *Muscles of the Larynx* table, under larynx.

infrasonic (in-frə-son′ik) [infra- + L. *sonus,* sound] Denoting those sounds with frequencies below the normal hearing range of the ear. Syn: subsonic.

infrasonic frequency See under frequency.

infraversion See under teeth malpositions.

inhalation (in-hə-lā'shən) [L. *inhalatus*, breathed in] Inspiration.

inhalation method See under speech, methods of esophageal speech.

inhibition (in-hə-bi'shən) [L. *inhibitus*, kept back] Curbing or restraining of natural or volitional acts; *e.g.*, fear of stuttering tends to restrain the stutterer's impulse or desire to speak.

initial consonant position See under consonant position.

initial lag See lag.

initial masking See under masking.

initial string See under *derivation* of a sentence.

initial teaching alphabet See under alphabet.

injection method See under speech, methods of esophageal speech.

innate (in-nāt') [L. *innatus*, born in (inborn)] Instinctive; inborn; not learned or acquired; does not imply that such a behavior is fully manifested without practice.

innateness theory Nativist theory. See under language theories.

inner ear See under ear.

inner language or **speech** See under language.

innervation (in-ėr-vā'shən) [in- + L. *nervus*, nerve] Distribution or supply of nerves to a structure.

in phase See phase.

input Amount of energy or effort deposited into a system; a signal fed into a receiver.

insert hearing protection device Earplugs. See under hearing protection device.

insertion (in-sėr'shən) [L. *insertio*, a planting in] Place of attachment of a muscle to the more movable part of the skeleton; *e.g.*, the sternocleidomastoideus muscle has its insertion in the mastoid process and its origin in the sternum. *Cf.* origin.

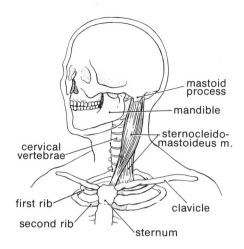

Insertion

Insertion of the sternocleidomastoideus muscle at the mastoid process.

insertion loss In audiology, the difference between the sound pressure level at the eardrum measured with the ear canal occluded by an earmold.

inspiration (in-spə-rā'shən) [L. *inspiratus*, breathed in] Act of drawing air into the lungs. Syn: inhalation. See also respiration.

inspiratory capacity (IC) See under respiratory capacity.

inspiratory reserve volume (IRV) See under respiratory volume.

inspiratory voice See under voice.

instantaneous power In acoustics, the rate at which sound energy is radiated at some given instant.

instinct (in'stiŋt) [L. *instinctus*, impulse] **1.** Any action or reaction as a result of an inner force or natural aptitude; a natural and unreasoning prompting to action. **2.** Native or hereditary factor in behavior.

instructional objective Performance objective.

instrumental See under parts of speech.

instrumental avoidance act theory See under learning theory, under stuttering theories.

instrumental conditioning Operant *conditioning*.

insufficient jaw grading See under jaw grading.

integration (in-tə-grā′shən) [L. *integratus*, made whole] **1.** State of being combined or the process of combining into a complete and harmonious whole. **2.** In language, combining of the data received through input modalities and processing the resulting input products; includes storing the information (temporarily or permanently), attaching and interpreting its meaning, comparing and correcting its content, and making decisions about the necessity for generating an output response.

integrative language Inner *language*.

integrative learning See under learning.

intelligence (in-tel′ə-jəns) [L. *intelligential*] **1.** Aggregate capacity to act purposefully, think rationally, and deal effectively with the environment, especially in relation to the extent of perceived effectiveness in meeting challenges. **2.** Global concept composed of factors such as cognitive skills, abstract verbal and numerical processing, and memory, and the ability to learn, solve problems, and engage in reasoning.

intelligence quotient (IQ) Estimate of intellectual status in terms of an index determined by dividing the mental age (MA) in months by the chronological age (CA) in months and reducing the result to a percentage; *i.e.*,

$$IQ = \frac{MA}{CA} \times 100$$

intelligible (in-tel′i-ji-bəl) Degree of clarity with which one's utterances are understood by the average listener; influenced by articulation, rate, fluency, vocal quality, and intensity. See also under speech.

intelligibility threshold Speech reception *threshold*.

intensity (in-ten′si-tē) [L. *intensus*, stretched out] **1.** Quantitative attribute of a sensation which is correlated with the strength of the stimulus, such as the brightness of a color or the loudness of a sound. **2.** Strength of any behavior or experience, such as the fervor with which an opinion or attitude is held or the magnitude of an emotional response. **3.** In acoustics, the power transmitted along a wave; involves the flow of energy (in ergs) carried by the sound waves through a unit area (square centimeters) in a unit of time (seconds), usually expressed in decibels. **4.** Magnitude of force, energy, power, or pressure acting to produce a sound wave, as measured by instruments. **5.** In speech, the rate at which energy is generated by the vocal folds; originates predominately as a function of (a) the level of subglottal air pressure produced by the thoracic-abdominal expiratory effort; (b) the rate of airflow past the vocal folds; and (c) the manner and amplitude of the vocal fold vibration pattern. **6.** Force or stress with which a sound is produced by a speaker, and the attribute of loudness of the sound to the listener.

intention semantics See under semantics.

intentional marker (I marker) Term used to represent semantic designs, the idea of what one wanted to say as opposed to what was actually said (linked to surface structure); *e.g.*, "baby doll" may mean "baby's doll," "baby wants the doll," or "give the doll to baby."

intentional tremor See under tremor.

inter- [L. *inter*, between] Prefix denoting between, among.

interaural attenuation See under attenuation.

interconsonantal vowel See under vowel.

intercostalis externus muscle See *Muscles of Respiration* table, under respiration.

intercostalis internus muscle See *Muscles of Respiration* table, under respiration.

interdental See linguadental under consonant, place or point of articulation.

interdental lisp Frontal *lisp.*

interference modification Linguistic retention.

interiorized stuttering See under stuttering.

interjection In stuttering, the insertion of extraneous sounds and words, usually in an attempt to avoid, postpone, or escape from a moment of stuttering; *i.e.*, uh, um, well, and ah you know. See under parts of speech.

intermediate string See under *derivation* of a sentence.

intermediate structure See under structure.

intermittent aphonia Aphonic episode.

intermittent reinforcement schedule See under reinforcement schedule.

intermodal transfer Cross-modality *perception.*

intermodulary distortion See under distortion.

intermodulation (in'tėr-mod-yu-lā'shən) [inter- + L. *modulari*, to properly measure off] Modification of the components of a complex (nonsinusoidal) wave by each other in a nonlinear system.

internal auditory canal Internal auditory meatus. See under inner *ear.*

internal auditory meatus See under inner *ear.*

internal juncture See under juncture.

International Organization for Standardization International Standards Organization.

International Phonetic Alphabet (IPA) See under alphabet.

International Standard Manual Alphabet See under alphabet.

International Standards Organization (ISO) Organization composed of members from various countries which develops and issues recommendations for standards in various fields, including acoustics. Also known as International Organization for Standardization. See also American National Standards Institute.

International Test for Aphasia See *Language Tests and Procedures* in appendices.

interneurosensory learning See under learning.

interoceptor (in-tėr-ō-sep'tėr) [inter- + L. *capio*, to take] Any of the sensory nerve cells within the viscera which convey internal stimuli to the central nervous system.

interoral speech aid Device which produces an electronically generated tone that is transmitted to the mouth of the user who modifies the tone into recognizable speech by movements of the tongue and lips, *i.e.*, by "mouthing the words." It may be used by individuals who cannot produce sound, *e.g.*, patients with laryngectomies, those on respirators, patients with emphysema.

Interpersonal Language Skills and Assessment (ILSA) See *Language Tests and Procedures* in appendices.

interrogative sentence See under sentence types.

interrupted See continuant under distinctive features.

interrupted tracings (I tracings) In audiology, impressions which result when pulsed tones are used in automatic audiometers.

interrupter device In stuttering, any sudden jerk, surge of tension, or irrelevant sound used by the stutterer to terminate the stuttering pattern because of pressures to complete communication.

intersensory transfer Cross-modality *perception.*

interstitial word Functor. See under word.

interverbal acceleration Abbreviation or omission of the essential pauses between words (indicated in writing by a comma or period); often symptomatic of cluttering, *q.v.*

intervocalic (in'tėr-vō-kā'lik) Denoting a consonant position between two vowel phonemes. See under consonant position.

in-the-ear hearing aid See under hearing aid.

intonation (in-tō-nā′shən) **1.** Linguistic system within a language which is concerned with pitch, stress, and juncture of the spoken language; a unit with specific communicative import, such as interrogation, exclamation, and assertion. **2.** Awareness of changes in the fundamental frequency of vocal fold vibration during speech production. **3.** Pattern of pitch and stress in the flow of speech.

intonation contour 1. Any change occurring in the fundamental frequency of vocal fold vibration over several consecutive segments. **2.** Shift of pitch and stress extending over several words in an utterance.

intoneme (in′tō-nēm) Working unit in a language which consists of various intonational elements; *e.g.*, negative intonation, questioning intonation, happiness intonation.

intra- [L. *intra*, within] Prefix denoting within.

intra-aural reflex Acoustic *reflex.*

intraneurosensory learning See under learning.

intraoral (in-trə-ô′rəl) [intra- + L. *os*, mouth] Within the mouth.

intraoral pressure Accumulation of air within the mouth creating the force necessary for voluntary expulsion of the air to aid in the production of specific sounds; often lacking in persons with cleft palate.

intrapleural (in-trə-plur′əl) [intra- + G. *pleura*, rib (pl. side)] Within the pleura, the membrane lining the lungs and the thoracic cavity.

intrapleural pressure Intrathoracic pressure.

intrapulmonic (in′trə-pùl-mon′ik) [intra- + L. *pulmo*, lung] Within the lung.

intrapulmonic pressure Pressure in the lungs and air passages. Syn: pulmonary pressure.

intrathoracic (in′trə-thôr-a′sik) [intra- + L. fr. G. *thōrax*, chest] Within the thorax.

intrathoracic pressure Pressure in the thorax outside of the pulmonary spaces. Syn: intrapleural pressure.

intraverbal acceleration Constriction of long words; often associated with cluttering, *q.v.*

intraverbal operant See under operant, verbal.

intrinsic (in-trin′sik) [L. *intrinsecus*, on the inside] Belonging to the part where located or acting. *Cf.* extrinsic.

intrinsic muscles of the larynx See *Muscles of the Larynx* table, under larynx.

intrinsic muscles of the tongue See *Muscles of the Tongue* table, under tongue.

intro- [L. *intro*, into] Prefix denoting in, into.

introversion (in-trō-vėr′zhən) [*intro-* + L. *versus*, turned] Preoccupation with oneself to the detriment of social intercourse and involvement with the external world. *Cf.* extroversion.

introvert (in′trə-vėrt) Person manifesting introversion.

intubation (in-tu-bā′shən) Introduction of a tube into a hollow organ, as into the trachea to keep it open or into the larynx during anesthesia.

inverse feedback Negative *feedback.*

inverse-square law In physics, a law that energy decreases in proportion to the square of the distance from the source; applicable to sound, light, heat, and odor.

inversion (in-vėr′zhən) [L. *inversus*, turned upside down, turned about] Reversal of phonemes which are in contact with one another within a word; *e.g.*, *aks* for *ask*.

involuntary (in-vol′ən-tār-ē) [in- + L. *voluntarius*, willing] Independent of the will; without intent or despite an attempt to prevent, as of an action or behavior.

involuntary whispering Aphonia. See under voice disorders of phonation.

ion (ī′on) [G. *iōn*, going] Atom or group of atoms carrying a charge of electricity by having gained or lost one or more electrons.

negative i. Atom having more than the normal number of electrons.

positive i. Atom which has lost electrons, and therefore has less than the normal number of electrons required for charge neutrality.

IPA International Phonetic Alphabet.

ipsilateral (ip-si-lat′ĕr-əl) [L. *ipse*, same + *latus*, side] Relating to the same side. *Cf.* contralateral (1).

ipsilateral frontal routing of signals (IFROS) Front routing of signals (FROS). See under contralateral routing of signals (CROS), under hearing aid.

ipsilateral routing of signals (IROS) See under contralateral routing of signals (CROS), under hearing aid.

IQ Intelligence quotient.

irony See under figure of speech.

IROS Ipsilateral routing of signals.

irritability (ir′i-tə-bil′ə-tē) [L. *irritabilitas*, excitable] Inherent property of protoplasm to react to a stimulus.

electric i. Response of nerve or muscle to the passage of an electric current.

myotatic i. Ability of a muscle to contract in response to the stimulus produced by a sudden stretching.

IRV Inspiratory reserve volume.

ISO International Standards Organization.

isochronal (ī-sok′rə-nəl) [G. *isos*, equal + *chronos*, time] Equal in rate, frequency, or time of occurrence; does not imply equal in duration.

isogloss (ī′sō-glos) [G. *isos*, equal + *glossa*, tongue] In linguistics: **1.** Geographical boundary of a linguistic trait. **2.** Linguistic feature shared by some but not all of the speakers of a dialect, language, or group of languages.

isolation (ī-sō-lā′shən) In articulation: **1.** Breaking up of the configuration of a word so that the target sound can be heard by itself. **2.** Presentation of a phoneme by itself for the purposes of discrimination and production.

isolation aphasia See under aphasia.

isthmus of fauces Fauces.

-itis [G. fem. adj. suffix agreeing with *nosos*, disease] Suffix denoting inflammation.

I tracing Interrupted tracing.

J Symbol for joule.

jacksonian seizure [J. H. Jackson, Eng. neurologist, 1835–1911] Convulsive movement beginning in one part of the body and progressing to other parts of the body; the entire body may eventually be affected.

Jackson's syndrome [J. H. Jackson, Eng. neurologist, 1835–1911] Unilateral paralysis of the soft palate, larynx, and sternocleidomastoideus and trapezius muscles and hemiatrophy of the tongue; results from lesions of the vagus, spinal accessory, and hypoglossal nerves (cranial nerves X, XI, and XII); similar to Mackenzie's syndrome, *q.v.*

James Language Dominance Test See *Language Tests and Procedures* in appendices.

jargon (jär′gən) [Fr. gibberish] **1.** Verbal behavior of children, beginning at about 9 months and ceasing at about 18 months, which contains a variety of syllables that are inflected in a manner approximating meaningful connected speech; in advanced stages, some true words may be heard. **2.** Speech impairment characterized by continuous but unintelligible speech, with little or no transmission of information; may be composed of standard linguistic units or nonlinguistic units. **3.** Terminology or language peculiar to a specific profession or field.

jargon aphasia See under aphasia.

jaw The mandible (lower jaw) or maxilla (upper jaw). See under bone.

jaw grading The ability to vary the extent of jaw depression in small amounts that are appropriate for biting foods of different thicknesses.

 insufficient j. g. The tendency of the infant and young child to use an easy full opening of the jaw for the spoon, cookie, or other finger food. The child's ability to use visual and kinesthetic cues to anticipate the appropriate amount of jaw opening needed does not appear to develop in the first year.

jaw stabilization Active, internal jaw control with minimal up and down jaw movements, especially significant in cup drinking; initially obtained by biting on the cup rim at about 13 to 15 months of age; gradually develops using active jaw musculature by 24 months of age.

jejunostomy See under feeding.

jejunum A portion of the digestive tract that is below the stomach; the middle portion of the small intestine.

Jena method (yā′nə) [Jena, Ger., where developed by K. Braukmann] Analytic method of speechreading which uses the rhythmic and kinesthetic aspects of talking and transfers them to listening. See also speechreading, under aural rehabilitation.

jitter 1. In voice, pitch disturbance; cycle-to-cycle variation in the periods of glottal cycles; used as basis for perceived roughness. See also shimmer. **2.** Variations in vocal frequency; often heard in dysphonic voices. **3.** Rhythmic variations in the frequency (Hz) of a sound. Syn: frequency jitter.

JND Just noticeable difference.

joint [L. *junctus*, joined] Place where two things are joined; the articulation of two or more bones. For various joints, see specific terms.

Joliet 3-Minute Speech and Language Screen—Revised edition See *Language Tests and Procedures* in appendices.

Jonah words [Jonah, Biblical personage] In stuttering, specific words which a stutterer fears because of previous unpleasant experiences with them.

joule (J) (jul) [J. P. Joule, Eng. physicist,

1818–1889] Unit of energy expended in one second by an electric current of one ampere against a resistance of one ohm.

J tube Jejunostomy tube. See under *feeding*.

jumbling See under teeth malpositions.

junctural feature That which may distinguish words from phrases or a phrase from a compound word, but not words from words; considered to be a phonemic contrast because it has a differential rather than a referential function.

juncture (jəŋk′chər) [L. *junctura*, a joining] **1.** Manner in which syllables join one another in contextual speech. **2.** Suprasegmental cue which enables the listener to differentiate between messages, as in "I scream" from "ice cream." **3.** Articulation, joint, or area of union between two parts.

   closed j. Juncture in which the transition between syllables is from vowel to consonant and the syllable is of the consonant-vowel type, as in "I scream." Syn: normal transition.

   internal j. Method of separating words in such a way as to control meaning; *e.g.*, differentiating "ice cream" from "I scream."

   open j. 1. Juncture in which successive syllables are not joined in the normal consonant-vowel pattern; rather, an effort has been made to retain the terminal consonant of a syllable, as in "ice cream." **2.** Contrasts in the transition of syllables which may be within a word or between words and are reflected by changes in the length, voicing, and degree of aspiration of the vowels and consonants involved; symbolized by / + /. Syn: plus juncture.

   plus j. Open *juncture.*

   terminal j. Any pause or inflection used to end phrases, clauses, or sentences; indicates whether more is to be said or the idea is complete, whether it is a statement or question. Syn: clause terminal; terminal contour.

just noticeable difference (JND) Difference limen *threshold.*

juvenile (ju′və-nīl) [L. *juvenilin*, youthful] Pertaining to or denoting youth, childhood, immaturity.

juvenile papillomatosis See under papillomatosis.

Kahn-Lewis Phonological Analysis—Second Edition See *Articulation Tests and Phonological Analysis Procedures* in appendices.

Kanner's syndrome [L. Kanner, Aus. psychiatrist, 1894–1981] Infantile *autism*.

Kaufman Assessment Battery for Children See *Psychological Measures and Tests* in appendices.

Kaufman Brief Intelligence Test See *Psychological Measures and Tests* in appendices.

kc Kilocycle.

K-complex Waveform which appears on an electroencephalogram as a result of a sound or other stimulus.

keratoma (kăr-ə-tō′mə) [G. *keras*, horn + *-oma*, tumor] **1.** A horny tumor. **2.** Cholesteatoma.

keratosis (kăr-ə-tō′sis) [G. *keras*, horn + *-osis*, condition] Any horny overgrowth on the skin. See also hyperkeratosis, under laryngeal anomaly.

kernel (kèor′nəl) [Ger. *kern*, kernel (nucleus)] **1.** Simplest possible fundamental structure. **2.** In linguistics, the basic part of a word or sentence.

kernel sentence See under sentence classification, transformational grammar.

key word method In articulation, utilization of a word in which a usually defective speech sound is made correctly to stabilize the correct pronunciation of that sound; serves as a standard of correctness or as a target.

kilocycle (kc) (kil′ə-sī-kəl) One thousand cycles per second.

Kindergarten Auditory Screening Test See *Auditory Tests and Procedures* in appendices.

Kindergarten Language Screening Test—Second Edition (KLST) See *Language Tests and Procedures* in appendices.

kinesics (ki-nē′ziks) [G. *kinēsis*, movement] Systematic study of body language, such as gestures, body movements and postures, and facial expressions.

kinesiology (ki-nē-zē-ol′ə-jē) [G. *kinēsis*, movement + *logos*, discourse] In speech, a study of the method of sound production in terms of muscle movement.

kinesthesia, kinesthesis (ki-nes-thē′-zē-ə, -thē′sis) [G. *kinēsis*, movement + *aisthēsis*, sensation] **1.** In speech, an awareness of the movement or position of the speech muscles and structures. **2.** Sense of movement originating from sensory end organs in muscles, tendons, joints, and sometimes the canals of the ear. See also feedback; proprioception.

kinesthetic (ki-nes-thet′ik) Pertaining to kinesthesia.

kinesthetic analysis In speech, the study of error sounds in terms of awareness of the movement patterns of the articulators.

kinesthetic cue In speech, the use of the awareness of the position of the articulators or their correct pattern of movements as an aid in teaching the correct production of a speech sound. Syn: kinesthetic technique.

kinesthetic feedback See under feedback.

kinesthetic method See under aural rehabilitation.

kinesthetic perception See under perception.

kinesthetic technique Kinesthetic cue.

kinetic (ki-net′ik) [G. *kinētikos*] Relating to movement or motion. *Cf.* kinesthetic.

kinetic analysis Analysis of what an individual is doing when articulating, *i.e.*, how he is producing the sounds.

kinetic energy See under energy.

Kinzie method [C. and R. Kinzie, U.S. teachers of deaf, early 20th century]

168

System of speechreading which, although basically a synthetic method, uses some of the features of the analytic method by concentrating on elements of the language before learning to read entire ideas. See also speechreading, under aural rehabilitation.

KLST Kindergarten Language Screening Test—Second Edition.

kymogram (kī′mə-gram) [G. *kyma*, wave + *gramma*, word] Tracing obtained from a kymograph.

kymograph (kī′mə-graf) [G. *kyma*, wave + *graphō*, to record] **1.** Instrument which graphically records the different articulatory movements of the tongue, lips, soft palate, and breath on blackened paper for analysis. **2.** Mechanical aid which can show differences of voicing, duration, aspiration, and nasality.

labeling (lā′bəl-iŋ) Naming, identifying, designating.

labial (lā′bē-əl) [L. *labia*, lips] Pertaining to the lips.

labial assimilation See under assimilatory phonological processes.

labial cleft Cleft lip.

labialization (lā′bē-əl-i-zā′shən) [see labial] **1.** Lip rounding; pursing or protrusion of the lips. **2.** See under substitution, under phonological processes.

labiodental (lā′bē-ō-den′təl) [L. *labia*, lips + *dentes*, teeth] Relating to the lips and teeth.

labiodental area See under consonant, place of articulation.

labioglossolaryngeal paralysis Bulbar *paralysis*.

labioversion Facioversion. See under teeth malpositions.

labyrinth (la′bə-rinth) [G. *labyrinthos*] System of interconnecting canals and cavities within the temporal bone which makes up the inner ear; consists of the cochlea, vestibule, and semicircular canals. See also inner *ear*.

   bony l. Actual hollowed out form, within the temporal bone, of a series of communicating canals and cavities that comprise the labyrinth. Syn: osseous labyrinth.

   membranous l. System of communicating membranous ducts and sacs contained within the larger bony labyrinth; contains the sensory receptors for both the auditory and vestibular systems.

   osseous l. Bony *labyrinth*.

labyrinthitis Inflammation of the labyrinthine canals of the inner ear which may result in abrupt vertigo; associated with tinnitus and sensorineural hearing loss.

lacrimal (lak′rə-məl) [L. *lacrima*, a tear] Relating to tears, their secretion, and involved structures.

lacrimal bone See under skull.

LAD Language acquisition device.

laddergram In audiology, a graph, resembling a ladder, which illustrates the results of a loudness balance test of recruitment (*e.g.*, alternating binaural loudness balance test).

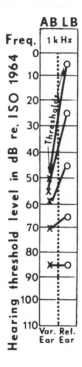

Laddergram

lag 1. Brief period of time following application of a stimulus during which it is not perceived (**initial lag**), and after removal of the stimulus during which it is still perceived (**terminal lag**). **2.** Space of time between the application of a stimulus and the resulting response.

-lalia [G. *lalia*, talk, talking] Combining form, usually a suffix, denoting talk, talking, speech.

lalling (läl′iŋ) [G. *laleō*, to prattle, chatter] **1.** Babbling, infantile form of speech. **2.** Articulatory disorder characterized by errors on sounds produced by elevating the tip of the tongue, specifically the /l/ and /r/; /t/ and /d/ may also be involved.

laminography (lam-i-nog′rə-fē) [L. *lamina*, layer + G. *graphō*, to write] Tomography.

language (laŋ′gwij) [L. *lingua*] **1.** Any accepted, structured, symbolic system for interpersonal communication composed of sounds arranged in ordered sequence to form words, with rules for combining these words into sequences or strings that express thoughts, intentions, experiences, and feelings; comprised of phonological, morphological, syntactic, semantic, and pragmatic components. **2.** Symbolic formulation, vocal or graphic, of ideas according to semantic and grammatical rules for communication of thoughts and feelings. **3.** Organized set of symbols used for communication; an interrelation of the reception, integration, and expression of information.

    automatic l. 1. Habitual use of words or phrases which because of overuse contain little, if any, semantic content; often the first words uttered by an individual after suffering central nervous system damage. **2.** Reflexive sounds made in the first several months of life.

    body l. Nonvocal, nonlinguistic bodily motions which aid in communication, often accompanying speech; *e.g.*, gestures, facial expressions, body movements. See also kinesics; paralanguage.

    computer l. Linguistic units used in communicating with computing machines; simpler than human (natural) languages and also finite (number of sentences is limited).

    confused l. Unconscious rambling from idea to idea; difficulty in maintaining focus in verbal interaction.

    delayed l. Failure to comprehend or produce language at the expected age; may be due to slow maturation, hearing impairment, brain injury, mental retardation, or emotional disturbances; may also be accompanied by multiple articulatory errors.

    deviant l. Language disorder.

    dominant l. Most powerful, influential, controlling, or ruling language; *e.g.*, in the United States, it is "standard" English, while in the homes of native speakers of ebonics it is Black English.

    egocentric l. 1. Early stage in a child's linguistic development during which verbalizations are controlled by the child's own needs and are insensitive to the needs of others. **2.** Utterances having no social reference or at least making no social demand, although they may be made in the presence of others; talking to one's self. Syn: egocentric speech.

    emergent l. Developmental processes of language acquisition in infancy and early childhood, including the comprehension and expression of speech.

    expressive l. 1. Use of conventional symbols to communicate one's perceptions, ideas, feelings, or intentions to others. **2.** Ability to communicate via the spoken or printed word. Syn: encoding.

    figurative l. Language that represents abstract concepts not always stated in a literal interpretation; *e.g.*, idioms, metaphors, similes, and proverbs.

    gesture l. Any visible bodily movement, without accompanying speech, that effectively communicates meaning. *Cf.* body *language*.

    home l. Dominant language in an individual's home environment.

    hypercorrect l. Adoption of the standard form of a language more strongly than the high-prestige group.

    implicit l. Inner *language*.

    inner l. 1. Transforming of experience into symbols (verbal and nonverbal) for purposes of self-awareness, thinking, and adjustment. **2.** Communicating with oneself; the relationships between concepts as experienced through the mediation of linguistic symbols by the central auditory recall and memory systems. **3.** Perceptual response to verbal stimuli which may or may not result in overt speech; a subliminal response to verbal stimuli. **4.** Process of thinking in word meanings; verbal thought. Syn: integrative or implicit language; inner speech.

integrative l. Inner *language.*

native l. One's first learned language.

nonspecific l. Language with low information content, including indefinite pronouns, such as "they" and "them," and nouns, such as "stuff," "thing," and "something," with no discernible referent point established.

nonstandard l. Verbal expressions differing markedly from the accepted norms of a particular language. Syn: substandard language.

oral l. Communication through spoken symbols. See also language.

prelinguistic l. Behaviors that are thought to precede the acquisition of true language; presumed by some to precede the first true word; *e.g.,* crying, cooing, babbling, echolalia. See also *Developmental Sequences of Language Behavior: Overview* in appendices.

protolanguage Phase of language learning in young children (between 9 and 15 months) which is thought by some to constitute a bridge between language precursors and the child's subsequent language development; during this phase children use words only to regulate social interaction.

receptive l. 1. Translation of sound patterns into their intended meaning. **2.** Words one understands; may be verbal or visual. **3.** Spoken or written messages received by the individual. Syn: decoding.

school l. Dominant language in an individual's school environment.

sign l. Means of communication for the deaf in which gestures perform the function of words; includes sign, pidgin sign English, and Sign or Manual English, *q.v.*

standard l. Accepted forms of a particular language.

subcultural l. Native language of a subgroup which functions as the effective means of communication within the subgroup located in a larger community.

substandard l. Nonstandard *language.*

true l. In children's language, intentional use of words or word approximations with behavior indicating anticipation of a response to the situation and what was said.

twin l. See idioglossia (3).

written l. Set of phonological, syntactic, and semantic rules represented by orthographic features.

language acquisition device (LAD) 1. One component of a total system of intellectual structures; its internal structure presumably is composed of various formal universals which provide a plan that is applied to incoming data so as to determine, in a restricted manner, the general form of the grammar that emerges on presentation of language samples from the environment. The grammar can change over time, since the individual continues to receive new linguistic data; *e.g.,* incoming data → LAD → grammar (output). **2.** Innate knowledge of grammatical relations which is the starting point for basic sentence structure from which all transformational operations stem; its internal structure corresponds to the fundamental human capacity for language. **3.** Inborn or innate capacity to acquire the rules underlying language. See also language theories; linguistic universals.

language and speech characteristics of cleft palate See cleft palate.

language arts Academic activities such as listening, speaking, reading, handwriting, and spelling.

Language Assessment, Remediation, and Screening Procedure See *Language Tests and Procedures* in appendices.

language boundary See isogloss (1).

language centers Any of the areas of the brain which are presumed to function in various aspects of spoken and written language; *e.g.*, Broca's area.

language clinician Speech and language pathologist.

language content What people talk about and what they understand of what other people say; concerned with what people know about objects and events, and the feelings and attitudes that they have about what they know. See also semantics; *Linguistic Components* table.

language development See *Developmental Sequences of Language Behavior: Overview; Mean Length of Utterance;* and *General Outline of Language Development From Birth to 11 Years,* in appendices.

language difference Individual who meets the norms of his or her primary linguistic community but who does not meet the norms of standard English.

language disorder 1. Any difficulty with the production or reception of linguistic units, regardless of environment, which may range from total absence of speech to minor variance with syntax; meaningful language may be produced, but with limited content; *e.g.*, reduced vocabulary; restricted verbal formulations; omission of articles, prepositions, or tense and plural markers; paucity of modifiers. **2.** Inability or limited ability to utilize linguistic symbols for communication. **3.** Any interference with the ability to communicate effectively in any community as

dictated by the norms of that community. Syn: deviant language; language impairment. See also communicative disorder; speech disorder.

language form or **structure** Units of sound (phonology), units of meaning that are words or inflections (morphology), and the ways in which units of meaning are combined with one another (syntax). See also *Linguistic Components* table.

language function or **use** Reason for talking; the socially and cognitively determined selection of behaviors according to the goals of the speaker and the context of the situation. See also pragmatics; *Linguistic Components* table.

language impairment Language disorder.

Language Modalities Test for Aphasia See *Language Tests and Procedures* in appendices.

language pathologist Speech and language pathologist.

language pathology Speech and language pathology.

language processing Process of hearing, discriminating, assigning significance to, and interpreting spoken words, phrases, clauses, sentences, and discourse.

Language Processing Test See *Language Tests and Procedures* in appendices.

Language Proficiency Test (LPT) See *Language Tests and Procedures* in appendices.

language sample Systematic collection and analysis of an individual's utterances used as part of a regular diagnostic procedure.

language structure See language form.

Language-Structured Auditory Retention Span Test (LARS) See *Auditory Tests and Procedures* in appendices.

language tests and procedures See appendices.

language theories Hypotheses concerning the origin of human language and why man talks as he does.

   biolinguistic theory Nativist theory (see below).

empiricist theory 1. Belief that language is acquired through pairing of verbal behavior with proper reward situations, thus ensuring continued usage of these verbal behaviors. **2.** Assumption that language is learned entirely through experience. Syn: learning theory.

innateness theory Nativist theory (see below).

learning theory Empiricist theory (see above).

mixture theory Attempt to bridge the gap between the empiricist and nativist theories by the proposition that the universals of language are accounted for by means of an innate mechanism; the principles of stimulus-response conditioning, with all its varieties, are seen as assisting in the individual's acquisition of an intricate language system.

nativist theory Belief that the acquisition of language is an innate, physiologically predetermined, genetically transmitted phenomenon; the function of experience is not to teach language directly, but to activate the innate capacity and turn it into linguistic competence; language maturation is explained in terms of certain properties of the human organism, not on the basis of experience and learning. Syn: biolinguistic, innateness, or rationalist theory.

rationalist theory Nativist theory (see above).

language therapist Speech and language pathologist.

language use See language function.

laryng- Combining form relating to the larynx.

laryngeal (lə-rin'jē-əl, -rin'jəl) Pertaining to the larynx.

laryngeal anesthesia See under laryngeal sensory *paralysis.*

laryngeal anomaly Pathologic condition of the vocal folds and related structures; vocal production is often affected. See also voice disorders.

chorditis (kôr-dī'tis) [G. *chordē*, string + *-itis*, inflammation] Inflammation of the vocal folds.

chorditis nodosa or tuberosa Vocal nodules (see below).

contact ulcer Benign bilateral ulceration of the vocal folds which occurs posteriorly over the vocal process of the arytenoid cartilages; usually the result of vocal abuse, and may result in hoarseness and laryngeal pain; more common in men than women, and only rarely seen in children.

granuloma (gran-yu-lō'mə) [L. *granulum*, granule + *-oma*, tumor] Localized nodule of inflamed tissue, commonly, the result of intralaryngeal intubation during surgical procedures but also associated with vocal ulcer; results in hoarseness.

hyperkeratosis (hī'pėr-kăr-ə-tō'sis) Benign mass of accumulated tissue which may grow on the inner glottal margins or on the vocal folds; occasionally, it may develop into a malignancy; voice is characterized by hoarseness, and dysphonia may be present.

hyperkinesia of the false folds Contraction and closure of the false vocal folds (normally completely open during phonation) over the vocal folds, with additional problems arising from the absence of protective tissue at the edges of the false vocal folds which leaves them highly vulnerable to vocal abuse; the voice may be almost continuously hoarse, or it may be normal in the morning and then deteriorate later in the day. Diagnosis is difficult because the larynx may appear normal on one inspection by laryngeal mirror, while subsequent inspection may reveal the abnormal actions of the false vocal folds.

laryngeal web Membranous tissue that extends across the glottis from one vocal fold to the other; usually located in the anterior part of the lar-

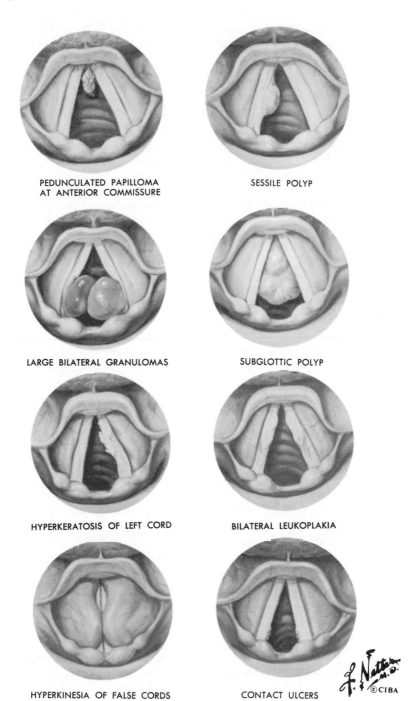

PEDUNCULATED PAPILLOMA
AT ANTERIOR COMMISSURE

SESSILE POLYP

LARGE BILATERAL GRANULOMAS

SUBGLOTTIC POLYP

HYPERKERATOSIS OF LEFT CORD

BILATERAL LEUKOPLAKIA

HYPERKINESIA OF FALSE CORDS

CONTACT ULCERS

Laryngeal Anomalies

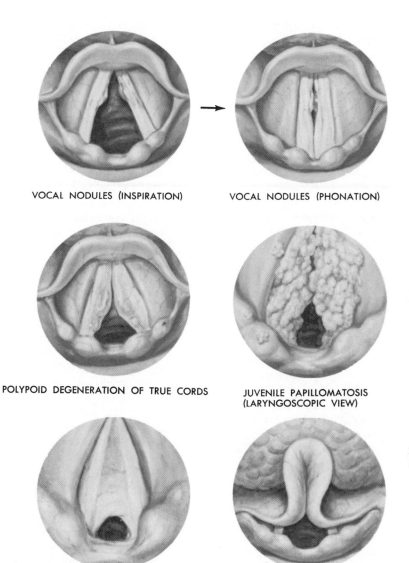

VOCAL NODULES (INSPIRATION)

VOCAL NODULES (PHONATION)

POLYPOID DEGENERATION OF TRUE CORDS

JUVENILE PAPILLOMATOSIS
(LARYNGOSCOPIC VIEW)

CONGENITAL WEB (INCOMPLETE)
VIEWED THROUGH LARYNGOSCOPE

LARYNGOMALACIA (CONGENITAL
LARYNGEAL STRIDOR)

Laryngeal Anomalies

ynx and varying in size from a small membrane filling the anterior commissure to a structure extending to the vocal processes of the arytenoid cartilages, thereby occluding most of the airway; webs may be congenital or the result of an injury, and may connect the ventricular folds or span the larynx subglottally; varying degrees of breathing difficulties are present, and surgical removal may be required.

laryngomalacia (lə-rin′jō-mə-lā′sē-ə, -riŋ′gō-) [laryngo- + G. *malakia*, softness] Presence of soft laryngeal cartilage; it is not fatal and usually clears at about two years of age; in extreme cases, severe breathing problems may be present.

leukoplakia (lu-kō-plā′kē-ə) [G. *leukos*, white + *plax*, plate] Benign growth of thick whitish patches which may be found on the vocal folds, most prominent anteriorly; characterized by hoarseness and a moderate cough and caused by chronic irritation, particularly from tars of tobacco smoke; considered to be a precursor of cancer.

nodularity (nod-yu-lar′i-tē) Thickening at the anterior third of the vocal folds; not a fully developed nodule.

papilloma, pl. **papillomas, papillomata** (pa-pi-lō′mə, -məz, -mä′tə) [L. *papilla*, nipple + G. *-oma*, tumor] Wartlike growth having a bumpy appearance, often spreading over a large surface of the vocal folds, laryngeal walls, or epiglottis; often described as mulberry-like nodular masses varying in color from pinkish-white to red. Varying degrees of dysphonia may result, but these growths may multiply rapidly and seriously interfere with the opening of the airway; periodic surgical removal may be required. Papillomas are perhaps the most common benign tumors of the larynx in childhood, and are referred to as juvenile papillomatosis.

polyp (pol′ip) [L. *polupus* fr. G. *polys*, many + *pous*, foot] Bulging enlargement occurring at the juncture of the anterior middle one third of the vocal fold, and more likely to be unilateral than bilateral; hoarseness usually accompanies this condition. When an extremely large polyp fills most of the glottis, dyspnea and stridor are present.

polypoid degeneration of the true folds Condition in which the true vocal folds become waterlogged, flabby, and almost jellylike as the result of heavy smoking or vocal overuse; voice is characterized by low pitch and hoarseness.

vocal nodules Benign, callus-like growth constituting an inflammatory reaction to frictional rubbing together of the vocal fold edges; such nodules are usually paired and opposite each other on the glottal margins approximately at the midpoint of the membranous portions of the vocal folds, which is also the junction of the anterior and middle thirds of the entire glottis (area of maximum pressure on contact); hoarseness, harshness, and occasional dysphonia are often present. In most cases nodules disappear following vocal rest or voice therapy, but surgical removal may be required. Syn: chorditis nodosa or tuberosa; singer's or speaker's nodules or nodes.

Polypoid vocal nodules are growths at the anterior third of the vocal folds characterized by having a peduncle or "neck" at their base attachment rather than the typical mound shape of a nodule.

Sessile vocal nodules are growths which appear swollen and watery, and have a broad base of attachment.

laryngeal atresia See under atresia.

laryngeal hyperesthesia See under laryngeal sensory *paralysis*.

laryngeal motor paralysis See under pa-ralysis.

laryngeal oscillation See under oscilla-tion.

laryngeal paralysis See under paralysis.

laryngeal paresthesia See under laryn-geal sensory *paralysis.*

laryngeal prominence Projection on the anterior aspect of the neck formed by the thyroid *cartilage, q.v.*

laryngeal reflex See under reflex.

laryngeal respiration See under respira-tion.

laryngeal sensory paralysis See under pa-ralysis.

laryngeal stuttering Spastic dysphonia. See under voice disorders of phona-tion.

laryngeal web See under laryngeal anomaly.

laryngectomee (lăr-ən-jek′tə-mē) One who has undergone a laryngectomy.

laryngectomy (lăr-ən-jek′tə-mē) [lar-yngo- + G. *ektomē*, excision] **1.** Total removal of the larynx; the most com-mon surgical procedure performed for carcinoma of the larynx. In this procedure, the larynx is removed, the trachea is brought forward and su-tured to the skin in the lower midline neck to create a permanent stoma, and the pharynx is closed as a sepa-rate tract for swallowing. This proce-dure is used to treat more advanced cancers. **2.** Surgical removal of part or all of the larynx. See also alar-yngeal *speech.*

    anterior partial l. Removal of an an-terior section of thyroid cartilage and the vocal folds.

    frontolateral l. Removal of one en-tire vocal fold and an anterior section of the thyroid cartilage.

    hemilaryngectomy (hem′i-lăr-ən-jek′

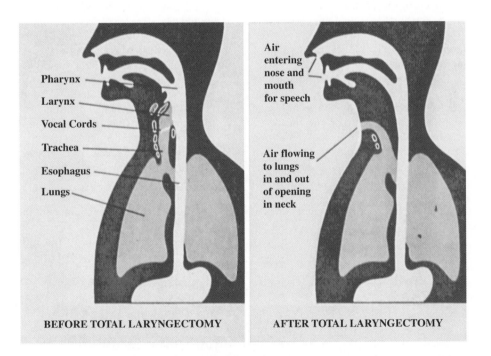

Pharynx
Larynx
Vocal Cords
Trachea
Esophagus
Lungs

Air entering nose and mouth for speech

Air flowing to lungs in and out of opening in neck

BEFORE TOTAL LARYNGECTOMY   **AFTER TOTAL LARYNGECTOMY**

Laryngectomy
From International Association of Laryngectomees: *Helping Words for the Laryngectomee,* 1964.
Courtesy of the American Cancer Society, Inc.

tə-mē) **1.** Surgical procedure in which larynx is divided in or near the midline vertically, and half of the larynx containing the tumor is removed. **2.** Removal of one side of the larynx. Syn: partial laryngectomy; vertical hemilaryngectomy.

subtotal l. Removal of one entire vocal fold and up to one third of the other.

supraglottic 1. Surgical procedure performed for patients with tumors limited to the supraglottic structures of the larynx: the epiglottis, the aryepiglottic folds, and false vocal folds. The larynx is divided horizontally through the laryngeal ventricles making indentations in the wall of the larynx just above the true vocal folds. The arytenoid cartilages are preserved as are the recurrent laryngeal nerves.

total l. Excision of the entire larynx from the trachea to the base of the tongue, often including the hyoid bone.

larynges (lə-rin′jēz) Plural of larynx.

laryngitis (lăr-ən-jī′təs) [laryngo- + G. -itis, inflammation] Inflammation of the mucous membrane of the larynx, often resulting in hoarseness or loss of voice; may be acute or chronic.

hyperplastic l. Chronic condition that is marked either by localized or diffuse enlargement of the mucous membrane, and which may have an injurious effect on the voice; it is secondary to acute laryngitis, vocal abuse, or dietary deficiencies, but the specific cause is unknown; it may occur in singers who use their voices incorrectly.

laryngo- [G. *larynx*] Combining form relating to the larynx.

laryngocele (lə-rin′gō-sēl, -rin′jə-) [laryngo- + G. *kēle*, hernia] Irregular air sac which connects with the cavity of the larynx and produces a tumorlike lesion which is visible on the outside of the neck.

laryngofissure (lə-rin′gō-fish′ĕr, -rin′jə-) Surgical procedure in which the larynx is directly exposed by dividing the thyroid cartilage in the midline; permits adequate exposure for the surgical handling of lesions which cannot be attacked satisfactorily via the oral route, yet are not sufficiently extensive to require total laryngectomy.

laryngograph Electroglottograph.

laryngology (lăr-in-gol′ə-jē) [laryngo- + G. *logos*, discourse] Science of the anatomy, physiology, and diseases of the larynx.

laryngomalacia See under laryngeal anomaly.

laryngopathy (lăr-in-gop′ə-thē) [laryngo- + G. *pathos*, suffering] Disease of the larynx.

laryngopharynx (lə-rin-gō-făr′inks, -rinjō-) [laryngo- + G. *pharynx*, throat] Inferior portion of the pharynx lying between the larynx and the oropharynx. Syn: hypopharynx. See also pharynx.

laryngoplasty (lə-rin′gō-plas-tē, -rin′jō-) [laryngo- + G. *plasso*, to form] Reparative or plastic surgery of the larynx.

laryngoscope (lə-rin′gō-skōp, -rin′jō-) [laryngo- + G. *skopeō*, to inspect] Any of several types of hollow tubes equipped with electrical lighting, used in examining or operating on the interior of the larynx through the mouth.

laryngoscopy (lăr-in-gos′kə-pē) Inspection of the interior of the larynx by means of a laryngoscope.

direct l. Examination of the interior of the larynx by direct vision with the aid of a laryngoscope.

indirect l. Examination of the interior of the larynx by means of a laryngeal mirror.

laryngostenosis (lə-rin′gō-stə-nō′sis, -rin′jō-) [laryngo- + G. *stenōsis*, a narrowing] Contraction or stricture of the larynx.

larynx, pl. **larynges** (lăr′inks, lə-rin′jēz) [G. *larynx*] Primary organ of phonation; a cartilaginous and muscular funnel-shaped structure situated at the

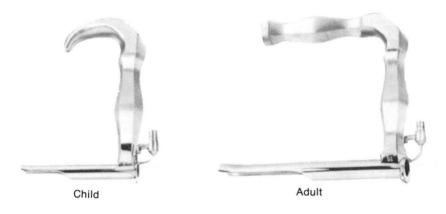

Child   Adult

Laryngoscope
Courtesy of American Hospital Supply Corporation.

top of the trachea and below the tongue roots and hyoid bone; sound is produced by vibration of its vocal folds and regulated by movements of its cartilages, which are activated by voluntary muscles controlled primarily by the vagus nerve (cranial nerve X). It is composed of three divisions, from above downward: (a) **vestibule** or **supraglottic region,** the space between the entrance to the larynx above and the ventricular folds below; (b) **ventricle, glottic region, ventriculus laryngis,** or **sinus of the ventri-**

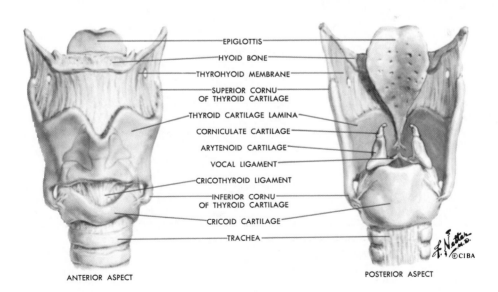

EPIGLOTTIS
HYOID BONE
THYROHYOID MEMBRANE
SUPERIOR CORNU OF THYROID CARTILAGE
THYROID CARTILAGE LAMINA
CORNICULATE CARTILAGE
ARYTENOID CARTILAGE
VOCAL LIGAMENT
CRICOTHYROID LIGAMENT
INFERIOR CORNU OF THYROID CARTILAGE
CRICOID CARTILAGE
TRACHEA

ANTERIOR ASPECT   POSTERIOR ASPECT

Larynx

MUSCLES OF THE LARYNX
Extrinsic Muscles

Suprahyoid Muscles (Elevators)

Muscle	Origin	Insertion	Innervation	Function
Digastric (paired)				
Anterior	Inner surface of mandible near symphysis	Lesser cornu of hyiod bone via facial sling	Nerve to mylohyoid	Elevates and fixes hyoid bone
Posterior	Mastoid process	Hyoid bone and intermediate tendon	Facial (VII) nerve	Elevates and retracts hyoid bone
Geniohyoid (paired)	Inferior genial tubercle of mandible	Body of hyoid bone	1st and 2nd cervical nerves with descending hypoglossal nerve	Elevates and draws hyoid bone forward
Mylohyoid (unpaired)	Inner surface of mandible	Hyoid bone	Nerve to mylohyoid	Elevates hyoid bone and supports floor of mouth
Stylohyoid (paired)	Styloid process	Hyoid bone	Facial (VII) nerve	Elevates and draws hyoid bone backward

Infrahyoid Muscle (Depressors)

Muscle	Origin	Insertion	Innervation	Function
Omohyoid (paired)				
Anterior	Intermediate tendon of clavicle	Hyoid bone	Descending cervical and hypoglossal nerves	Depresses hyoid bone
Posterior	Superior margin of scapula	Intermediate tendon		
Sternohyoid (paired)	Manubrium of sternum	Hyoid bone	Descending cervical and hypoglossal nerves	Depresses hyoid bone
Sternothyroid (paired)	Manubrium of sternum	Thyroid cartilage	Descending cervical and hypoglossal nerves	Depresses larynx
Thyrohyoid (paired)	Thyroid cartilage	Hyoid bone	1st and 2nd cervical nerves with descending hypoglossal nerve	Draws thyroid and hyoid bones toward each other

MUSCLES OF THE LARYNX—*Continued*
Intrinsic Muscles

Muscle	Origin	Insertion	Innervation	Function
Aryepiglottic	Apex of arytenoid cartilage	Lateral margin of epiglottis	Recurrent laryngeal nerve of vagus (X) nerve	Closes inlet of larynx
Arytenoid Oblique	Dorsal aspect of muscular process of arytenoid cartilage	Apex of opposite arytenoid cartilage	Recurrent laryngeal nerve of vagus (X) nerve	Approximates arytenoid cartilages
Transverse		Becomes continuous with thyroarytenoid muscle		
Cricoarytenoid Lateral	Lateral surface of cricoid cartilage	Muscular process of arytenoid cartilage	Recurrent laryngeal nerve of vagus (X) nerve	Approximates vocal folds
Posterior	Dorsal surface of criocoid cartilage			Separates vocal folds
Cricothyroid	Arch of cricoid cartilage	Lamina of thyroid cartilage	External branch of superior laryngeal nerve of vagus (X) nerve	Stretches vocal folds
Thyroarytenoid	Lamina of thyroid cartilage	Muscular process of arytenoid cartilage	Recurrent laryngeal nerve of vagus (X) nerve	Shortens vocal folds; closes vestibule of larynx
Thyroepiglottic	Lamina of thyroid cartilage	Epiglottis	Recurrent laryngeal nerve of vagus (X) nerve	Closes inlet of larynx
Vocalis (vocal)	Thyroid cartilage	Vocal process of arytenoid cartilage	Recurrent laryngeal nerve of vagus (X) nerve	Adjusts vocal folds

cle, the middle division which extends from the ventricular folds above to the flat superior surface of the vocal folds below; and (c) **infraglottic, inferior, hypoglottic,** or **subglottic region,** the lowest division which includes the space between the vocal folds above and the inferior border of the cricoid cartilage below.

Muscles of the larynx are of two types: (a) **extrinsic,** two groups of muscles which support the larynx and change its vertical position, and have at least one attachment to a structure outside the larynx: **suprahyoid muscles** or **elevators,** attached to the upper part of the hyoid bone and involved in elevating it, and **infrahyoid muscles** or **depressors,** inferior to the hyoid bone and involved in pulling it downward; (b) **intrinsic,** those muscles which control phonation and have their origins and insertions within the larynx. See *Muscles of the Larynx* table.

laser (lā′zėr) [acronym for light amplification by stimulated emission of radiation] Device which transforms light of various frequencies into an extremely intense, narrow, and nearly nondivergent beam of monochromatic radiation. It is capable of concentrating immense heat and energy to burn away in a brief flash a precise area which would otherwise be excised by traditional surgical instruments; sometimes used successfully with cancer and papilloma involving the larynx.

lateral [L. *lateralis,* fr. *later-, latus,* side] **1.** Away from the median or midline; opposite of medial. **2.** See under consonant, manner of formation.

lateral adenoidectomy See under adenoidectomy.

lateral canal See semicircular canals, under inner *ear.*

lateral dominance Laterality (1).

lateral incisor teeth See incisor *teeth.*

laterality 1. Preferential use of organs or members of one side of the body, such as the right ear, eye, hand, and leg **(dextrality)** or the left ear, eye, hand, and leg **(sinistrality).** Syn: lateral dominance. See also cerebral *dominance.* **2.** Awareness of the two sides of one's body and the ability to correctly identify them as left or right.

    crossed l. 1. Tendency to perform some actions with the right side of the body and others with the left side; *e.g.,* pitching a baseball with the left hand, but writing with the right hand. **2.** Preferential use of heterolateral members of the different pairs of organs or limbs; *e.g.,* the left hand coordinated with the right eye. Syn: mixed laterality.

    mixed l. Crossed *laterality.*

laterality theory of stuttering See cerebral dominance and handedness the-

ory, under breakdown theory, under stuttering theories.

lateral lisp See under lisp.

lateral sulcus See under sulcus.

lateral trim of the adenoid Lateral *adenoidectomy.*

latissimus dorsi muscle See *Muscles of Respiration* table, under respiration.

lax consonant See under consonant.

lax phoneme See under phoneme.

lax vowel See under vowel.

LD Learning disability.

learning 1. Acquisition of any relatively permanent change in behavior as a result of practice or experience. **2.** That which evolves from a sensation (or awareness of a stimulus) which is refined through perception, imagery, and generalization, and finally terminates in conceptualization **3.** Process of acquiring responses as a result of special practice.

    integrative l. Acquisition of knowledge or of a skill in which all modality systems function simultaneously, working together as a unit; the process of incorporating input stimuli with previously learned information.

    interneurosensory l. Learning resulting from the interrelated function of two or more systems in combination; *e.g.,* copying a square involves visual and kinesthetic modalities.

    intraneurosensory l. Acquisition of knowledge or of a skill which takes place predominantly through one sensory modality; *e.g.,* phonics, primarily an auditory skill.

    serial list l. Response to a previously presented word list in which an attempt is made to repeat the word that follows the stimulus word.

learning disability (LD) 1. "Specific learning disability" means a disorder in one or more of the basic psychological processes involved in understanding or in using language, spoken or written, which may manifest itself in an imperfect ability to listen, think, speak, read, write, spell, or perform mathematical calculations. The term includes such conditions as perceptual handicaps, brain injury, minimal brain dysfunction, dyslexia, and developmental aphasia. The term does not include children who have learning problems which are primarily the result of visual, hearing, or motor handicaps, of mental retardation, of emotional disturbance, or of environmental, cultural, or economic disadvantage [Public Law 94–142–121a.5]. **2.** Generic term that refers to a heterogeneous group of disorders manifested by significant difficulties in the acquisition and use of listening, speaking, reading, writing, reasoning, or mathematical abilities. These disorders are intrinsic to the individual and are presumed to be due to central nervous system dysfunction. Even though a learning disability may occur concomitantly with other handicapping conditions (*e.g.*, sensory impairment, mental retardation, or social and emotional disturbance) or environmental influences (*e.g.*, cultural differences, insufficient or inappropriate instruction, or psychogenic factors), it is not the direct result of those conditions or influences [Legislative Council Report, *ASHA*, 1982, p. 200].

learning theory 1. Empiricist theory. See under language theories. **2.** See under stuttering theories.

Lengthened-Off-Time (LOT) See *Audiometric Tests and Procedures* in appendices.

lenis consonant Lax *consonant.*

lenis phoneme Lax *phoneme.*

Lermoyez syndrome [M. Lermoyez, Fr. otolaryngologist, 1858–1929] Tinnitus and deafness preceding an attack of vertigo and thereafter subsiding.

lesion (lē′zhən) [L. *laesus*, injured] A wound, injury, or area of pathologic change in tissue.

leukoplakia (lu-kō-plā′kē-ə) [G. *leukos*, white + *plax*, plate] Disease characterized by a whitish patchy thickening of the epithelium of a mucous membrane. See also under laryngeal anomaly.

levator costae muscle See *Muscles of Respiration* table, under respiration.

levator veli palatini muscle See *Muscles of the Palate* table, under palate.

level Any plane, standard, position, status, or rank in a graded series of values, as of sensory efficiency, motor performance, intellectual capacity, etc.

lexical (lek′sə-kəl) [G. *lexikos*, or words] **1.** Any element that relates to the total stock of linguistic signs or morphemes in a language. **2.** Relating to words, word formatives, and vocabulary, as distinct from grammatical forms and constructions. See also word.

lexical categories Classes of objects, actions, or properties that words in general represent, rather than a specific object, action, or property; *e.g.*, furniture (chair, table, etc.); action (touch, bite, etc.); colors (red, blue, etc.).

lexical cohesion See under cohesive devices.

lexical meaning Semantic intent of words. See also word.

lexical morpheme See under morpheme.

lexical word Content *word.*

lexicography (lek-sə-kog′rə-fē) [G. *lexikos*, of words + G. *graphō*, to write] Listing and describing of the words or morphemes of a language, with respect to meaning and derivation.

lexicon (lek′sə-kon) [G. *lexikon* fr. *lexikos*, of words] **1.** Total accumulation of linguistic signs, words or morphemes, or both, in a given language; the list of all the words in a language. **2.** Dictionary, in the sense of being a collection of words available in a given vocabulary or language. **3.** Vocabulary of a language.

LF Low frequency.

light contact 1. In stuttering, loose or nontensed contacts of the lips or tongue on plosive sounds, which are optimal for the production of speech sounds. **2.** In voice, the easy contact of the vocal folds for the production of vowel sounds.

light lateral See lateral, under consonant, manner of formation.

light voice Falsetto. See under voice disorders of phonation.

light vowel Neutral *vowel*.

limen (lī′mən) Latin word for threshold.
  difference l. (DL) See under threshold.

limit [L. *limes*, boundary] **1.** First or last value or score in a distribution of scores or in a step interval. **2.** End of any continuum, such as the limit of the range of hearing.

limited range audiometer See under audiometer.

limited range speech audiometer See under audiometer.

Lindamood Auditory Conceptualization Test See *Auditory Tests and Procedures* in appendices.

linear (lin′ē-ėr) [L. *linea*, line] **1.** Pertaining to or resembling a line. **2.** Pertaining to continuous, as opposed to discrete, functions. **3.** Amplifies sound equally through all intensity levels.

lingua-alveolar (liŋ′gwə-al-vē′ə-lėr) Pertaining to the tongue and the alveolar process.

lingua-alveolar area Alveolar area. See under consonant, place of articulation.

linguadental (liŋ′gwo-den′təl) Pertaining to the tongue and teeth.

linguadental area See under consonant, place of articulation.

linguagram (liŋ′gwə-gram) [L. *lingua*, tongue + G. *gramma*, a drawing] Photograph or other graphic representation of the tongue, showing what areas have touched the palate during the making of a palatogram.

lingual (liŋ′gwəl) [L. *lingua*, tongue] Pertaining to the tongue.

lingual frenum See under frenum.

lingual hypoplasia See under hypoplasia.

lingual lisp Frontal *lisp*.

lingual paralysis See under paralysis.

lingual raphe Median lingual *sulcus*.

linguist (liŋ′gwist) [L. *lingua*, tongue] **1.** One who specializes in the study of the form and structure of language. **2.** Person accomplished in languages; one who speaks several languages.

linguistic (liŋ-gwis′tik) **1.** Of or pertaining to language. **2.** Of or pertaining to linguistics.

linguistic aspects All of the known levels involved in the analysis of language; these include the distinctive sound elements (phonological), the word meaning units of sound combinations (morphological), the rules for sentence structure (syntactic), the meaning mediated through the language (semantic), and the connotative meaning conveyed or actually experienced (affective and pragmatic).

linguistic competence 1. Knowledge of the rules of syntax, meaning, and sound that make possible the performance of language. **2.** Knowledge a native speaker of a language must possess to understand and to produce any of the infinite number of grammatical sentences of his language.

linguistic component One of the aspects of grammar, *i.e.*, phonological, morphological, syntactic, semantic, and pragmatic. See *Linguistic Components* table.

  morphological Component of grammar concerned with the formation of words, the smallest or elementary meaningful unit in a language, as a bridge between phonology and syntax.

  phonological Component of grammar determining the meaningful combination of sounds; concerned with the relationship between linguistic elements and their production.

  pragmatic The functional use of language in context.

  semantic Component of grammar concerned with word meanings and meaningful sentences; in transforma-

LINGUISTIC COMPONENTS	
	Form
Phonological ↕	Sentences defined in terms of sound patterns
Morphological ↕	Combination of minimal units of grammatical structure that have meaning
Syntactic ↕	Grammatically well-formed sentences
	Content
Semantic ↕	Meaningfully well-formed sentences
	Function
Pragmatic	The functional use of language in context

tional grammar, describes the way in which an utterance is used and understood.

syntactic Component of grammar concerned with grammatically well-formed structures; associates a grammatical structure with each sentence to indicate how the information in that sentence is organized.

linguistic determinism Theory that language dictates thought, based on the premise that all higher levels of thinking are dependent on language. See also Whorf's hypothesis.

linguistic intrusion Linguistic retention.

linguistic performance 1. Overt expression of linguistic competence in the activities of listening, speaking, reading, and writing. 2. Speaker's actual use of language.

linguistic phonetics Phonology.

linguistic relativity Belief held by some that because languages appear to differ substantially the world is experienced differently by native speakers of various languages; people with the same language think in similar ways. See also Whorf's hypothesis.

linguistic retention Occurrence of definite structural aspects of a speaker's native language when attempting to speak another language which is structurally different. Syn: linguistic intrusion; interference modification. See also accent (2).

linguistic universals 1. Theory that all languages contain some linguistic similarities and that the study of these similarities may provide the links between languages and cultures. 2. Structural feature that is common to all languages.

formal universals 1. Belief that the grammar of any language must meet certain specified conditions; concerned with the formulation of grammatical rules. 2. Constraints on the possible form of language, which may be similar in all languages; the general form and organization of grammars and the rules which comprise them.

substantive universals 1. Universals pertaining to the content of a language rather than to the form, such as that all languages have nouns, verbs, and adjectives. 2. Particular contentive elements which may appear in all languages, *e.g.*, noun, verb, and sentence. See also content *word*.

linguistic variation Differences existing linguistically (phonemes, morphemes, syntax, semantics, pragmatics) which affect production relative to the differences in speech situations, speakers, or both, *e.g.*, differences between an *ing* ending pronounced as *ing* /ŋ/ (walking) or as *in* /n/ (walkin).

linguistics (liŋ-gwis′tiks) [L. *lingua*, tongue] 1. Scientific study of the nature and function of language; the use of scientific methodology to bring precision and control to the study of language. **2.** Scientific investigation of the origin, form and structure, and modifications of language; includes phonology, morphology, syntax, and semantics. **3.** Study of man's speech habits.

anthropological l. Study of languages as part of the investigation of their associated cultures.

applied l. Application of the findings resulting from research in all areas of linguistics (descriptive, general, historical, etc.) to practical usage, particularly in the area of language teaching.

comparative l. Study of the relationships among different languages; may be **synchronic,** dealing with relationships at one point in time among different languages having a common origin, or **diachronic,** comparing different forms of one language at different points in time.

contrastive l. Study, when learning a new language, of the differences between the dominant language and the target language.

descriptive l. **1.** Systematic study of a language, or of one or more languages and dialects; attempts to explain languages and dialects, not to prescribe correct usage. **2.** Study of sounds (phonemes) and sound groups (morphemes, words) of a language to arrive at a detailed and comprehensive explanation about the expression system of a specific language.

general l. Investigation of the theories and description of language; includes the search for the most universal features of human languages in order to describe language simply, exactly, and objectively. Syn: theoretical linguistics.

historical l. Study of the changes that occur in a language through time.

structural l. Investigation and analyzation of the structure of a language.

theoretical l. General *linguistics*.

linguoversion See under teeth malpositions.

linking verb Copula.

lip One of the two fleshy folds which form the opening of the mouth cavity.
cleft l. See cleft lip.

lipreading Speechreading. See under aural rehabilitation.

lip rounding Production of a sound with the lips forming a semicircle; *e.g.*, rule. See also vowel and subentries.

liquid See under consonant, manner of formation.

lisp Defective production of one or more of the six sibilant consonants /s/, /z/, /ʃ/, /ʒ/, /tʃ/, and /ʤ/, usually caused by improper tongue placement or by abnormalities of the articulatory mechanism; the /s/ and /z/ phonemes are the most commonly involved phonemes. Syn: parasigmatism; sigmatism.

dental l. Type of frontal lisp in which the tongue is positioned against the upper or lower central incisors during production of /s/, /z/, /ʃ/, and /ʒ/.

frontal l. Substitution of the *th* /θ/ or *th* /ð/ phonemes or approximations of these phonemes for a sibilant phoneme; produced by obstruction of the narrow channel of air by placing the tongue tip too far forward either against the teeth or between the teeth, or by pressing the tongue tip against the alveolar ridges instead of allowing it to be free; *e.g.*, *th*oup for soup; *th*oo for *z*oo. Syn: interdental, lingual, protrusion, or substitutional lisp.

interdental l. Frontal *lisp*.

lateral l. Defective production of the sibilant sounds due to excessive escape of air and saliva over or around the sides of the tongue, producing a sound similar to *sh* /ʃ/; may be the result of dental malocclusion; *e.g.*, *sh*un for *s*un.

lingual l. Frontal *lisp*.

nasal l. Substitution of a snorted unvoiced /n/ for a sibilant sound; the tongue is sluggish, the lips are lax, and the air is deflected backward and escapes through the nose; commonly heard in cleft palate speech.

occluded l. Substitution of /t/ or /d/ for a sibilant sound; *e.g.*, *tit*ter for sister.

protrusion l. Frontal *lisp.*

strident l. Misarticulation in which /s/ or /z/ assumes a whistling quality.

substitutional l. Frontal *lisp.*

listening (lis'en-iŋ) **1.** Reception and utilization of information transmitted via acoustic events; influenced by numerous factors, such as motivation, length of presentation of information, relevance of information, distracting influences, and psychological integrity of the listener. **2.** Hearing with thoughtful attention.

literal paraphasia See under paraphasia.

litotes (lī'tə-tēz) Understatement. See under figure of speech.

live voice audiometry See under audiometry.

load In electricity, the device to which signal power is delivered; the recipient of the work output of an electrical or mechanical device.

lobe (lōb) [G. *lobos*] Globular part of an organ separated by boundaries. For lobes of the brain, see under cerebrum, under brain.

lobule (lob'yul) [L. *lobulus*, dim. of *lobus*, lobe] **1.** Anatomical landmark of the auricle of the ear. See auricle, under external *ear.* **2.** Small lobe or subdivision of a lobe.

localization (lō-kəl-i-zā'shən) **1.** Limitation to a definite area. **2.** Ability to identify a place on the surface of the body which has been stimulated. See *Auditory Processes* table, under auditory processes.

    auditory l. Ability to describe the location of a sound source exclusively with auditory information.

    cerebral l. Assumption that there are areas of the brain which are essential for particular functions, such

as articulation, speech, perception, reading, and writing.

localization audiometry See under audiometry, visual reinforcement

localized amnesia See under amnesia.

locative See under parts of speech.

locomotion (lō-kə-mō'shən) [L. *locus*, place + *motio*, movement] Act or power of moving from place to place.

locutions (lō-kyu'shənz) [L. *locutus*, spoke] **1.** Acts that are required for the production of speech, such as constructing propositions and uttering sounds. **2.** Actual verbal utterance and the proposition or content it contains. *Cf.* illocution; perlocution.

loft register A falsetto voice. See also falsetto, under voice disorders of phonation.

logarithm (log'ə-rith-əm) Exponent which indicates the power to which a number is raised; the number of times that a number (the base) is multiplied by itself.

logarithmic graph Graph which records proportionate steps and is extremely sensitive to the doubling and tripling of numbers; used to record speech responses.

logical method Analytic method. See aural rehabilitation.

logical operations See cognitive development stages, Period III.

logopedics (lo-gə-pē'diks) [G. *logos*, word, speech + *pais (paid-)*, child] Primarily European term for speech and language pathology.

logopedist (lo-gə-pē'dist) Primarily European term for speech and language pathologist.

logorrhea (lo-gə-rē'ə) [G. *logos*, word, speech + *rhoia*, a flow] Mental aberration characterized by continuous, incoherent talking.

Lombard Test See *Audiometric Tests and Procedures* in appendices.

longitudinal cerebral fissure See under fissure.

longitudinalis inferior muscle See *Muscles of the Tongue* table, under tongue.

longitudinalis superior muscle See *Muscles of the Tongue* table, under tongue.

longitudinal wave See under wave.

long-term memory See under memory.

loop induction auditory trainer See under auditory training units.

loquacity (lō-kwas′i-tē) [L. *loquax*, talkative] Extreme talkativeness; propensity to speak often and at length.

LOT Lengthened-Off-Time.

loudness 1. Subjective sensation of the effect of amplitude or intensity; determined partly by the number of auditory nerve fibers activated by the sound and partly by the number of impulses carried by each nerve fiber; may be arranged on a scale from soft to loud; unit of measurement is the sone. **2.** Perceptual attribute of the amount of sound a given speech sound makes; relates to the stress, or amount of muscular energy involved in every articulatory movement, and to the acoustic attribute of intensity. **3.** Sensation related to the amplitude of molecular motion of the sound wave; controlled primarily by the vibrator but varies directly with air pressure. **4.** Psychological response to the intensity of a physical stimulus, which also varies somewhat with frequency.

loudness level In audiometry, the intensity above the reference level for a 1000-Hz tone that is subjectively equal in loudness; measured in phons.

loudness unit See sone.

loudspeaker See transducer.

low See under distinctive features.

low fence Medicolegal term referring to the lower limit of hearing impairment, expressed as an average of 500, 1000, and 2000 Hz.

low frequency (LF) See under frequency.

low-pass filter See under band-pass *filter*.

low tone deafness See under deafness.

low vowel See under vowel.

lung [A.S. *lungen*] One of a pair of irregularly conical viscera occupying the thoracic cavity and functioning as the organ of respiration; usually, the right lung is slightly larger than the left and is divided into three lobes, while the left has but two lobes.

lung capacity Respiratory capacity.

lung volume Respiratory volume.

MA Mental age.

Mackenzie's syndrome [Sir S. Mackenzie, Eng. physician, 1844–1909] Associated unilateral paralysis of the tongue, soft palate, and vocal fold with resulting hoarseness, partial aphonia, and dysphagia; results from lesion of the hypoglossal nerve (cranial nerve XII), ambiguous nucleus, or branches of the vagus nerve (cranial nerve X); similar to Jackson's syndrome. *q.v.*

macro- [G. *makros*, large] Combining form meaning large, long.

macrocephaly (mak-rō-sef′ə-lē) [macro + G. *kephalē*, head] Abnormal largeness of the head, as from imperfect development of the cranium. *Cf.* microcephaly.

macrocheilia, macrochilia (mak-rō-kī′lē-ə) [macro- + G. *cheilos*, lip] Permanent swelling of the lips. *Cf.* microcheilia.

macroglossia (mak-rō-glo′sē-ə) [macro + G. *glōssa*, tongue] Abnormal enlargement of the tongue.

macrognathia (mak-rō-na′thē-ə) [macro- + G. *gnathos*, jaw] Abnormal enlargement or elongation of the jaw.

macrophonia See under voice disorders of phonation.

macrostomia (mak-rō-stō′mē-ə) [macro- + G. *stoma*, mouth] Abnormally large and wide mouth; may result from an incomplete fusion of the mandibular and maxillary processes. *Cf.* microstomia.

MAF Minimum audible field.

magnetic resonance angiography A radiologic procedure used to study arteries. Using an MRI scanner, a contrast material is injected into a vein to evaluate arteries throughout the body.

magnetic resonance imaging (MRI) A procedure that involves creating cross-sectional images of body organs and structures. MRI exposes the patient to a magnetic field while he or she lies inside a large magnet structure. Images are created when the body's hydrogen ions move (the movement is caused by exposure to radio waves), producing a radio signal that is detected and changed by computer to an image. Body tissue that contains a large amount of hydrogen will produce a bright image. Body tissue that contains little or no hydrogen is dark. No radiation is used in MRI.

main clause See under clause.

mainstreaming Educational attempt to serve children with learning or adjustment problems in the regular school environment with the aid of supportive personnel such as consulting, itinerant, or resource teachers; an effort to provide the most appropriate education for every child in the least restrictive setting.

maintenance In conditioning, administration of occasional reinforcement to keep an already-acquired response at some frequency of occurrence; additional reinforcement may result in a further increase in frequency (assuming the response is not already at a maximum), and less reinforcement may produce extinction.

maladaptive response See under response.

malar bones Zygomatic bones. See under skull.

malignant (mə-lig′nənt) [L. *malignus*, wicked, malicious] Denoting a neoplasm (tumor) characterized by uncontrollable growth and dissemination, and which invades and destroys neighboring tissue; it is likely to recur after removal; usually used in reference to cancer. *Cf.* benign.

malinger (mə-liŋ′gèr) [Fr. *malingre*, poor, weakly] To feign illness or disability, especially to avoid work, obtain compensation, or arouse sympathy.

malleus (mal'ē-əs) [L. hammer] First and largest bone of the ossicular chain in the middle ear. See also under *middle ear.*

malocclusion (mal-ə-klu'zhən) Any deviation from normal occlusion. See teeth malocclusion.

mand See under operant, verbal.

mandible See under skull.

mandibular (man-dib'yu-lėr) Relating to the mandible or to the lower jaw.

mandibular hypoplasia Micrognathia.

mandibular restriction Limited movement of the mandible.

mandibulofacial dysostosis (man-dib'y-ulō-fa'shəl dis-os-tō'sis) [G. *dys-*, difficult + *osteon*, bone + *-osis*, condition] Hereditary disorder of embryonic development characterized by ocular anomalies, defects or hypoplasia of the malar and zygomatic bones and mandible, micrognathia, macrostomia, high-arched or cleft palate, malposition and malocclusion of teeth, deformities of the external ear, conductive hearing loss, occasional pits or clefts between the mouth and ear, and atypical hair growth; the incomplete form of this syndrome is referred to as Treacher Collins syndrome. Syn: Franceschetti's syndrome.

manic reaction See under reaction.

manometer (mə-nom'ə-tėr) [G. *manos*, thin, skanty + *metron*, measure] Instrument used to measure the amount of air pressure exerted in respiration or intraoral pressure; air blown into a tube is measured by either elevation of a liquid in a tube or a dial calibrated in ounces per square inch connected to a diaphragm.

manometric flame (mə-nom'ə-trik) Instrument that displays visibly the sound wave from a voiced sound; consists of a jet of burning gas, the pressure of which varies as the pressure of the sound wave varies.

manual alphabet See American Manual *Alphabet.*

manual English Sign English.

manual method See under aural rehabilitation.

manual volume control See under volume control.

manubrium, pl. **manubria** (mə-nu'brē-əm, brē-ə) [L. handle] Handle of the malleus which extends from the head of the malleus along the medial surface of the tympanic membrane to the umbo.

MAP Minimum audible pressure.

marked falling curve Sharply falling curve. See under audiogram configurations.

markedness theory Binary principle.

masking **1.** Noise of any kind that interferes with the audibility of another sound. **2.** In stuttering, an interference with perception of a sound or pattern of sounds by simultaneously presenting another sound of a different frequency, intensity, quality, or pattern in one or both ears of the subject; may result in increased but temporary fluency. **3.** In audiology, noise used in an attempt to eliminate the participation of one ear while the opposite ear is being tested. See also noise and its subentries.

    In the critical band concept, the only components of the noise having a masking effect on the pure tone are those frequencies included in a restricted band with the test tone as its center; when the pure tone is just audible in the presence of the noise, the acoustic energy in the restricted band of frequencies is equal to the acoustic energy of the test tone.

    backward m. Phenomenon by which a test tone is masked by a noise which is presented after the test tone.

    central m. Elevation in threshold in the test ear as a result of the introduction of a masking noise in the nontest ear; the noise is not of sufficient intensity to cross the skull to the test ear.

effective m. Minimum amount of noise required to mask a signal (under the same earphone) at a given hearing threshold level, *e.g.*, 50 dB effective masking will mask a 50-dB hearing threshold signal.

forward m. Phenomenon by which a sound continues to be masked (not heard) for a brief period after the masking noise is discontinued.

initial m. Lowest level of effective masking presented to the nontest ear. In air conduction testing, this level is equal to the threshold of the masked ear; in bone conduction testing, it is masked ear plus the occlusion effect at that frequency.

maximum m. Highest level of noise that can be presented to one ear via an earphone before the noise crosses the skull and shifts the threshold of the opposite ear.

overmasking Masking noise of such a high level which when presented to the nontest ear may cross over and elevate the threshold of the test ear.

peripheral m. Elevation of the hearing threshold when the signal and the masking noise are in the same ear.

undermasking Insufficient intensity of masking to prevent the better ear from participating in the test.

upward m. Phenomenon by which the less intense high-frequency consonants are masked by more intense low-frequency vowel formants.

masking efficiency Relationship between the overall intensity level and the magnitude of the threshold shift produced by a noise; *e.g.*, when three noises are presented to an ear at equal overall sound pressure levels, the noise producing the greatest threshold shift in that ear could be regarded as the most efficient.

masking level difference Phenomenon that occurs after a tone and masking noise (sufficient to mask the tone) are presented binaurally in phase, and then either the tone or the noise is presented out of phase to the accompanying tone or noise, making the tone once again audible; may be accomplished for speech thresholds as well.

masking techniques Methods used in audiology to eliminate the participation of one ear while the opposite ear is being tested.

Hood technique [J. D. Hood, 1960] Procedure for ensuring masking without overmasking; if a threshold shift is noted after an original threshold is obtained, the masking noise is increased in 10-dB steps, with a redetermination of threshold at each noise level until the threshold shows no further increase in masking over a range of at least 20 to 30 dB of masking noise. Syn: plateau, shadowing, or threshold shift method.

plateau method Rainville technique (see below).

Rainville technique [M. J. Rainville, contemporary Fr. audiologist] Bone-conduction test involving a comparison of the air- and bone-masking intensities required to mask an air-conducted pure-tone threshold; this procedure helps determine the conductive loss by comparing the masking effect on air-conducted tones produced by bone-conducted noise at the mastoid process.

SAL test Sensorineural acuity level technique (see below).

sensorineural acuity level technique- Modification of the Rainville technique in which masking presented at a fixed level is introduced through a bone-conduction oscillator placed in the center of the forehead; the sensorineural acuity level is computed by subtracting the change of threshold produced by the noise from the designated amount of threshold change occurring with normal ears. Syn: SAL test.

shadowing method Rainville technique (see above).

Studebaker technique [G. A. Studebaker, U.S. audiologist, *1932] Method used to determine the amount of hearing participation of each ear. After an unmasked threshold is obtained, a noise is presented at an effective level of 40 dB above bone-conduction thresholds of the opposite ear, and the noise is increased by an amount equal to any observed threshold shift. If a sizable air-bone gap is observed in the masked ear, a threshold shift procedure is used with the calculated noise level as the starting point. Threshold is then presented at a level which does not shift on masking application or masking level increase.

threshold shift method Rainville technique (see above).

mastication (mas-ti-kā′shən) [L. *mastico*, pp. *-atus*, to chew]. The act of chewing food in preparation for swallowing and digestion.

mastoidectomy (mas-toi-dek′tə-mē) [mastoid (process) + G. *ektomē*, excision] Surgical procedure involving the removal of the air cells of the mastoid process.

   modified radical m. Mastoidectomy to eliminate the disease process without sacrificing any of the middle ear structures.

   radical m. Mastoidectomy in which the eardrum and middle ear structures are removed, with resulting marked hearing loss.

mastoiditis Inflammation within the air cells of the mastoid process; often the result of complications from otitis media.

mastoid process (mas′toid) [G. *mastos*, breast + *eidos*, resemblance] Bony protuberance behind and below the external ear, a portion of which is hollowed out into a number of air cells

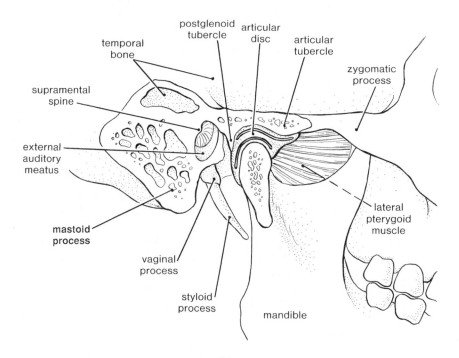

Mastoid Process

resembling a honeycomb; the superior and anterior parts, which communicate with the tympanic cavity, contain air, and are lined by a prolongation of the mucous membrane of the tympanic cavity.

mathetic function of language (mə-thet′ik) [G. *mathēsis*, acquisition of knowledge] Use of language for learning about the world.

mathetic text See under text.

matrix, pl. **matrices** (mā′triks, -trə-sēz) Main *clause.*

matrix sentence See under sentence classification, transformational grammar.

maturation (ma-chu-rā′shən) [L. *maturatio*, a ripening] Developmental changes leading to maturity; includes physiologic, neurologic, and psychologic growth.

maturational lag Delay in specific aspects of the developmental processes in relation to chronological age.

mature (mə-tur′) [L. *maturus*, ripe] **1.** Denoting an organism, or part or aspect of an organism, which has achieved full development. **2.** To develop completely.

maxilla See under skull.

maxillary (mak′sə-lãr-ē) Denoting the maxilla.

maximal contrasts Bisyllables containing two vowels with widely different lingual postures and markedly different acoustic characteristics; *e.g.,* /bi ba/. *Cf.* minimal contrasts.

maximum acoustic output See under output.

maximum amplitude See under amplitude.

maximum duration of phonation Greatest amount of time a sound can be sustained after inhaling as much air as possible.

maximum duration of sustained blowing Greatest length of time an oral flow of air can be maintained.

maximum frequency range Highest and lowest frequencies that can be pho-

nated in the frequency ranges of vocal fry, modal level, and falsetto.

maximum masking See under masking.

maximum power output (MPO) Maximum acoustic *output.*

MBD Minimal brain dysfunction (syndrome).

McCarthy Scales of Children's Abilities See *Psychological Measures and Tests* in appendices.

MCL Most comfortable loudness.

MCLR Most comfortable loudness range.

mean Central value of a set of measurements computed by addition of all scores and division of the sum by the number of scores. *Cf.* average; central tendency.

meaning Concept which a symbolic act denotes.

mean length of response (MLR) Average number of words used in a number of separate utterances, which may be words, phrases, or sentences; determined by dividing the number of words by the number of utterances.

mean length of utterance (MLU) Average length of oral expressions as measured by a representative sampling of oral language; usually obtained by counting the number of morphemes per utterance and dividing by the number of utterances. See also *Mean Length of Utterance* and *Language Tests and Procedures* in appendices.

mean relational utterance (MRU) Number of grammatical relations utilized during a representative sampling of speech; obtained by dividing the number of grammatical relations by the number of utterances.

mean sentence length (MSL) Average number of words used in a sentence as measured by a representative sampling of oral language; obtained by dividing the number of words used by the number of sentences uttered.

meatus, pl. **meatus** (mē-ā′təs) [L. a passageway] **1.** Any natural anatomical passageway or space between confining walls. **2.** Passage from the auricle to the tympanic membrane and through the petrous portion of the temporal bone.

 external auditory m. See under external *ear.*

 internal auditory m. See under internal *ear.*

medial (mē′dē-əl) [L. *medialis*, middle] **1.** In or near the middle; opposite of lateral. **2.** In phonetics, situated within a word, but not beginning or ending it; *e.g.,* pre*tend*ing. **3.** See under consonant position.

medial nasal concha See nasal conchae, under skull.

medial turbinated bone Medial nasal concha. See nasal conchae, under skull.

median (mē′dē-ən) [L. *medianus*, middle] **1.** Midline, or in the middle. **2.** In statistics, that point on a scale of measurement above which are exactly half of the scores, and below which are the other half. *Cf.* mean; central tendency.

median cleft lip See under cleft lip.

median lingual sulcus See under sulcus.

median longitudinal raphe Median lingual *sulcus.*

median sagittal plane See under plane.

medulla oblongata See under brainstem, under brain.

mel Unit describing tone pitch relationships; equals about 1/1000 of the pitch of a tone of 1000 Hz at 40 dB above threshold; *e.g.,* a 1000-Hz tone at a level of 40 dB is said to have a pitch of 1000 mel.

melody of speech See prosody (2).

membrane [L. *membrana*, skin or membrane] Thin layer or sheet of pliable tissue which serves as a covering of a part, lining of a cavity, partition, or connection of two structures.

 basilar m. Membrane extending the entire length of the cochlea, separating the scala tympani from the scala media and supporting the organ of Corti. See also under inner *ear.*

 mucous m. Any mucous-secreting lining or surface of an organ or struc-

ture, as of the mouth, nose, esophagus, tympanic cavity, tongue, etc. Syn: mucosa.

 Reissner's m. [E. Reissner, Ger. anatomist, 1824–1878] Vestibular *membrane.*

 vestibular m. Membrane of the cochlea which separates the scala vestibuli from the scala media. Syn: Reissner's membrane. See also cochlea, under inner *ear.*

membranous labyrinth See under labyrinth.

memory (mem′ə-rē) [L. *memoria*] Assimilation, storage, and retrieval of previously experienced sensations and perceptions when the original stimulus is no longer present; may be auditory or visual. Syn: recall (1). See also auditory memory in *Auditory Processes* table, under auditory processes.

 long-term m. Memory retained for an indefinite time period.

 rote m. Storage and retrieval of information without comprehension; *e.g.,* memorization and recitation of a poem without understanding its meaning.

 sequential m. Storage and retrieval of information requiring a specified order of input and recall; *e.g.,* counting, days of the week, months of the year, words in a sentence. See also *Auditory Processes* table, under auditory processes.

 short-term m. Memory retained for only a relatively brief time period.

memory span Number of items that can be recalled from stimulation; includes immediate and delayed recall of digits, words, sentences, and paragraphs; may be auditory or visual.

Ménière's disease or **syndrome** [P. Ménière, Fr. physician, 1799–1862] Condition confined to the inner ear, with a sensorineural type of hearing loss; symptoms may include tinnitus, vertigo, and hearing loss, and may be episodic, lasting for a few minutes or several days. Syn: endolymphatic or vestibular hydrops.

meniscus, pl. **menisci** (men-is′kəs, -kī) [G. *mēniskos*, crescent] **1.** Normal fluid level in the middle ear cavity as seen through the tympanic membrane. **2.** Any crescent-shaped structure.

mental (men′təl) [L. *mens (ment-)*, mind] Relating to the mind.

mental age (MA) Intellectual age as determined by performance on a standardized test; usually expressed in months.

mental retardation 1. Significantly subaverage general intellectual functioning existing concurrently with deficits in adaptive behavior and manifested during the developmental period. "Significantly subaverage" refers to an IQ more than two standard deviations below the mean for the test. **2.** Mental retardation described according to the level of support a person needs. The level of support can be identified once an individual receives a diagnosis of mental retardation and his need for support is classified (the diagnosis of mental retardation is made if the individual is 18 years or younger with an

IQ score below 70–75 and has significant disability in two or more adaptive skill areas. Classification of an individual's need for support is based on intellectual functioning and adaptive skills, psychological and emotional considerations, health and physical considerations, and environmental considerations.) See *Mental Retardation—Levels of Support* table.

Merrill Language Screening Test See *Language Tests and Procedures* in appendices.

mesioclusion See under teeth malocclusion.

mesioversion See under teeth malpositions.

metacognition (met′ə-kog-ni′shən) Ability to reflect on thinking in general, *i.e.,* thinking about thinking.

metacommunication (met′ə-kə-myu-nə-kā′shən) Messages accompanying language communicating such things as how the speaker feels about what he or she is saying, how he or she feels about the listener, or how the message is to be interpreted (*e.g.,* a joke, seriously, ironically); includes eye contact, body posture, intonation, and pitch. See also paralanguage.

metalinguistic (met′ə-liŋ-gwis′tiks) **1.** An aspect of language competence that goes beyond the ability to understand word meanings and learn grammar. It is the conscious awareness and use of language as a tool. Metalinguistics encompasses the ability to recognize and interpret multiple meanings in words and sentences; to make multiple inferences; to perceive and interpret figurative usage; to plan and organize for production at sentence, paragraph, and discourse levels; and to identify effective strategies for memorizing. Metalinguistic ability emerges during the elementary and secondary school years. **2.** Ability to think about language and to comment on it, as well as to produce and comprehend it. **3.** Language awareness; a temporary

MENTAL RETARDATION—LEVELS OF SUPPORT

1. Intermittent	The individual only requires support on a short-term basis for special circumstances, such as help in finding a new job.
2. Limited	The individual has a consistent need for certain supports, such as handling finances or job training.
3. Extensive	The individual requires consistent support in certain aspects of daily living, such as long-term job support.
4. Extensive	The individual requires constant support for all aspects of life.

From the American Association on Mental Deficiency.

shift in attention from what is being said to the language used to say it; *e.g.*, noticing a particular word because it was incorrectly produced, or produced with an unfamiliar accent. **4.** Ability to reflect on language.

metaphor See under figure of speech.

metapragmatic (met′ə-prag-mat′ik) **1.** Ability to talk about whole speech acts or coordinates of a given speech act; *e.g.*, "You can't say that." It includes mastery of elements that refer indirectly to preceding discourse, tying the present utterance to what has gone before; *e.g.*, "Yes, but . . . " **2.** Speech about acts of speech; *e.g.*, "I said, 'You are pretty.' " **3.** Conscious awareness of pragmatic rules which allows an individual to consciously decide what to talk about and how to phrase it, based on a knowledge of the listener's mood or physical condition.

metastasis, pl. **metastases** (mə-tas′tə-sis, -sēz) [G. a removing] **1.** Shifting of a disease or its local manifestations from one part of the body to another. **2.** In cancer, the appearance of neoplasms in parts of the body remote from the site of the original tumor.

metastasize (mə-tas′tə-sīz) To spread or invade by metastasis, said usually of a cancer.

metathesis (mə-tath′ə-sis) [G. transposition] Transposition of sounds or syllables in a word. See also under phonological processes.

method See the specific term.

methods of esophageal speech See after *speech* subentries.

metonymy See under figure of speech.

Metz Test for Loudness Recruitment See *Audiometric Tests and Procedures* in appendices.

MI Mentally impaired.

micro- [G. *mikros*, small] **1.** Prefix denoting smallness. **2.** Prefix denoting one-millionth of any unit.

microbar (mī′krō-bar) In acoustics, the basic measurement of sound pressure; represents the amount of energy re-

quired to move a mass of one gram a distance of one centimeter in a time period of one second.

microcephaly (mī-krō-sef′ə-lē) [micro- + G. *kephalē*, head] Abnormal smallness of the head, as from imperfect development of the cranium. *Cf.* macrocephaly.

microcheilia, microchilia (mī-krō-kī′lē-ə) [micro- + G. *cheilos*, lip] Abnormal smallness of the lips. *Cf.* macrocheilia.

microglossia (mī-krō-glo′sē-ə) [micro- + G. *glōssa*, tongue] Abnormally small tongue.

micrognathia (mī-krō-na′thē-ə) [micro- + G. *gnathos*, jaw] Unusually small lower jaw, usually accompanied by recession of the chin. Syn: mandibular hypoplasia.

microorganism (mī′krō-ôr′gan-iz-əm) [micro- + G. *organon*, tool, organ] Minute living body imperceptible to the naked eye, such as a bacterium, virus, and protozoon.

microphone (mī′krō-fōn) [micro- + G. *phōnē*, sound] Transducer that converts acoustic signals (sound pressure waves) into electrical energy.

    directional m. Microphone that is more responsive to sound approaching from a certain direction.

    nondirectional m. Microphone that picks up sound almost equally from any location. Syn: omnidirectional microphone.

    omnidirectional m. Nondirectional *microphone.*

microphonics (mī-krō-fon′iks) Audio-frequency noise caused by mechanical vibration of elements in a system; *e.g.*, vibration of the elements within an electron tube.

microstomia (mī-krō-stō′mē-ə) [micro- + G. *stoma*, mouth] Abnormal smallness of the mouth. *Cf.* macrostomia.

microtia (mī-krō′shē-ə) [micro- + G. *ous*, ear + *-ia*, condition] Congenital abnormal smallness of the external ear.

midbrain See under brainstem, under brain.

middle ear See under ear.

middle ear muscle reflex Acoustic *reflex*.

middle latency response See under response.

middle pharyngeal constrictor See *Muscles of the Pharynx* table, under pharynx.

mid vowel See under vowel.

migration (mī-grā′shən) See metathesis, under phonological processes.

mild hearing impairment or **loss** See hearing impairment degrees.

milk scanning A delivery device used in barium swallow evaluations in which the barium is mixed with milk; generally used with the pediatric population.

mimic speech Echolalia.

MINICROS See under contralateral routing of signals (CROS), under hearing aid.

minimal brain dysfunction syndrome (MBD) Obsolete term for attention deficit/hyperactivity disorder.

minimal contrasts Bisyllables containing two vowels with only slightly different lingual positions and acoustic characteristics; *e.g.*, /bi bɪ/, /bu bʊ/. *Cf.* maximal contrasts.

minimal pair Words that are alike in sound, except for a single phonetic feature; *e.g.*, pear-bear, fat-vat.

minimum acceptable skill See under skill.

minimum audible field (MAF) Threshold of hearing measured under controlled sound field conditions.

minimum audible pressure (MAP) Threshold of hearing measured using earphones.

Minimum Auditory Capabilities Test (MAC) See *Audiometric Tests and Procedures* in appendices.

Minnesota Preschool Scales See *Psychological Measures and Tests* in appendices.

Minnesota Test for Differential Diagnosis

of Aphasia See *Language Tests and Procedures* in appendices.

misarticulation (mis′är-tik-yu-lā′shən) Any phoneme spoken with insufficient accuracy and precision.

misphonia (mis-fō′nē-ə) Distorted or unusual voice quality.

mispronunciation (mis′prō-nən-sē-ā′shən) Distortion of a correct word pattern by adding, omitting, or transposing sounds.

mitigated echolalia See under echolalia.

mixed deafness See under deafness.

mixed laterality Crossed *laterality*.

mixed nasality See under voice disorders of resonance.

mixture theory See under language theories.

MLR Mean length of response.

MLU Mean length of utterance.

Möbius syndrome [P. J. Möbius, Ger. physician, 1853–1907] Congenital bilateral facial paralysis associated with neurologic, ocular, and musculoskeletal anomalies; characterized by mask-like expression, open mouth with drooling at the corners, micrognathia, paralysis of the soft palate and muscles of mastication, atrophy of the tongue, and middle ear defects; due to lesions of the oculomotor, trigeminal, abducent, facial, and hypoglossal nerves (cranial nerves III, V, VI, VII, and XII).

modal or **modal auxiliary** In transformational grammar, a type of verb conveying mood and tense but which does not have the bound morpheme /-s/, a distinguishing characteristic of all other verbs; there is no infinitive form for a true modal verb; *e.g.*, can, may, shall, will, must.

modal frequency or **tone** Habitual *pitch*.

modality (mō-dal′ə-tē) [See mode] **1.** Any sensory avenue through which information may be received; *e.g.*, visual, auditory, olfactory, tactile, and taste. **2.** In case grammar, a term referring to words which indicate tense, aspect, mood, negation, etc.

mode (mōd) [L. *modus*, a measure, quantity] **1.** Point on a scale of measurement with the maximum frequency in a distribution. **2.** That measurement which occurs most frequently *Cf.* central tendency.

model (mod′əl) **1.** Stimulus to be imitated. **2.** In speech and language training, a form of verbally demonstrating a desired verbal response; *e.g.*, Clinician: "Say, 'I go home.' " Client: "I go home."

modeling In speech: **1.** Intervention procedure in which models are provided. **2.** Emulation or following the example of another.

moderate hearing impairment or **loss** See hearing-impairment degrees.

moderately severe hearing impairment or **loss** See hearing-impairment degrees.

modification (mod-ə-fə-kā′shən) [L. *modificatus*, changed, measured] **1.** Change in the frequency at which a response occurs, either by increasing it, as with reinforcement, or by decreasing it, as with extinction. **2.** Change in the form of a response by changing the frequency of one or more of its components.

modified barium swallow See under barium swallow.

modified radical mastoidectomy See under mastoidectomy.

modifier (mod′ə-fī-ėr) In traditional grammar, any word or group of words which describes or qualifies another element in a sentence; may indicate how, where, when, which, under what conditions, or despite what conditions the action took place.

    nonrestrictive m. Modifier that adds information to the sentence, but does not limit the meaning to the degree that it cannot be removed from the sentence without changing its meaning; considered parenthetical and is set off from the rest of the sentence by commas. See also parenthetical expression.

    restrictive m. Modifier that limits the meaning of the sentence so sharply that it cannot be removed from the sentence without altering the intended meaning; not separated from the rest of the sentence by punctuation.

modular theory In cognition, an expansion of connectionistic theory of neurocognitive organization which proposes that there are many separate but interrelated cognitive systems within the human brain with subcomponents which are activated in parallel for information processing.

modulation (mod-yu-lā′shən) [L. *modulatus*, measured off] **1.** Alteration of the vocal quality and volume during speech. **2.** In acoustics, the process whereby some characteristic (amplitude, frequency, phase, etc.) of one wave is varied in accordance with another wave. For types of modulation, see specific term.

modules In cognition, neuroanatomical cognitive subcomponents which are theorized to process information within a cognitive system parallel.

molar teeth See under teeth.

monaural (mon-är′əl) [mono- + L. *auris*, ear] **1.** Designating one ear, as opposed to both ears. **2.** Hearing with one ear.

monaural hearing aid See under hearing aid.

Monaural Loudness Balance Test (MLB) See *Audiometric Tests and Procedures* in appendices.

mongolism (moŋ′gə-li-zəm) [refers to facial appearance like that of a Mongol] Down's syndrome.

monitored live voice audiometry Live voice *audiometry*.

monitoring (mon′ə-tėr-iŋ) **1.** Observing or recording, as in checking the output of speech or measurement of hearing. **2.** In stuttering, a self-observation technique used by an individual to become highly aware of the behaviors which characterize his habitual pattern of stuttering.

monitoring audiometry See under audiometry.

mono- [G. *monos*, single] Prefix denoting single, one; equivalent of Latin *uni-*.

monoplegia (mon-ō-plē'jē-ə) [mono- + G. *plēgē*, a stroke] Paralysis of one extremity. *Cf.* diplegia; hemiplegia; paraplegia; quadriplegia; triplegia.

monosyllabic word See under word.

monotone See under voice disorders of phonation.

mood Property of verbs which indicates the speaker's attitude toward a verbal idea as a fact, contrary to fact, a command, or a possibility.

    imperative m. Mood indicating a command; *e.g.*, "Sit down."

    indicative m. Mood indicating a statement of fact; *e.g.*, "It is cold."

    subjunctive m. Mood indicating a statement contrary to fact *(e.g.*, "If I were you . . . "), granting of a concession *(e.g.*, "Be it as you say . . . "), or statement of an improbability *(e.g.*, "If this were the case . . . ").

Moro's reflex See under reflex.

morpheme (môr'fēm) [G. *morphē*, form + *phēmē*, voice] Smallest meaningful unit of language having a differential function.

    bound m. Morpheme which must be joined to a free morpheme to convey meaning; frequently a grammatical inflection which may indicate singularity and plurality in nouns, tense in verbs, degree in adjectives, negation, possession, and the various parts of speech one word can assume; *e.g.*, cat*s;* walk*ed;* soft*ness; un*happy; boy*'s;* play*ed,* play*er,* play*ing,* play*ful.*

    free m. Morpheme which can stand alone and designate meaning; *e.g.*, cat; walk; soft. Syn: free form.

    grammatical m. 1. Inflection on nouns, verbs, and adjectives which signals different kinds of meaning: *e.g.*, the morpheme /-s/ when added to a noun such as "dog" indicates plu-

rality; when added to a noun such as "Mommy" can indicate possession; when added to a verb such as "go," indicates present or habitual action. **2.** Morpheme which expresses subtle modulations of meaning rather than naming places, things, or processes; *e.g.*, articles, prepositions, conjunctions, auxiliary words, inflections, and affixes. See also functor, under word. **3.** A morpheme serving a grammatical function.

    lexical m. Substantive or contentive aspects of an utterance. See also content *word.*

    zero m. (Ø) Variation of the plural bound morpheme which indicates the absence of a change from singular to plural form; *e.g.*, sheep (singular and plural).

morpheme structure rule Sequence of phonemes in a specific language which allows the production of new words; *e.g.*, *bloot* but not *bnoot.*

morphographemic rule (môr'fō-grə-fēm'ik) [G. *morphē*, form + *grapho*, to write + *phēmē*, voice] Guideline indicating how a sentence is written or how terminal strings are produced into actual sentences; also directs the spelling or pronunciation of a word after a bound morpheme has been added to the base form of the word.

morphological (môr-fə-loj'i-kəl) **1.** Pertaining to morphology (1). **2.** Anatomical. **3.** See under linguistic component.

morphology (môr-fol'ə-jē) [G. *morphē*, form + *logos*, discourse] **1.** Study of how morphemes are put together to form words; indicates how words are formed and provides a bridge between phonology and syntax. See also linguistic components. **2.** Science of the forms and structures of organized beings.

morphophonemic component That which allows for the rewriting of morphemic representations into a proper string of morphemes with rules of the form X → Y.

morphophonemics (môr′fō-fə-nēm′iks) [G. *morphē*, form + *phonēma*, a voice] **1.** Rules of pronunciation; indicate how words in a sentence are to be pronounced, as opposed to how they appear in a written form. **2.** Sound changes that result from the joining of one morpheme with another; *e.g.*, when the morpheme *ity* is added to the morpheme *divine*, the second vowel in *divine* changes from /aɪ/ to /ɪ/. **3.** Building words from phonemes (sound) and morphemes (meaning).

morphotactics (môr-fō-tak′tiks) [G. *morphē*, form + *taktikos*, fit for arranging] Rules which define the permissible sequences of morphemes in a particular language; *e.g.*, *catch-dogger* for *dogcatcher* is a morphotactic violation in English.

most comfortable loudness (MCL) See under threshold.

most comfortable loudness range (MCLR) See under threshold.

mother method Synthetic method. See aural rehabilitation.

motility (mō-til′ə-tē) [L. *motio*, movement] Range and speed of motion.

motivating operation Use of a certain stimulus as a reinforcer if a certain condition has occurred; *e.g.*, food is a better reinforcer after food deprivation.

motivation (mō-tə-vā′shən) [L. *motivus*, moving] Internal or external stimulation which results in an action, such as an idea, need, emotion, or organism state.

motokinesthetics (mō′tō-ki-nes-thet′-iks) [motor + kinesthetic] In speech, a system of speech training used to teach placement of sound; touch and manipulation of the various articulators are accompanied by auditory stimulation and visual demonstrations.

motor (mō′tėr) [L. a movement] **1.** Pertaining to a nerve or nerve fiber which passes from the central nervous system to a muscle and, by the impulse which it transmits, causes movement.

2. Involving or pertaining to muscle movement.

fine m. Pertaining to skillful, discrete, spatially oriented movements requiring use of small muscle sets, as in speech and the grasping and use of small objects. See also *Developmental Sequences of Motor Behavior* in appendices.

gross m. Pertaining to movements of large refined muscles for activities such as locomotion and balance. See also *Developmental Sequences of Motor Behavior* in appendices.

motor aphasia See under aphasia.

motor area See frontal lobe, under cerebrum, under brain.

motor neuron Motor *nerve*.

motor speech disorders **1.** Denotes a collection of communication disorders involving the retrieval and activation of motor plans for speech. **2.** The execution of movements for speech production. See also apraxia; dysarthria.

mouth See oral cavity.

MPO Maximum power output.

MR Mentally retarded.

MRA Magnetic resonance angiography.

MRI Magnetic resonance imaging.

MRU Mean relational utterance.

MSL Mean sentence length.

mucoid (myu′koid) [mucus + G. *eidos*, resemblance] Resembling mucus, especially mucin, the chief component of mucus.

mucoid otitis media See under otitis.

mucosa (myu-kō′sə) [L. fem. *mucosus*, mucous] Mucous *membrane*.

mucous (myu′kəs) [L. *mucosus*] Pertaining to, relating to, or secreting mucus.

mucous membrane See under membrane.

mucous otitis Mucoid *otitis* media.

mucus (myu′kəs) [L.] Viscous fluid secreted by a mucous membrane.

Mueller-Walle method [J. Mueller-Walle, Ger. educator of deaf, *c.* 1886] Analytic method of teaching speechreading which emphasizes rapid and rhythmic syllable drills; sounds are taught first in isolation, then combined into words, phrases, and sentences. See also speechreading, under aural rehabilitation.

muffled voice See under voice.

multi- [L. *multus*, much] Prefix denoting multiplicity; corresponds to Greek prefix *poly-*.

MULTICROS See under contralateral routing of signals (CROS), under hearing aid.

multiple sclerosis (sklə-rō'sis) [G. *sklērōsis*, hardening] Progressive and deteriorating muscular disability produced by overgrowth of the connective tissue surrounding the nerve tracts, especially the spinal cord; muscle tremors, paralysis, and speech disturbances are associated, but symptoms vary depending on the site of the lesions.

multiply handicapped See handicapped.

multisensory (məl'tē-sen'sôr-ē) Denoting those training procedures which simultaneously utilize more than one sense modality.

Muma Assessment Program (MAP) See *Language Tests and Procedures* in appendices.

munching The earliest form of chewing. A flattening and spreading of the tongue combined with an up and down movement of the jaw. The body of the tongue may elevate slightly and make contact with the hard palate. The jaw makes a definite biting or chewing rhythm. There is no lateral movement of the tongue to transfer food to the teeth for real chewing.

muscle (məs'əl) [L. *musculus*] Fibrous contractile organ attached at each extremity (origin and insertion) by a tendon to a bone or other structure, and which produces motion on stimulation; classified as skeletal, smooth (as of internal organs), and cardiac (heart). When stimulated, it functions only by contracting and tends to draw the attached structures toward each other; to return the attached structures to their original positions, an op-

posing muscle must contract. See also tissue. For various muscles, see specific term.

muscles of respiration See *Muscles of Respiration* table, under respiration.

muscles of the larynx See *Muscles of the Larynx* table, under larynx.

muscles of the palate See *Muscles of the Palate* table, under palate.

muscles of the tongue See *Muscles of the Tongue* table.

muscular dystrophy See under dystrophy.

mutation (myu-tā'shən) [L. *mutatus*, changed] **1.** Any basic alteration in form, quality, or some other characteristic. **2.** In genetics, a permanent transmissible change in genetic material of a chromosome which produces a new individual basically unlike its parents.

mutation voice Adolescent *voice*.

mutism (myu'tiz-əm) [L. *mutus*, mute] **1.** Condition of being unable to speak; may be the result of an organic or structural disability such as paralysis or deafness. **2.** Inability to produce speech due to hysteria, abnormal inhibition, or emotional involvement. Syn: elected or voluntary mutism.

    elected m., voluntary m. Mutism (2).

myasthenia (mī-əs-thē'nē-ə) [G. *mys*, muscle + *astheneia*, weakness] Any generalized weakness of muscle.

myelination, myelinization (mī-ə-li-nā'shən, -ni-za'shən) Covering of the nerve fibers with a protective sheath (myelin); recognized as being correlated with physiologic maturation and the development of control of function; myelinated nerve fibers transmit impulses more precisely than those which are not completely myelinated.

mylohyoid muscle See *Muscles of the Larynx* table, under larynx.

myoclonus Sudden contraction of a limb or muscle group; usually characterized by rapid, synchronous up and down movement; occurs irregularly and usually involves a muscle of a limb.

myoelastic-aerodynamic theory of phonation (mī′ō-ə-las′tik ār′ō-dī-nam′ik) Theory that the vocal folds are subject to well-established aerodynamic principles and are set into vibration by the airstream from the lungs and trachea, and that the frequency of vibration is dependent on their length in relation to their tension and mass. These factors are primarily regulated by the interplay of the intrinsic laryngeal muscles. *Cf.* neurochronaxic theory of phonation.

myofunctional mī-ō-fəŋk′shən-əl) **1.** Pertaining to muscular function. **2.** In speech, denoting the action of muscle groups related to facial development and tongue function.

myofunctional therapy Method of restoring to normal the action of the muscle groups related to tongue function and swallowing. Syn: tongue thrust therapy.

myology The science or branch of anatomy dealing with muscles.

myopathic (mī-ō-path′ik) [G. *mys*, muscle + *pathos*, suffering] Relating to myopathy, an abnormal condition or disease of muscle.

myopathic paralysis See under paralysis.

myopathy Any disease of muscular tissue.

myotatic (mī-ō-ta′tik) [G. *mys*, muscle + *tasis*, a stretching] Relating to myotasis, a stretching of muscle.

myotatic irritability See under irritability.

myotatic reflex Stretch *reflex.*

myringitis (mir-iŋ-jī′tis) [L. *myringa*, drum membrane + G. *-itis*, inflammation] Inflammation of the tympanic membrane. Syn: tympanitis.

myringoplasty (mir-iŋ′gō-plas-tē) [L. *myringa*, drum membrane + G. *plasso*, to form] Surgical procedure in which the tympanic membrane is restored through a skin graft. Syn: tympanoplasty.

myringostomy (mir-iŋ-gos′tə-mē) [L. *myringa*, drum membrane + G. *stoma*, mouth] Surgical placement of small drainage tubes by single or double myringotomy to promote continued drainage and aeration of the tympanic air space.

myringotomy (mir-iŋ-got′ə-mē) [L. *myringa*, drum membrane + G. *tomē*, excision] Surgical incision into the tympanic membrane to allow drainage of fluid from the middle ear. Syn: paracentesis (2); tympanotomy.

myrinx (mī′riŋks) [L. *myringa*, drum membrane] Tympanic membrane. See under external *ear.*

AaBbCcDdEeFfGgHhIiJjKk
kLlMmNnO-PpQqRrSsTtUu
UuVvWwXx N AaBbCcDd
EeFfGgHhIiJjKkLlMmNnOo

N Newton.

nares (năr′ēz) Plural of naris.

nares constriction Closing of the nostrils to prevent the emission of air pressure; normally occurs at the velopharyngeal port. It may appear as though the nostrils are being flared, but actually the nasal alae are being constricted posterior to the nares.

naris, pl. **nares** (năr′is, -ēz) [L.] Anterior opening of either side of the nasal cavity. Syn: nostril.

narrative (năr′ə-tiv) [L. *narrativus*] Orderly continuous account of an event or series of events.

narrative speech See under speech.

narrow-band noise See under noise.

narrow range audiometer See under audiometer.

narrow transcription Phonetic *transcription*.

narrow vowel High *vowel*.

nasal (nā′zəl) [L. *nasus*, nose] **1.** Pertaining to the nose or to the nasal cavities together with the structures contained within them. **2.** See under consonant, manner of formation. **3.** See under distinctive features.

nasal alae (ā′lē) [L. wings] Wings of the nostrils; the flaring cartilaginous expansion which forms the outer sides of the nostrils.

nasalance (nāz′ə-ləns) Degree of nasal resonance as compared to the degree of oral resonance.

nasal bone See under bone.

nasal cavity Passageway to the pharynx from the nostril; strictly, there are two principal nasal cavities, right and left, separated by the nasal septum.

nasal conchae See under skull.

nasal consonant See under consonant, manner of formation.

nasal coupling Condition in which the velum is lowered to allow air to pass directly through the nose. See also hy-

pernasality, under voice disorders of resonance.

nasal emission or **escape** Airflow through the nose, usually measurable or audible and heard most frequently during the production of voiceless plosives and fricatives; usually indicative of an incomplete seal between the nasal and oral cavities, and is typical of cleft palate speech. Nasal emission differs from nasal resonance in that the former refers principally to the release of air through the nose, whereas the latter refers to phonated sound. See also hypernasality, under voice disorders of resonance.

nasality (nā-zal′ə-tē) **1.** Reference to speech sounds delivered wholly via the nares, such as /m/, /n/, and /ŋ/. See also under consonant, manner of formation. **2.** General symptom classification that includes all voices that acoustically have an excessive nasal component. Syn: rhinolalia; rhinophonia.

  assimilated n. See under voice disorders of resonance.

  mixed n. See under voice disorders of resonance.

nasalization (nā′zəl-ə-zā′shən) **1.** Quality given to any vowel when adjacent to a nasal sound. **2.** Lowering of the velum to leave the nasal cavity accessible to the air stream, resulting in production through the nose of nonnasal sounds; may be the result of (a) the absence of sufficient structure to make an appropriate velopharyngeal closure, or (b) an inability to manipulate the velar structure.

nasalization of vowels See under assimilatory *phonological processes*.

nasal lisp See under lisp.

nasal port Passageway from the oropharynx to the nasopharynx; it is opened by the action of the velum and superior pharyngeal constrictor. Syn: nasal tract.

nasal resonance See under resonance.

nasal respiration See under respiration.

nasal rustle Nasal pharyngeal sound which accompanies the production of voiceless pressure sounds in the speech of some individuals with cleft palate.

nasal septum [L. *saeptum*, a partition] Partition of bone and cartilage separating the right and left nasal cavities.

nasal snort Substitution of what may be referred to as an unvoiced /n/ for fricative or plosive sounds; usually accompanied by overt nasal constrictions and facial grimacing. See also nasal emission.

nasal tract Nasal port.

nasal turbulence See under turbulence.

nasal twang 1. Vocal quality often thought to result from incomplete velopharyngeal closure, but which may also result from various pharyngeal and tongue postures emphasizing the higher frequency harmonics; may occur in conjunction with nasality, but may also have a different physiologic origin; often associated with various dialects and professions. **2.** In linguistics, a secondary feature of articulation that differs from the distinctive feature of nasality, which is used to mark a class of sounds.

nasal uncoupling Condition in which the velum is raised at all times, thus preventing any air from passing through the nose; opposite of nasal coupling. See also hyponasality, under voice disorders of resonance.

naso- [L. *nasus*, nose] Combining form relating to the nose.

nasogastric tube (NG tube) See under feeding, nonoral.

naso-ocular (nā-zō-ok′yu-lėr) Pertaining to the nose and eye.

naso-oral (nā-zō-ôr′əl) Relating to the nose and mouth.

nasopalatine (nā-zō-pal′ə-tēn) Pertaining to the nose and palate.

nasopharyngeal (nā′zō-fə-rin′jē-əl, -rin′ jəl) Relating to the nose or nasal cavity and the pharynx or nasopharynx.

nasopharyngoscope (nā′zō-fə-rin′jə-skōp, -riŋ′gō-) [naso- + G. *pharynx*, throat + *skopeō*, to view] Electrically lighted telescopic instrument used for examination of the nasal passages and the nasopharynx.

nasopharynx (nā-zō-fār′iŋks) [naso- + G. *pharynx*, throat] That part of the pharynx above the level of the soft palate and which opens anteriorly into the nasal cavity. See also pharynx.

natal (nā′təl) [L. *natalis*, born] Pertaining to birth.

native Inborn; innate.

native language See under language.

nativist theory See under language theories.

natural frequency See under frequency.

natural method Synthetic method. See under aural rehabilitation.

natural phonological processes Sound changes in a language which purportedly represent a universal phonemic simplification system. Such sound changes must satisfy two conditions: (a) *simplification*, a more complex articulatory structure at the underlying level is changed to a less complex structure at the surface level; and (b) *universality*, the process is attested in a sufficient number of sound change phenomena in natural languages of the world. See also phonological processes.

natural pitch See under pitch.

NDT 1. Neurodevelopmental treatment. **2.** Noise detection threshold.

necrosis (ne-krō′sis) [G. *nekrōsis*, death] Pathologic death of a portion of a tissue or organ resulting from irreversible damage.

negation (nə-gā′shən) **1.** Denoting denial or refusal; not positive. **2.** In linguistics, denial or refusal which may be noted in syntax or semantics. In early language, the negative forms are *no* and *not; e.g., no* hit me; cat *no* chase dog; this is a cat, *no* (syntactic constructions). Semantically, the meaning of *no* and *not* are learned from statements made by others; *e.g.*, do *not* hit (semantic construction).

negative correlation See under correlation.

negative emotion All-inclusive term used to generally describe fear, anxiety, guilt, stress, and similar responses without distinction among them. See also negative *response*.

negative feedback See under feedback.

negative practice Therapy technique using, intentionally and voluntarily, a previously learned incorrect or abnormal behavior to make the behavior more vivid in the mind of the individual and thus to help extinguish it.

negative reinforcer See under reinforcer.

negative response See under response.

negative spikes See under electroencephalogram.

negative spike-waves See under electroencephalogram.

neoglottis (nē-ō-glo′tis) [G. *neos*, new + *glottis*, aperture of larynx] Vibratory segment or area that functions for vocal phonation in the absence of the glottis; some consider the area to be the pharyngoesophageal (PE) junction, while others consider the area to include fibers from the inferior pharyngeal constrictor muscle and the superior esophageal sphincter muscle. Syn: pseudoglottis.

neologism (nē′ə-lō-jiz-əm, nē-ol′ə-) [Fr. *néologisme*] **1.** Invented word, one for which there is no authority in the generally accepted code of language, but which appears to serve a linguistic function. **2.** Conventional word which is replaced by a new one, the meaning of which is not apparent in the utterance; occurs often in the language of the aphasic; *e.g.*, *spork* as the evoked word for *spoon* and *fork*.

neonatal (nē-ō-nā′təl) [L. *neonatus*, newborn] Relating to the period immediately following birth and continuing through the first month of life.

neonatal auditory response cradle See under audiometry.

neonatal period The first four weeks of life.

neonate (nē′ō-nāt) A baby during the first four weeks of life. Syn: newborn.

neonatology 1. The study of the newborn; a subspecialty related to obstetrics, pediatrics, and fetal biology. **2.** Diagnosis and treatment of disorders of the newborn infant.

neoplasm (nē′ə-plaz-əm) [G. *neos*, new + *plasma*, thing formed] Abnormal mass of tissue that grows more rapidly than normal and continues to grow after the stimuli which initiated the new growth cease; may be benign or malignant. Syn: tumor.

nerve [L. *nervus*, sinew] Cordlike structure comprised of a bundle of myelinated or unmyelinated nerve fibers, most often mixtures of both, together with accompanying connective tissue and blood vessels, which conducts electrical impulses to and from the central nervous system on stimulation. Characteristically, a nerve (a) is composed of cellular units called neurons, which are linked together by synaptic junctions to form conduction pathways for electrical impulses; (b) transmits electrical impulses at different speeds and intensities, but with total potential; (c) is fatigable, and the neurons cannot be stimulated immediately after an impulse; (d) possesses varying thresholds of response; and (e) exhibits the phenomena of recruitment. See also cranial nerves; tissue. For individual nerves not listed below, see specific term.

  afferent n. Nerve that conveys impulses from the periphery to the central nervous system; *e.g.*, in the ascending nerve pathways. See also sensory *nerve*.

  efferent n. Nerve that conveys impulses from the central nervous system to muscles and glands; *e.g.*, in the descending neural pathways. See also motor *nerve*.

motor n. Efferent nerve that conveys an impulse from the central nervous system to stimulate muscle contraction. Syn: motor neuron.

sensory n. Afferent nerve that conveys an impulse from a sense organ to the central nervous system.

nerve cell Neuron.

nerve deafness See sensorineural *deafness*.

nerve fiber See under fiber.

nerve force Ability of nerve fibers to transmit stimuli.

nerve loss See sensorineural *deafness*.

nervous system Entire nervous apparatus of the body, including the brain, brainstem, spinal cord, cranial and peripheral nerves, and ganglia.

autonomic n. s. One of the chief divisions of the nervous system, consisting of a large outflow of peripheral efferent fibers that regulate visceral and glandular responses. Syn: visceral nervous system.

central auditory n. s. (CANS) Anatomical regions in the brainstem and brain where auditory fibers may be found. May include pons, midbrain, thalamus, primary auditory reception area (Brodmann 41), parietal lobe, temporal lobe, and the corpus callosum.

central n. s. (CNS) The brain, brainstem, and spinal cord; that part of the nervous system to which sensory impulses are transmitted and from which motor impulses are transmitted.

peripheral n. s. (PNS) Autonomic nervous system and the cranial nerves; that portion of the nervous system conducting impulses to and from the central nervous system.

visceral n. s. Autonomic *nervous system*.

neurilemoma, neurinoma (nu'ri-lə-mō'-mə, -ə-nō'mə) [neuro- + G. *eilema*, closely adhering sheath + *-oma*, tumor] Benign encapsulated neoplasm of a nerve sheath; it may originate from a peripheral, sympathetic, or cranial nerve (especially cranial nerve VIII). Syn: schwannoma.

acoustic n. Benign neoplasm of the intracranial segment of the eighth cranial nerve, which produces cerebellar, lower cranial nerve, and brainstem signs and symptoms. Syn: acoustic neurinoma; eighth nerve tumor.

neuro- [G. *neuron*, nerve] Combining form denoting a nerve or relating to the nervous system.

neuroaudiology (nu'rō-ô-dē-ôl'ə-jē) Study of hearing that centers on assessments of the eighth nerve and central auditory pathways.

neurochronaxic theory of phonation (nu'rō-krō-nak'sik) Theory that each new vibratory cycle is initiated by a nerve impulse transmitted from the brain to the vocalis muscle via the recurrent branch of the vagus nerve; the frequency of vocal fold vibration is dependent on the rate of impulses delivered to the laryngeal muscles. *Cf.* myoelastic-aerodynamic theory of phonation.

neurodevelopmental treatment (NDT) Bobath method.

neurolinguistics (nu'rō-liŋ-gwi'stiks) Medical science branch concerned with the neuroanatomical basis of speech and its disorders.

neurologic, neurological (nu-rō-loj'ik, -i-kəl) [neuro- + G. *logos*, discourse, study] Pertaining to the nervous system in both its normal and diseased states.

neurological dysfunction Term for a brain impairment which is a problem of altered processes, not of a generalized incapacity to learn. Individuals having such an impairment usually experience perceptual and integrative organizational differences from the norm, and therefore tend to learn differently than normal individuals; may be congenital or acquired. See also learning disability; attention deficit/hyperactivity disorder.

neuromotor (nu-rō-mō′tėr) Pertaining to efferent nerve impulses.

neuromuscular (nu-rō-məs′kyu-lėr) Pertaining to any process that is a combined function of the muscles and nerves.

neuron (nu′ron) [G. nerve] Basic structural unit of the nervous system by means of which impulses are received, transmitted, and processed. It consists of (a) **axon,** a branched nerve fiber that conveys impulses away from the nerve cell body; (b) **cell body,** the center of the neuron which encloses the nucleus and various masses; (c) **den-**

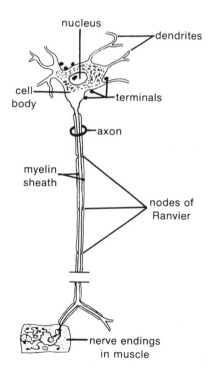

Neuron
Diagram of a motor neuron based on the site of impulse origin rather than location of the cell body. From Carpenter, MB, and Sutin, J. *Human Neuroanatomy,* 8th ed. Baltimore: Williams & Wilkins, 1982.

drite, a branched filament at the end of the myelinated sheath which conveys impulses toward the cell body (sensory neurons have a single dendrite, motor neurons have many); and (d) **terminals,** button-shaped structures that form synapses with other neurons. Syn: nerve cell.

    motor n. Motor *nerve.*

neuronal circuit Transmission of impulses by chains of neurons linked at junction points where synapses with other neurons occur; patterns of organization of such chains differ according to their function.

    convergence circuit Neuronal circuit having two or more distinct input channels that join to control a single neuron.

    divergence circuit Neuronal circuit that has a single input channel and serves as the primary source of stimulation for multiple output neurons.

neuropathy Any disease of the nervous system.

neurophonia (nu-rō-fō′nē-ə) [neuro- + G. *phōnē,* voice] Spasm or tic of the muscles of phonation causing involuntary sounds or cries.

neurophrenia (nu-rō-frē′nē-ə) [neuro- + G. *phrēn,* mind] Behavior symptoms resulting from central nervous system impairment. See also minimal brain dysfunction syndrome.

neurosis, pl. **neuroses** (nu-rō′sis, -sēz) [neuro- + G. *-osis,* condition] Psychological or behavioral disorder in which anxiety, anticipation, tension, and irritability are the primary characteristics; usually there is no gross distortion of reality or disorganization of personality. Defense mechanisms or any phobia are adjustive techniques learned in order to cope with the condition. *Cf.* psychosis.

neurotic (nu-ro′tik) Relating to or suffering from a neurosis.

neurotic profit Defect or handicap used unconsciously to gain attention, control environment, or relieve guilt; *e.g.,* child with laryngitis not having to do his written homework. Syn: secondary gain.

neurotic theory of stuttering See repressed need theory, under stuttering theories.

neutralization (nu'trə-li-zā'shən) **1.** Opposing of one force or condition with an opposite force or condition to such a degree as to cause a counteraction that allows neither to dominate. **2.** In linguistics, a phonological fusion of two or more forms. **3.** In linguistics, a temporary suspension of an otherwise distinctive feature of two sounds; *e.g.*, /t/ in *tie* and /d/ in *die* serve different functions, but /t/ in *wetting* often acquires the sound of /d/ in *wedding*, making these words sound the same. **4.** See under substitution, under phonological processes. Syn: obscuration. See also assimilation.

neutral stimulus See under stimulus.

neutral vowel See under vowel.

neutroclusion See under teeth malocclusion.

newborn Neonate.

newton (N) (nu'tən) [I. Newton, Eng. physicist, 1642–1727] Unit of measurement used to determine how much force will be necessary to accelerate one kilogram of mass at one meter per second; 1 N = 100,000 dyne.

NG tube nasogastric tube. See under feeding.

NIL Noise interference level.

ninth cranial nerve See *Cranial Nerves* table, under cranial nerves.

Nitchie method [E. B. Nitchie, U.S. educator of deaf, 1876–1916] Synthetic method of speechreading technique which emphasizes the positive attitude of the speech reader and the training of the mind in intuition, synthesis, quickness, alertness, and concentration; stresses teaching speechreading of whole paragraphs of material before learning to read sentences or words. See also speechreading, under aural rehabilitation.

node (nōd) [L. *nodus*, knot] **1.** Knob or circumscribed swelling of tissue. See also nodule. **2.** In transformational grammar, dots used in a branching tree diagram, *q.v.* **3.** In acoustics, a point in a standing wave which has no amplitude. **4.** Point in a vibrating system which is free of vibration.

  n. of Ranvier [L. A. Ranvier, Fr. pathologist, 1835–1922] Points between successive segments of the myelin sheath of the axon of a neuron.

  singer's n. Vocal nodule. See under laryngeal anomaly.

nodularity (nod-yu-lār'i-tē) Nodule that is not fully developed. See under laryngeal anomaly.

nodule (nod'yul) [L. *nodulus*, dim. *nodus*, knot] A small node.

  polyploid vocal n. See vocal nodules, under laryngeal anomaly.

  singer's n. Vocal nodules. See under laryngeal anomaly.

  vocal n. See under laryngeal anomaly.

no-echo chamber Anechoic chamber.

noise (noiz) **1.** Complex sound wave having aperiodic or irregular vibrations to which no definite pitch can be assigned; may be broken down into a number of sinusoidal curves, but the higher partials are not multiples of the lower partials; the frequencies are not in mutual harmonious relation. **2.** Sensory effect of irregular or aperiodic sound waves, generally considered as unpleasant or undesired sound. **3.** Unwanted additions to a signal not arising at its source; *e.g.*, 60-cycle frequency wave in a radio transmission. See also masking.

  ambient n. Sounds of the environment or in an amplifying system which are not part of the desired signal. Syn: extraneous noise.

  background n. Extraneous undesired sounds, such as static, heard with the intended sounds.

  complex n. Noise with a fundamental frequency of about 120 Hz, with numerous harmonics for masking at frequencies below 1000 Hz.

extraneous n. Ambient *noise.*

gaussian n. [J. F. K. Gauss, Ger. physicist, 1777–1855] White *noise.*

narrow-band n. White noise selectively filtered and presented in restricted frequency bands; often used in masking.

pink n. 1. Irregular sound similar to white noise but whose spectrum level decreases with increase in frequency to provide constant energy per octave of bandwidth below 2000 Hz. **2.** Sound whose sound power unit frequency is inversely proportional to frequency over a specified range.

random n. Complex sound wave whose instantaneous amplitudes vary in time according to a normal distribution curve; it has energy distributed over a band of frequencies; *e.g.*, noise from ventilating systems, jet engines, blowers.

sawtooth n. Noise composed of a complex tone, usually with a fundamental frequency of 120 Hz and including in random phase harmonics of the fundamental frequency to 10,000 Hz; often used in masking.

sixty-cycle hum Type of noise heard as a buzz which occurs in electrical appliances, especially radios and television, at the frequency of 60 Hz; often used in masking.

speech n. Any type of noise within the speech frequencies (500–2000 Hz); often used in masking.

thermal n. White *noise.*

white n. Signal containing energy at all frequencies in the audible spectrum and presented at approximately equal intensities; often used in masking. Syn: gaussian, thermal, or wideband noise.

wide-band n. White *noise.*

noise analyzer Instrument designed to determine frequency components of a particular noise; it may range in effectiveness from the analysis of sound levels in a one-octave range to only $\frac{1}{30}$ of an octave width. Syn: noise exposure meter.

noise detection threshold (NDT) See under threshold.

noise exposure meter Noise analyzer.

noise generator Noise-producing source used clinically and experimentally, as in masking, to simulate various types of noise.

noise-induced deafness See under deafness.

noise interference level (NIL) In audiology, the point at which an individual can no longer repeat the speech spondees presented because of the intensity of the noise presented in conjunction with the spondees. Syn: speech interference level.

noise limiter See peak clipping.

noise pollution Noise in the environment at a loudness level that may be annoying or damaging to hearing.

nomenclature (nō-men-klā′chër) [L. *nomenculator*, name-caller] System or set of terms or symbols used in a particular science, discipline, or art.

nominal 1. In grammar, a word, phrase, or clause that is equivalent to a noun in its structural role. See also noun, under parts of speech. **2.** Being such in name only; trifling or minor in comparison.

nominal aphasia See under aphasia.

nominal compound Combination of words which produces nominals. It may include three types: (a) subject-verb combination, *e.g.*, The *toes* (subject) *twinkle* (verb). = *twinkle toes;* (b) subject-predicate, *e.g.*, The *girl* (subject) is a *friend* (predicate). = *girlfriend;* (c) verb-prepositional object, *e.g.*, The *fountain* (subject) is for *drinking* (prepositional object). = *drinking fountain.*

nominative case See case.

non- [L. not] Prefix used in compound

terms to denote negation, opposite of, absence of, or omission.

nonavoidance therapy In stuttering, a technique used to reduce avoidance tendencies within an individual and to increase approach tendencies in ways that do not increase anxiety or fear.

noncontrastive distribution Complementary *distribution.*

nondirectional microphone See under microphone.

nondistinctive features Characteristics of sounds which occur in all manners of distribution, usually with a limit to their variability; a gross acoustic feature.

nonfluency (non-flu′ən-sē) Dysfluency.

nonfluent aphasia See under aphasia.

nonkernel sentence See derived sentence, under sentence classifications, transformational grammar.

nonlinear distortion Harmonic *distortion.*

nonnasal sound Any sound that does not require the passage of air through the nose; any English sound except /m/, /n/, and /ŋ/.

nonobtrusive text See under text.

nonoccluding earmold Open earmold.

nonoral communication Augmentative *communication.*

nonorganic deafness Functional *deafness.*

nonperiodic wave Aperiodic *wave.*

nonpropositional speech See under speech.

nonpurulent (non-pyur′ə-lənt) [non- + L. *purulentus,* pus-forming] Nonsuppurative.

nonreduplicated babbling See under babbling.

nonreinforcement (non′rē-in-fôrs′-mənt) Counter *conditioning.*

nonrestrictive modifier See under modifier.

nonsense syllable See under syllable.

nonsense word See under word.

nonsonorant Sibilant. See under consonant, manner of formation.

nonspecific language See under language.

nonspeech sounds 1. Sounds considered to be environmental in nature. **2.** Sound effect recordings sometimes used to obtain hearing threshold estimates in children.

nonstandard language See under language.

nonsuppurative (non-səp′yə-rā-tiv) [non + L. *suppuratus,* pus-forming] Not containing, forming, or discharging pus. Syn: nonpurulent.

nonsuppurative otitis media See under otitis.

nonsyllabic speech sounds See under consonant.

nonverbal Without oral language.

nonverbal test Any examination, evaluation, or measurement procedure that does not utilize verbal material; may be administered without using words; *e.g.,* Leiter International Performance Scale.

nonvocal (non-vō′kəl) Denoting individuals who have not developed functional oral communication skills; includes nonvocal hearing-impaired individuals (NVHI), nonvocal mentally retarded individuals (NVMR), nonvocal autistic individuals (NVA), and nonvocal severely physically handicapped individuals (NVSPH).

nonvocal communication Augmentative *communication.*

norm Set standard or pattern derived from a representative sampling of median achievement of a large group; offers a range of values against which individual comparisons may be made.

normal [L. *normalis,* according to pattern] **1.** Reference to some region of a distribution arbitrarily designated as not extreme. **2.** Condition at or near average in any measurable structure, function, or trait. **3.** Not pathologic; may be equated with health as the "average" or generally "expected" condition.

normal curve Normal *distribution.*

normal distribution See under distribution.

normal probability curve Normal *distribution.*

normal swallowing habit Swallowing in which the tongue does not push against or protrude past the upper central incisors. The tip of the tongue presses against the rugae behind the upper anterior teeth; the midpoint of the tongue rises to meet the hard palate, with the posterior part of the tongue tipped against the pharyngeal wall; the teeth are closed; and the lips may be sealed. Swallowing is accomplished with negative intraoral pressure. See also tongue thrust, swallow.

normal transition Closed *juncture.*

normative phonetics See under phonetics.

norm-referenced tests Standardized tests.

Northampton charts [orig. Clark School for the Deaf, Northampton, Mass., 1867] In aural rehabilitation, a method used in which the letters of the English alphabet are arranged to give phonetic significance. The charts arrange symbols in columns and rows according to the method of production of the sounds; *e.g.*, /p/, /b/, and /m/ are in the same row because the lips are initially shut in the production of all three, but they are in different columns because /p/ is voiceless, /b/ is voiced, and /m/ is nasal. See also aural rehabilitation.

Northwestern University Children's Perception of Speech Test See *Auditory Tests and Procedures* in appendices.

nose 1. That part of the face that bears the nostrils and covers the anterior part of the nasal cavity. **2.** The olfactory organ.

nose cleft See atypical *cleft.*

nostril (nos′trəl) Naris.

notched waves See under electroencephalogram.

noun See under parts of speech.

novel stimulus See under stimulus.

noxious stimulus (nok′shəs) Negative *reinforcer.*

noy Unit for a subjective measure of perceived noisiness indicated in terms of how loud a sound appears to a listener; *e.g.*, 1 noy is assigned the perceived noisiness of a band of frequencies from 910 to 1090 Hz presented at a sound pressure level of 40 dB; values of 0.5 noy and 2 noy are assigned respectively to noises half as loud and twice as loud as this reference noise level.

NU Auditory Test Lists 4 and 6 See *Audiometric Tests and Procedures* in appendices.

nucleus, pl. **nuclei** (nu′klē-əs, -ī) [L. little nut, pit, kernel] **1.** Central part or core about which other parts are grouped. **2.** Spherical specialized mass of protoplasm encased in a membrane within a cell that forms an essential element in the functions of the cell.

null In transformational grammar, an indicator that a position is empty of any change in a form of the word in a particular position in a particular sentence; indicated by Ø (zero morpheme); *e.g.*, sheep (singular), sheep (plural); the plural form is indicated by sheep Ø. See also zero morpheme.

numerical cipher method In aural rehabilitation, a primitive form of speechreading based on the concept that the sounds of English are revealed in 16 facial configurations.

nystagmus (nis-tag′məs) [G. *nystagmos*, a nodding] Oscillatory motion of the eyes; may be congenital or acquired.

Ø Zero morpheme.

OAE otoacoustic emissions.

object (ob′jekt) **1.** In grammar, a noun or pronoun used as a noun that completes the meaning of a transitive verb or follows a preposition. **2.** Any part of the environment, such as a material thing, a person, or an abstraction, of which one is aware. **3.** That which serves as a stimulus to elicit a response.

object concept or **constancy** Object permanence.

objective [L. *objectus*, thrown before] **1.** Independent of error of human judgment and bias; scientifically precise; opposite of subjective. **2.** A goal to be achieved. **3.** Proposed change indicating an expected behavior. See also performance objective. **4.** See under parts of speech.

objective case See case.

objective complement See complement.

objective quantity See under quantity.

objective test 1. Measure whose validity and reliability have been demonstrated and which requires specific responses; a standardized test; *e.g.*, Stanford-Binet Intelligence Test. **2.** In hearing, a measure of hearing sensitivity that does not depend on a voluntary response from the person being measured, *e.g.*, acoustic impedance audiometry.

object permanence 1. Awareness that an object is relatively permanent and is not destroyed if removed from the visual field; *e.g.*, an individual is still present even if his face is covered by his hands. **2.** Tendency for an object to remain perceptually the same regardless of a variation in the conditions of observation; *e.g.*, a table is a table whether viewed upright, upside down, or on its side. Syn: object concept or constancy.

obligatory occurrence Any instance in which a specific rule has to be applied for the sentence to be considered grammatical; *e.g.*, "I have three cats," the plural ending is obliged to be there by the rules of standard English.

obliquus abdominis externus muscle See *Muscles of Respiration* table, under respiration.

obliquus abdominis internus muscle See *Muscles of Respiration* table, under respiration.

obscuration (ob-skyu-rā′shən) Neutralization (3).

obscure vowel Neutral *vowel.*

observation (ob-sėr-vā′shən) [L. *observo*, to watch] Purposeful or intentional examination, such as evaluation of responses which can be perceived, counted, and recorded.

obsessive compulsive reaction See under reaction.

obstruent See under consonant, manner of formation.

obstruent omission Deletion of initial consonant. See under syllable structure, under phonological processes.

obtrusive text See under text.

obturator (ob-tə-rā′tėr) [L. *obturatus*, occluded or stopped up] **1.** Any structure which occludes an opening. **2.** Prosthetic appliance, similar to a dental plate, that forms an artificial palate to cover a cleft palate, designed so that the musculature of the palate and pharynx are able to contract around it, yet not interfere with nasal breathing, pronunciation of nasal consonants, or swallowing; also helps provide intraoral pressure. See also palatal lift.

OC Oral communication.

occipital (ok-sip′ə-təl) [L. *occipitalis*] Relating to the occiput, the back of the head.

occipital bone See under skull.

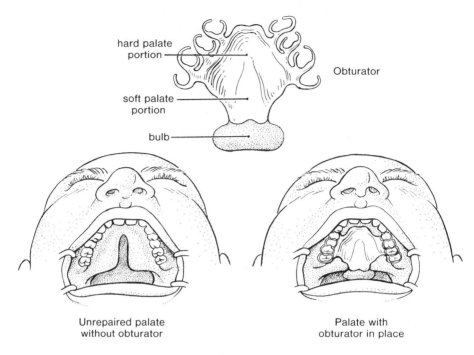

hard palate portion

Obturator

soft palate portion

bulb

Unrepaired palate without obturator

Palate with obturator in place

Obturator

occipital lobe See under cerebrum, under brain.

occluded lisp See under lisp.

occlusion (ə-klu′zhən) [L. *occlusus*, closed up] **1.** Act of closing or the state of being closed, as in the obstruction of the breath passage in the buccal cavity in the articulation of various sounds. **2.** Relationship between the various surfaces of the maxillary and mandibular teeth when they are in contact; may refer to (a) alignment of the teeth in the lower and upper arches; (b) relationship of the dental arches to each other; (c) axial inclination of the individual teeth; and (d) biting height of the teeth when the jaws are in contact. See also teeth malocclusion.

occlusion effect Increase in the loudness of tones of 1000 Hz and below when the ears are tightly covered during bone-conduction testing; this effect is seen in normal hearers and in patients with sensorineural hearing losses, but is absent in patients with conductive hearing losses.

occult (ə-kəlt′) [L. *occultus*, covered over, concealed] Hidden from view; not readily observable.

occult cleft palate Submucosal *cleft palate*.

occupational deafness Noise-induced *deafness*.

Occupational Safety and Health Act (OSHA) Federal legislation (1970) that sets minimum standards for industrial hearing conservation programs and extends the applicability of acceptable noise exposure levels to all industries participating in interstate commerce.

octave (ok′tiv) [L. *octava*, eighth] **1.** Interval between two frequencies, one of which is twice as large as the other (a ratio of 2:1). **2.** Frequency span extending to a tone having twice (or half) as many vibrations per second as the one taken as a reference point; the pitch interval between these two tones is such that the tone may be regarded as duplicating the other at the nearest possible higher (or lower) pitch.

octave band analyzer See under noise analyzer.

octave-band filter See under band-pass *filter.*

octave twist In stuttering, a device used by some stutterers in which the fundamental pitch shifts upward one octave as a reaction to the moment of stuttering.

ocular (ok′yu-lėr) [L. *oculus,* eye] Pertaining to the eye.

oculomotor (ok′yu-lō-mō′tėr) Relating to or causing movement of the eye.

oculomotor nerve See *Cranial Nerves* table, under cranial nerves.

odd-even method Split-half *reliability coefficient.*

off effect Sudden increase in activity in the auditory system when a sustained tone ends.

off-glide Movements of the articulators as they travel away from the most prominent adjustment for production of any of the sounds; differentiated from glide, a class name for certain sounds *e.g.,* the repositioning of the tongue from /s/ to /k/ in the /sk/ blend. Syn: after-glide. *Cf.* on-glide. See also release.

Ohio Tests of Articulation and Perception of Sounds (OTAPS) See *Articulation Tests and Phonological Analysis Procedures* and *Auditory Tests and Procedures* in appendices.

ohm (ōm) [G. S. Ohm, Ger. physicist, 1787–1854] **1.** Practical unit of electrical resistance; the resistance of any conductor allowing one ampere of current to pass under the electromotive force of one volt. **2.** In acoustics, a unit of measurement marking the resistance to the flow of sound pressure waves through a medium; one ohm equals a pressure amplitude of one

dyne per square centimeter per second of flux amplitude.

Ohm's law [G. S. Ohm, Ger. physicist, 1787–1854] **1.** In acoustics, a theory that a complex sound stimulus (contains many pure tones) can be analyzed into its frequency components; thus, each tone can be perceived individually. **2.** In electricity, a relationship between current voltage and resistance in an electrical circuit; the strength of the current in an electrical circuit is directly proportional to the applied voltage and inversely proportional to the resistance of the circuit.

olfactory (ol-fak′tôr-ē) [L. *olfactus,* smell] Pertaining to the sense of smell (olfaction).

olfactory nerve See *Cranial Nerves* table, under cranial nerves.

oligodontia (ol′i-gə-don′shē-ə) [G. *oligos,* few + *odous,* tooth] Condition in which there are fewer than the normal number of teeth in the mouth, usually only a few.

omission See under articulation disorder.

omnidirectional microphone Nondirectional *microphone.*

omohyoid muscle (ō-mō-hī′oid) See *Muscles of the Larynx* table, under larynx.

on effect Phenomenon in which the initial response of the auditory system to a sustained tone is its most vigorous response.

on-glide Movements of the articulators as they travel toward a position necessary for producing any particular sound; differentiated from glide, a class name for certain sounds; *e.g.,* repositioning of the tongue from /ɔ/ to /g/ in *dog.* Syn: fore-glide. *Cf.* off-glide.

onomatopoeia (on-ə-mät-ə-pē′ə) [G. *onoma,* name + *poiēsis,* making] Word so formed that it suggests its meaning through its sound *e.g.,* hiss, buzz, boom.

ontogenesis or **ontogeny** (on-tō-jen′ə-sis, on-toj′ə-nē) [G. *ōn,* being + *genesis,* origin] Developmental change that occurs in an individual, as opposed to phylogenesis or phylogeny, which is concerned with the development of the species.

open-bite See under teeth malpositions.

open class **1.** See under parts of speech. **2.** See also pivot *grammar.*

open earmold See under earmold.

open juncture See under juncture.

open quotient Time ratio of a vocal fold vibratory cycle during which the glottis is open, as compared with the duration of the entire open-closed-open cycle.

open-set tests Tests in which the listener has an unlimited number of response possibilities; no response alternatives are provided. See also closed-set tests.

open syllable See under syllable.

open vowel Low *vowel.*

open word See under word.

operant (op′ẻr-ənt) In conditioning, the target behavior or response chosen by the conditioner. See operant *conditioning.*

operant, verbal Verbal response for which there is no observable stimuli.

  autoclitic o. Manipulation of verbal thinking; includes assertions and various sentence structures.

  echoic o. Response that generates sound patterns similar to those of prior stimuli. See also echolalia.

  intraverbal o. Verbal response to verbal stimuli; *e.g.,* the response "four" in answer to the verbal stimulus "two plus two."

  mand o. Command or question in which a response is required by consequences and is, therefore, under the control of pertinent conditions which may include deprivation or adverse stimuli; *e.g.,* "Put it down or I will spank you."

  tact o. [fr. contact] **1.** Response emitted and strengthened by the presence of an object or event; *e.g.,* seeing rain, the child says, "It's raining." **2.** Behavior involving naming, describing, and pointing which does

not necessarily demand a response from another person.

  textual o. Verbal response to written stimuli; *e.g.,* talking about a newspaper article read.

operant behavior See under operant *conditioning.*

operant behavior theory See under learning theory, under stuttering theories.

operant conditioning See under conditioning.

operant learning See operant *conditioning.*

operant level Baseline.

operant procedures See operant *conditioning.*

operant therapy See operant *conditioning.*

operational objectives Performance objectives.

opposite phase See phase.

opposition breathing See opposition *respiration.*

opposition respiration See under respiration.

optic nerve See *Cranial Nerves* table, under cranial nerves.

optimal pitch Natural *pitch.*

OR Orienting reflex.

oral (ôr′əl) [L. *os (or-)*, mouth] Pertaining to the mouth.

Oral and Written Language Scales See *Language Test and Procedures* in appendices.

oral apraxia See under apraxia.

oral atresia Astomia.

oral-aural method See under aural rehabilitation.

oral cavity In speech, the mouth as it communicates with the pharynx through the fauces. The peripheral boundary is marked by the alveolar process and the teeth; the roof is marked by the hard palate; the floor is covered by the tongue; and the posterior wall is marked by the dependent portion of the soft palate; may also include the buccal cavity, which is bounded externally by the lips and cheeks and internally by the outer aspects of the teeth and gums.

oral communication (OC) A process by which meanings are exchanged between individuals by talking. See also under aural rehabilitation, oral-aural method.

oral form recognition Oral *stereognosis*.

oral inaccuracy or **inactivity** See general oral inaccuracy, under articulation disorder.

oralism (ôr′ə-liz-əm) Method of deaf education which emphasizes the use of verbal communication among the deaf to the exclusion of fingerspelling or the use of signs.

oral language See under language.

oral manometer See manometer.

oral peripheral examination Inspection of the mouth to determine its structural and functional adequacy for speech. It includes (a) *lips:* size, symmetry, mobility, and possible presence of scars; (b) *jaws:* symmetry, position at rest, and rate of movement; (c) *teeth:* occlusion while at rest and general condition; (d) *tongue:* size relative to the rest of the mouth, swallowing patterns, symmetry while at rest and in motion, and mobility and rate of mobility for protrusion, retraction, elevation, depression, and lateral movements; (e) *hard palate:* shape, width, height, and possible scarring; (f) *soft palate and velopharyngeal closure:* size, symmetry, movement up, back, and laterally, and possible scarring; and (g) *fauces:* status of tonsils, width of isthmus, scarring, and general condition of oropharynx.

oral respiration See under respiration.

oral stereognosis See under stereognosis.

orbit [L. *orbita*, wheel-track, fr. *orbis*, circle] Socket for the eyeball, formed by parts of seven cranial and facial bones.

organ (or′gən) [G. *organos*, a tool, organ] Any part of the body that has a specific function. For various organs, see specific terms.

organic (or-gan′ik) [G. *organikos*] **1.** Relating to an organ or structure. **2.** Denoting any impairment resulting from a structural alteration or weakness; includes genetic variations, biochemical irregularities, perinatal brain trauma, or the results of illnesses and injuries sustained.

organic articulation disorder See under articulation disorder.

organization (ôr′gən-i-zā′shən) **1.** Arrangement of data in such a manner as to reveal relationships among the constituents. **2.** Differentiation of parts and functions, and their integration into a systematic interconnected whole.

organ of Corti [A. Corti, It. anatomist, 1822–1888] Sensory part of the cochlea containing the essential sensory elements of hearing (hair cells). Syn: end organ of hearing. See also under inner *ear*.

orientation (ôr′ē-ən-tā′shən) [Fr. *orienter*, to set toward the East (in a definite position)] **1.** Mental awareness of spatial, temporal, practical, or circumstantial situations. **2.** Assuming a physical position in space with reference to external stimulation; having direction.

orienting reflex (OR) See under reflex.

orifice (ôr′i-fis) [L. *orificium*] Aperture or opening, usually said of an anatomical structure.

origin (ôr′i-jin) [L. *origo*, source, beginning] As applied to a muscle, the relatively fixed or less movable of its attachments; *e.g.*, the sternocleidomastoideus muscle has its origin in the sternum and its insertion in the mastoid process. *Cf.* insertion.

orofacial (ôr-ō-fā′shəl) Relating to the mouth and face.

orofacial muscle imbalance Tongue thrust.

orolingual (ôr-ō-lin′gwəl) Relating to the mouth and tongue.

oromotor (ôr-ō-mō′tėr) **1.** Relating to the

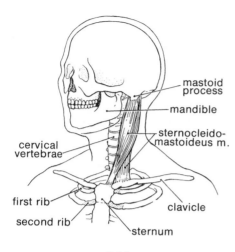

Origin

Origin of the sternocleidomastoideus muscle at the sternum and clavicle.

muscles or nerves of the mouth. **2.** Oral articulators.

oronasal (ôr-ō-nā′zəl) Relating to the mouth and nose.

oro-ocular (ôr-ō-ok′yu-lėr) Relating to the mouth and eye(s).

oropharynx (ôr-ō-făr′iŋks) [L. *os (or-)*, mouth + G. *pharynx*, throat] That part of the pharynx extending from the soft palate to the level of the hyoid bone; opens through the fauces into the oral cavity. See also pharynx.

orthodontics (ôr-thə-don′tiks) [G. *orthos*, correct, straight + *odous*, tooth] That specialty of dentistry concerned with the correction and prevention of irregularities and malocclusion of the teeth and jaws.

orthographic (ôr-thō-graf′ik) Denoting orthography.

orthography (ôr-thog′rə-fē) [G. *orthos*, correct, straight, + *graphē*, a writing] **1.** Part of language study concerned with letters and spelling. **2.** Representation of the sounds of a language by written or printed symbols; the writing system of a language. **3.** Art of writing words with the correct letters according to the standard usage of a particular language.

orthopsychiatry (ôr′thō-sī-kī′ə-trē) [G. *orthos*, correct, straight + *psychē*, mind, soul + *iatreia*, medical treatment] Field of psychiatry especially concerned with mental disorders during childhood and adolescence.

Orzeck Aphasia Evaluation See *Language Tests and Procedures* in appendices.

oscillation (os-i-lā′shən) [L. *oscillatio*, swinging] **1.** To and fro motion of a body about its rest position. **2.** Rhythmic repetitive movements; repetition of a sound or syllable. **3.** In stuttering, the tremulous vibration or repetition of speech musculature temporarily blocking speech. See also vibration.

   laryngeal o. Vibration of the vocal folds.

oscillator (os′i-lā-tėr) [see oscillation] Electronic device for producing sound vibrations.

oscilloscope (o-sil′ə-skōp) [L. *oscillo*, to swing + G. *skopeō*, to inspect] Instrument similar to a television tube which makes sound waves visible; may demonstrate differences between pure tones and complex tones, and measure peak amplitudes of waves. See also electrical measurements of speech production.

OSHA Occupational Safety and Health Act.

-osis [G.] Suffix, properly added only to words formed from Greek, denoting a process, condition, or state, usually abnormal or diseased.

osseotympanic bone conduction See under conduction.

osseous labyrinth Bony labyrinth. See under labyrinth.

ossicles (os′i-kəlz) [L. *ossiculum*, dim. of *os*, bone] Small bones; specifically, the bones of the middle ear (incus, malleus, and stapes) which, considered

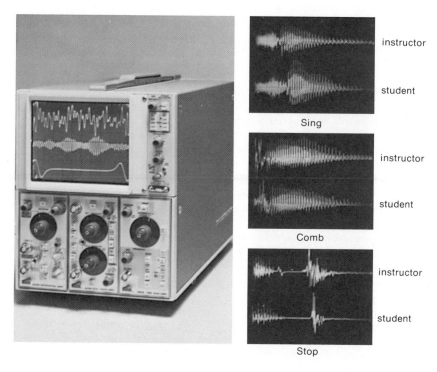

Oscilloscope
Storage oscilloscope with speech waveforms as shown on the oscilloscope for the words *sing, comb,* and *stop.* Courtesy of Tektronix, Inc.

collectively, are referred to as the ossicular chain. See also under middle *ear.*

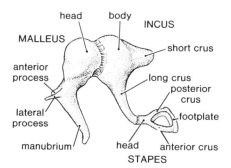

Ossicles

ossicular chain Incus, malleus, and stapes considered collectively; these smallest bones in the body are secured

in the middle ear by eight ligaments and two muscles. See incus, malleus, and stapes, under middle *ear.*

ossiculoplasty Reconstruction of the ossicular chain.

osteoma, pl. **osteomas, osteomata** (ostē-ō′mə, -məz, -ō-mä′tə) [G. *osteon,* bone + *-oma,* tumor] Of the ear: benign neoplasm of the external auditory meatus at the juncture of the cartilaginous and bony parts, composed of connective tissue that forms new bone; similar to an exostosis except that it tends to be unilateral and single, rarer in occurrence, and more likely to be associated with obstruction, infection, and hearing loss.

-ostomy [G. *stoma,* mouth] Suffix denoting incision or cutting into a structure to form an opening.

ot- [G. *ous*, ear] Combining form relating to the ear.

otitis (ō-tī′təs) [ot- + G. -*itis*, inflammation] Inflammation of the ear; may refer to otitis externa or otitis media.

   acute o. media Inflammation of the middle ear that begins with a rapid onset and usually runs its full course within a three-week period.

   adhesive o. media Fusion of the ossicles and the remnant of the tympanic membrane to the walls of the middle ear space as the result of scarring from chronic suppurative otitis media.

   chronic suppurative o. media Otitis media characterized by persistent infection in the middle ear cavity for a prolonged period of time; accompanied by a discharge of pus that has a foul odor.

   mucoid o. media Inflammation of the middle ear, with accumulation of a thick mucous fluid. Syn: glue ear; mucous otitis.

   mucous o. Mucoid *otitis* media.

   nonsuppurative o. media Those conditions in which fluid present within the middle ear cavity is noninfected, including serous otitis media and mucoid otitis media.

   o. externa Inflammation of the external ear occurring when changes in the skin lining the external auditory meatus allow growth of bacteria or fungi; accompanied by considerable swelling of the canal walls.

   o. media Inflammation of the middle ear.

   purulent o. media Suppurative *otitis* media.

   serous o. media (SOM) Inflammation of the middle ear, with the presence of serous fluid which impedes the movements of the ossicular chain, often resulting in reduced auditory acuity of a conductive nature; usually caused by prolonged blockage of the eustachian tube. Syn: secretory otitis media.

suppurative o. media Condition in which fluid is present in the middle ear and becomes infected (pus formation). Syn: purulent otitis media.

oto- [G. *ous*, ear] Combining form relating to the ear.

otoacoustic emissions (OAE) Sounds generated by the outer hair cells of a normal cochlea which may be either spontaneous or evoked.

   distortion product o. e. (DPOAE) These emissions are elicited by the simultaneous presentation of two tones closely spaced in frequency. A third tone (the distortion product) is produced by the basilar membrane indicating normal outer hair cell function in that region. See also audiometry, electrophysiologic.

   spontaneous o. e. (SOAE) Otoacoustic emissions that occur without external stimulation; consists of energy at one or more frequencies emitted by the normal ear and recorded in the ear canal with a sensitive microphone.

   stimulus-frequency o. e. (SFOAE) Sounds are evoked with a constant pure-tone stimulus presented at a low intensity level, and usually change slowly across a region of frequencies.

   transient evoked o. e. (TEOAE) Stimuli are evoked with clicks or tone bursts that activate the cochlea simultaneously from the basal to the apical regions of the basilar membrane. Their exact prevalence is unknown.

otocup (ō′tō-kəp) In audiology, an earphone enclosure used in audiological evaluations which allows the standard cushion to fit against the auricle of the ear; also helps attenuate ambient noise through an outer plastic case with a conforming seal that fits around the edge of the case and contacts the side of the head; used to supplement sound-treated test booths to reduce background noise. See also hearing protection devices.

otolaryngologist (ō′tō-lär-iŋ-gol′ə-jist) Physician specializing in otolaryngology.

otolaryngology (ō′tō-lär-iŋ-gol′ə-jē) [oto- + G. *larynx*, larynx + *logos*, discourse] Medical science and specialty concerned with diseases of the ear and larynx, often including disorders of the upper respiratory tract and many of the head, neck, and esophagus; commonly referred to as ear, nose, and throat (ENT). Syn: otorhinolaryngology.

otological screening See screening *audiometry*.

otology (ō-tol′ə-jē) [oto- + G. *logos*, study, discourse] Branch of medical science concerned with the study, diagnosis, and treatment of diseases of the ear and related structures.

-otomy [G. *tomē*, incision] Suffix denoting incision or cutting into.

otorhinolaryngology (ō′tō-rī′nō-lär-iŋ-gol′ ə-jē) [oto- + G. *rhis*, nose + *larynx*, larynx + *logos*, study, discourse] Otolaryngology.

otosclerosis (ō′tō-sklə-rō′sis) [oto- + G. *sklērosis*, hardening] Formation of spongy bone affecting the middle ear capsule, around the stapes and oval window; the weblike bone impedes the movement of the stapes into the oval window and results in a gradual loss of hearing; may be surgically corrected. The cause is unknown, but an inherited predisposition seems to be present.

otoscope (ō′tə-skōp) [oto- + G. *skopeō*, to view] Instrument for visual examination of the external ear canal and tympanic membrane.

otoscopy (ō-tos′kə-pē) [See otoscope] Inspection of the ear, especially the tympanic membrane, as with an otoscope.

ototoxic (ō-tō-toks′ik) [oto- + G. *toxikon*, poison] Poisonous to the ear; use of some drugs may cause a severe hearing loss or toxic deafness.

out of phase See phase.

outer ear See external *ear*.

output Power, energy, or sound pressure released by an instrument after the input signal has been increased or changed by electronic circuits. See also expressive *language*.

  HAIC o. Average maximum acoustic output at 500, 1000, and 2000 Hz (former standard); usually applies to a hearing aid.

  high-frequency average saturation sound pressure level (HF average SSPL 90) Average of 1000, 1600, and 2500 Hz values of saturation sound pressure level for 90-dB input sound pressure level; the current ANSI standard for measuring average output, replacing HAIC output.

  maximum acoustic o. Greatest amount of sound energy that can be provided by an amplifier regardless of the intensity of the original signal fed into it. Syn: maximum power output; saturation output; saturation sound pressure level. See also HAIC *output*.

  maximum power o. (MPO) Maximum acoustic *output*.

  saturation o. Maximum acoustic *output*.

  saturation sound pressure level Maximum acoustic *output*.

oval window See under middle *ear*.

overall sound level Total acoustic pressure when more than one frequency is present.

overbite See under teeth malpositions.

overeruption (ō′ver-i-rəp′shən) Projection of a tooth beyond the normal line of occlusion.

overextension (ō′ver-eks-ten′shən) **1.** Movement of a limb or any of its segments beyond what is normal or intended; *e.g.*, reaching beyond or to the side of an object when attempting to pick it up. Syn: overflow. **2.** In language, the extended use and often misapplication of a single word to represent a variety of objects; commonly found in a child's language as a result of his or her using less than the full set of features as the meaning of the same word; *e.g.*, use of *doggie* for all four-legged animals.

overflow Overextension (1).

overjet See under teeth malpositions.

overlapping Beginning of a second response before the first is completed. See also assimilation.

overlearning Practice or repetition of a skill past the point necessary for retention or recall; permits the response to become automatic or internalized, and permits a shift from the representational level (conscious or cognitive) to the subconscious or habitual level; *e.g.*, syntax and language must be automatic if they are to be used effectively.

overload **1.** Distortion of a sound signal by the ear when the intensity of the sound exceeds the limit of its mechanism. **2.** Distortion of a sound through an amplifier because of an input intensity greater than the amplifier can tolerate.

overmasking See under masking.

overrecruitment Hyperrecruitment. See under recruitment.

overrestriction (ō′vėr-ri-strik′shən) Underextension.

overstatement See under figure of speech.

overt (ō′vėrt) Clearly visible or audible, as opposed to covert.

overtone **1.** Multiple of a fundamental frequency in which the first overtone is the second harmonic. **2.** Pattern of distribution of energy of a sound wave among various frequencies that comprises the total complex of a tone; determines the quality of a tone. Its structure is a physically measurable aspect of tone. See also harmonics.

overt response See under response.

pain [L. *poena*, fine, penalty] Impression on the sensory nerves causing discomfort, distress, or agony; may be organic or psychogenic.

pain threshold *Threshold* of discomfort.

paired associate learning Method of teaching which uses a series of word pairs, with the first member of each pair being a stimulus and the second member a response; when the subject sees the stimulus word, he attempts to respond with the associated response word; *e.g.*, *th*an-*d*an; *r*ed-*b*ed. See also minimal pair.

paired syllables See under syllable.

palatal (pal'ə-təl) Pertaining to the palate.

palatal area See under consonant, place of articulation.

palatal fronting See under substitution, under phonological processes.

palatal insufficiency Velopharyngeal insufficiency.

palatal lift Prosthetic device which forms an upper dental plate in the mouth and extends back to push upward on the soft palate; effective in reducing nasal resonance in cases of palatal paralysis or velopharyngeal insufficiency. See also obturator.

palatal paralysis See under paralysis.

palate (pal'it) [L. *palatum*] **1.** Roof of the mouth; includes the anterior portion (hard palate) and the posterior portion (soft palate or velum). **2.** Structures lying posterior to the incisive foramen. Syn: secondary palate.

> **Muscles of the palate** assist in elevating, depressing, and tensing of the velum and tongue. See *Muscles of the Palate* table.
>
> **cleft p.** See cleft palate.
>
> **hard p.** Bony anterior part of the roof of the mouth.
>
> **primary p.** Prepalate.

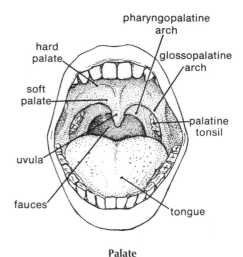

Palate

> **secondary p.** Palate.
>
> **soft p.** Velum.

palatine (pal'ə-tīn) Relating to the palate.

palatine bones See under skull.

palatine raphe See under raphe.

palatine tonsil See under tonsil.

palatization See under substitution, under phonological processes.

palato- [L. *palatum*, palate] Combining form relating to the palate. See also urano-.

palatoglossus muscle See *Muscles of the Palate* table, under palate; *Muscles of the Tongue* table, under tongue.

palatogram (pal'ə-tə-gram) [palate- + G. *gramma*, a drawing] Impressions made by the tongue on the artificial palate in palatography.

palatography (pal-ə-tog'rə-fē) (palato- + G. *graphō*, to record] Procedure for determining tongue placement and height by placing an artificial palate covered with chalk or powder in the mouth; after the desired sound or group of sounds has been pronounced,

MUSCLES OF THE PALATE

Muscle	Origin	Insertion	Innervation	Function
Glossopalatine or palatoglossus	Inferior surface of soft palate	Side of tongue	Spinal accessory nerve (cranial nerve XI) via pharyngeal plexus	Elevates tongue and constricts anterior fauces; draws side of soft palate down
Levator veli palatini	Apex of petrous part of temporal bone and cartilaginous part of eustachian tube	Aponeurosis of soft palate	Spinal accessory nerve (cranial nerve XI) via pharyngeal plexus	Raises uvula
Pharyngopalatinus or palatopharyngeus	Soft palate	Aponeurosis of pharynx and posterior border of thyroid cartilage	Spinal accessory nerve (cranial nerve XI) via pharyngeal plexus	Elevates pharynx and larynx; depresses soft palate
Tensor veli palatini	Scaphoid fossa; spine of sphenoid bone; cartilaginous part of eustachian tube	Aponeurosis of soft palate	Mandibular nerve of trigeminal nerve (cranial nerve V)	Tenses soft palate; opens eustachian tube
Uvular	Posterior nasal spine	Aponeurosis of soft palate	Spinal accessory nerve (cranial nerve XI) via pharyngeal plexus	Raises uvula; shortens uvula

the artificial palate is removed and a determination can be made concerning which parts have been touched by the tongue.

palatopharyngeal (pal'ə-tō-fə-rin'jē-əl) [palato- + G. *pharynx*, pharynx] Velopharyngeal.

palatopharyngeus muscle See *Muscles of the Palate* table, under palate.

palilalia (pa-li-lā'lē-ə) [G. *palin*, again + *lalia*, talking] Speech disorder in which a word, phrase, or sentence may be repeated several times with increasing rapidity and decreasing distinctness, so that the latter part of the utterance may become almost inaudible; often occurs in association with postencephalic Parkinson's disease and pseudobulbar palsy. Syn: paliphrasia.

paliphrasia (pa-li-frā'zē-ə) [G. *palin*, again + *phrasis*, speaking] Palilalia.

palpate (pal'pāt) [L. *palpatus*, touched, stroked] **1.** To obtain knowledge of a structure from touch and pressure. **2.** To stimulate action of a structure by touch or pressure.

palsy (päl'zē) [corruption of paralysis] Paralysis, often with a connotation of partial paralysis (paresis).

panendoscope (pan-en'də-skōp) [G. *pan*, all + *endon*, within + *skopeō*, to view] Instrument, resembling a penlight, which can be inserted directly into a patient's mouth to allow a view of the movement of the velum and the posterior pharyngeal wall; it also can be rotated to afford a view of lateral wall movement.

panendoscopy (pan-en-dos'kə-pē) Examination of the velum and posterior pharyngeal wall with a panendoscope.

papilloma, pl. **papillomas, papillo-**

mata (pa-pi-lō′mə, -məz, -mä′tə) [L. *papilla*, nipple + G. *-oma*, tumor] Benign tumor derived from epithelium; may arise from skin, mucous membrane, or glandular ducts. See also under laryngeal anomaly.

papillomatosis (pap′ə-lō-mə-tō′sis) Development of multiple papillomas.

> **juvenile p.** Papillomas of the larynx in children. See papilloma, under laryngeal anomaly.

para- [G. alongside of, near] **1.** Prefix denoting beside, along with, or involvement of two like parts. **2.** Prefix denoting a departure from the normal.

paracentesis (par′ə-sen-tē′sis) [para- + G. *kentēsis*, puncture] **1.** Surgical technique to remove fluid from a cavity. **2.** Myringotomy.

paracusis (par-ə-ku′sis) [para- + G. *akousis*, hearing] Any abnormality in the sense of hearing.

> **false p.** *Paracusis* willisi.
>
> **p. localis** Inability to determine the direction of a sound; usually occurs with unilateral hearing impairments or when the ears hear unequally.
>
> **p. willisi** or **Willis′ p.** [T. Willis, Eng. physician, 1621–1675] Auditory phenomena in which an individual with a conductive hearing loss hears speech better in a noisy environment. Syn: false paracusis.

paradigm (par′ə-dim) [L. *paradigma*, pattern] **1.** An example to be emulated; a model or design. **2.** In grammar, a set of related words containing a common base and all the affixes that may be attached to it; a complete set of all the various conjugational or declensional forms of a word; *e.g.*, go, gone, goes; man, man's, men, men's, manly. **3.** In phonemics, the listing of all the phonemes of a language in series, orders, and isolated elements.

paradigmatic (par-ə-dig-mat′ik) Pertaining to a paradigm.

paradigmatic response See under response.

paradigmatic shift Developmental shift that occurs at about 7 years of age in word-association tasks; younger children give syntagmatic responses (place the stimulus word into a syntactic context), whereas individuals over 7 years old give paradigmatic responses (response words are from the same category as the stimulus word).

paradigmatic word See under word.

paralalia (par-ə-lā′lē-ə) [para- G. *lalia*, talking] Substitution of one speech sound for another; occasionally used to mean "any speech disorder." See also articulation disorder.

paralanguage (par-ə-laŋ′gwij) Features that are not part of the formal language system but that are important in the comprehension and expression of that system; includes body postures, facial expressions, hand gestures, stress, intonation, volume, and phrasing. Syn: paralinguistics.

paralinguistics (par′ə-liŋ-gwis′tiks) Paralanguage.

parallel distribution See under distribution.

parallel talk In speech: **1.** Technique in which the clinician provides a verbal account of what the client is doing, perceiving, or probably feeling. **2.** Exact repetition by the clinician of what is said by the client.

paralysis, pl. paralyses (pə-ral′i-sis, -sēz) [G. fr. para- + *lysis*, loosening] Loss or impairment of muscle power or function, or of sensation (anesthesia), due to lesions of the neural or muscular mechanism.

> **abductor p.** See under laryngeal motor *paralysis*.
>
> **adductor p.** See under laryngeal motor *paralysis*.
>
> **Bell's p.** See Bell's palsy.
>
> **bilateral abductor p.** See abductor paralysis, under laryngeal motor *paralysis*.
>
> **bilateral adductor p.** See adductor paralysis, under laryngeal motor *paralysis*.

bilateral laryngeal p. Impairment of both vocal folds.

bulbar p. Impairment and atrophy of the muscles of the lips, tongue, mouth, pharynx, and larynx as a result of lesions in the motor centers of the medulla oblongata. Syn: labioglossopharyngeal or labioglossolaryngeal paralysis.

cricothyroid p. See under laryngeal *paralysis.*

facial p. Impairment of the facial and lip muscles, usually the result of injury to the facial nerve (cranial nerve VII); may be bilateral or unilateral.

flaccid p. Loss of tonus and absence of reflexes in the affected parts producing a weak, flabby, and relaxed condition, generally the result of superior laryngeal nerve impairment. *Cf.* spastic *paralysis.*

labioglossolaryngeal or **labioglossopharyngeal p.** Bulbar *paralysis.*

laryngeal p. Loss or impairment of muscle function, or of sensation (anesthesia), in the larynx; may be motor or sensory.

laryngeal motor p. Loss of laryngeal movements; may follow lesions of the upper motor neurons; the recurrent laryngeal nerve is primarily involved, and the involvement may be abductor, adductor, or tensor.

> **Abductor p.** Inability to separate the vocal folds due to the lack of motor impulses normally transmitted by the recurrent laryngeal nerve; it may involve one or both folds. In **bilateral abductor paralysis,** both vocal folds remain fixed in the midline position and cannot be abducted (opened); in **unilateral abductor paralysis,** the involved vocal fold remains fixed in a central adducted (closed) position while the other fold functions normally.

> **Adductor p.** Inability to bring together the vocal folds as a result of

involvement of the recurrent laryngeal nerve; it may involve one or both folds. In **bilateral adductor paralysis,** both vocal folds are fixed in an abducted (open) position and cannot be adducted (closed), thus impairing phonation; in **unilateral adductor paralysis,** one vocal fold functions normally and reaches the midline while the involved fold remains in a fixed position.

> **Cricothyroid p.** Paralysis in which vocal fold tension is impaired, and the folds elongate in phonation.

laryngeal sensory p. Impairment or loss of sensation and reflex function in the larynx; often caused by impairment of the trunk or internal branch of the superior laryngeal nerve.

> **Laryngeal anesthesia** Insensibility to pain or the absence of sensation in the larynx.

> **Laryngeal hyperesthesia** Increased or excessive sensitivity of the larynx.

> **Laryngeal paresthesia** Condition in which sensations such as prickling or heat are felt in the larynx.

lingual p. Impairment of the mobility of the tongue, usually the consequence of injury to the hypoglossus nerve (cranial nerve XII); may be bilateral or unilateral.

myopathic p. Impairment of muscular function as the result of disease; *e.g.,* of the intrinsic laryngeal muscles.

palatal p. Impairment of the mobility of the soft palate, usually as a result of damage to the vagus nerve (cranial nerve X).

pseudobulbar p. Impaired swallowing, articulation, and chewing movements as a result of disease of both hemispheres of the brain; resembles bulbar paralysis as the result of lesions of the medulla oblongata.

pseudolaryngeal p. Loss of voice, which is psychogenic in nature. See also aphonia, under voice disorders of phonation.

spastic p. Disability marked by rigidity and heightened tendon reflexes. *Cf.* flaccid *paralysis.*

unilateral abductor p. See abductor paralysis, under laryngeal motor *paralysis.*

unilateral adductor p. See adductor paralysis, under laryngeal motor *paralysis.*

unilateral p. Paralysis affecting only one side; *e.g.*, muscles attached to the arytenoid cartilage on one side.

vocal fold p. Inability of one or both vocal folds to function because of lack of innervation to particular intrinsic muscles of the larynx; may be of central or peripheral nervous system origin, but is often the result of injury to the neck, affecting the recurrent laryngeal nerve. See also laryngeal *paralysis.*

paramedical (par-â-med'i-kəl) Having some connection with or relation to the science or practice of medicine; adjunctive to the practice of medicine in the maintenance or restoration of health and normal functioning, such as physical, occupational, and speech therapy.

parameter (pə-ram'ətėr) [para- + G. *metron*, measure] **1.** Dimensions; any given constant or element whose values characterize one or more of the variables entering into a system of expressions, functions, etc.; *e.g.*, pitch and volume are dimensions of sound. **2.** Quantity that describes a statistical population.

paranoia (par-ə-noi'ə) [G. derangement, madness] Mental disorder characterized by systematized delusions, often persecutory or abusive in nature, but usually without gross distortion of personality; paranoics typically feel that they are the special object of persecution or abuse by others as a result of the latter's envy or jealousy.

paranoid reaction See under reaction.

paraphasia (par-ə-fā'zē-ə, -fā'zhə) [para- + G. *phasis*, speech] **1.** Any error of commission modifying a specific word (sound and morpheme substitution) or of word substitution in the spoken or written production of a speaker or writer. **2.** Condition characterized by fluent utterance of speech sounds in which the production of unintended syllables, words, or phrases are prominent during the effort to speak.

extended jargon p. Paraphasia in which speech flows smoothly, but neologisms and senseless words are prominent; the speaker is generally unaware of his errors.

literal p. Paraphasia in which the production of sounds and syllables are properly articulated but which may be extraneous, transposed, or substituted; some phonemic features, usually the vowels and the number of syllables of the intended words, are preserved.

verbal p. Unintended substitution of one word for another; the substituted word is often in the same class as the intended word; *e.g.*, *mother* for *daughter; cat* for *dog.*

paraplegia (par-ə-plē'jē-ə) [para- + G. *plēgē*, a stroke] Paralysis of both legs, and generally the lower trunk, but without involvement of the arms. *Cf.* diplegia; hemiplegia; monoplegia; quadriplegia; triplegia.

parasigmatism (par-ə-sig'mə-ti-zəm) [para- + G. *sigma*, letter S] Lisp.

paradoxic vocal cord dysfunction See under voice disorders of phonation.

parenthetical expression Any word, phrase, or clause which does not vitally modify the sentence or which is out of its normal order in the sentence; it does not specifically belong to the words to which it is adjacent and so is set off by commas; *e.g.*, Rudolf, the reindeer with the red nose, led the parade. Types include absolute constructions, appositives, and nonrestrictive modifiers.

paresis (pə-rē'sis) [G. a slackening] Partial or incomplete paralysis. See also palsy; paralysis.

paresthesia (par-es-thē′zē-ə, -thē′zhə) [para + G. *aisthēsis*, sensation] Abnormal spontaneous sensation, such as of prickling, tingling, or burning.
  laryngeal p. See under laryngeal sensory *paralysis.*

parietal (pə-rī′i-təl) [L. *parietes*, pl. of *paries*, wall] Relating to the wall of any cavity.

parietal bones See under skull.

parietal lobe See under cerebrum, under brain.

Parkinson's disease [J. Parkinson, Eng. physician, 1755–1824] Degenerative and progressive nervous system disease characterized by tremors, mask-like face, slowing of voluntary movements, peculiar posture, creeping type of walk, and general muscular weakness. Syn: parkinsonism.

parkinsonian dysarthria See under dysarthria.

parkinsonism (par′kin-sən-izm) Parkinson's disease.

partial cleft palate Incomplete *cleft palate.*

partial laryngectomy hemilaryngectomy.

partial recruitment See under recruitment.

partial reinforcement See under reinforcement.

partial tone See under tone.

participle See verbal, under parts of speech.

particle (pär′ti-kəl) [L. *particula*, dim. of *pars*, part] **1.** Minute portion of matter. **2.** In linguistics, a function word (such as up, down, on, off, in, out, over, under) that is associated with a verb. To distinguish between a verb particle and a preposition, transpose the word to the right of the object noun: if it is a particle, the sentence will remain grammatical; if it is a preposition, the sentence will be ungrammatical; *e.g.*, he *jumped over* the fence; he *jumped* the fence *over.*

particle velocity See under velocity.

particular grammar See under grammar.

parts of speech System of classifying words into grammatical forms and of explaining their general usage in sentences; the schemes separate words into categories and seek to describe the operations of a language. *Cf.* word classes.

  adjective In transformational and traditional grammars, a word or phrase used to modify (describe or make more definite) a noun or pronoun; may tell what kind (*blue* eyes), which one (*this* man), or how many (*several* players). See also article; comparison; determiner; modifier; qualifier; quantifier.

  adverb In transformational and traditional grammars, a word or phrase used to modify a verb, adjective, or another adverb; may tell how (they walked *slowly*), when (they walked *immediately*), where (they walked *there*), or to what extent (they walked *far*). See also comparison; modifier; qualifier.

  agenitive (ə-jen′i-tiv) In case grammar, typically an animate perceived as the instigator of action; *e.g., John* opened the door; the door was opened by *John.*

  conjunction (kən-juŋk′shən) or **conjoiner** (kən-join′ér) In transformational and traditional grammars, a word which serves to join two or more grammatical units; may join units which are either equal (and, but) or unequal (because, if) in construction; some must appear in pairs (either . . . or, not only . . . but also).

  dative (dā′tiv) **1.** In case grammar, the animate affected by the state or action named by the verb; *e.g., Adam* sees John; Bob gave the book to *Bill.* **2.** Recipient of action.

  factitive (fak′tə-tiv) In case grammar, the object or being resulting from the state or action named by the verb; *e.g.*, the boy created a *statue;* Bill built a *chair.*

gerund See under verbal (below).

infinitive See under verbal (below).

instrumental (in-strə-men′tal) In case grammar, the inanimate force or object causally involved in the state or action named by the verb; *e.g.*, the *key* opened the lock; he opened the lock with the *key*.

interjection (in-tėr-jek′shən) In transformational and traditional grammars, a word used near the beginning of a sentence to express emotion and which has no grammatical relation to other words in the sentence; usually an exclamatory word or phrase generally followed by an exclamation mark; *e.g.*, "ouch!," "my goodness!" See also expletive.

locative (lō′kə-tiv) In case grammar, the location or spatial orientation of the state or action named by the verb; *e.g.*, the hat is on the *chair; Chicago* is windy.

noun In transformational and traditional grammars, a word used to name a person (Abraham Lincoln), place (New York), thing (chair), idea (beauty), or collection (the class); may be singular or plural (cat-cats, man-men), show possession (cat's-cats', man's-men's), and be classified as to whether it is masculine (boy), feminine (girl), neuter (table), animate (cow), or inanimate (car).

objective (ob-jek′tiv) In case grammar, the semantically most neutral case; anything representable by a noun whose role in the state or action named by the verb depends on the meaning of the verb itself; *e.g.*, John sees *Mary;* the *hat* is on the table; Bill opened the *door.*

open In pivot grammar, the name assigned to a class of words used by children at the two-word stage of linguistic development; typified by many words infrequently used; usually includes nouns, verbs, and sometimes adjectives. See also pivot *grammar.*

participle See under verbal (below).

pivot (piv′ət) In pivot grammar, the name assigned to a class of words used by children at the two-word stage of linguistic development; typified by a small number of words each frequently used. See also pivot *grammar.*

preposition (pre-pa-zi′shən) In transformational and traditional grammars, a word used to show the relation of a noun or pronoun to some other word in the sentence; it may modify nouns, adjectives, or adverbs; in English, 36 are accepted as being the most commonly used; *e.g.*, in, on, under, between, for, to.

pronoun (prō′noun) In transformational and traditional grammar, a word that takes the place of a noun or any word used as a noun; it may refer to a person or thing and its possession (I, mine, we, ours), intensify or reflect meaning (myself, themselves), introduce or join clauses (who, that, which), introduce questions (whose, which, what), point out persons or things (this, that, these, those), or refer to a general group or a quantity (all, someone, neither, one). See also case.

    Exophoric or **anaphoric pronoun** is a pronoun which occurs in relative proximity to the noun to which it refers and which was previously mentioned in a particular sentence; *e.g.*, I wrote with the pencil and broke *it.*

verb 1. In transformational and traditional grammar, a word that expresses action (play, run) or helps make a statement (am, is, was, seem) performed by or to the subject or noun phrase of a sentence. Various endings and forms indicate number of persons, voice, mood, aspect, and tense; some connect the noun phrase to the verb phrase, others are complete without any direct connection with the subject. **2.** In case grammar, although recognized, little or no elaboration is made to distinguish among the various types of verbs as is done in transformational or traditional grammars. For types of verb, see specific term. See also aspect; mood; tense; voice.

verbal (vėr′bəl) In transformational grammar, although not a separate part of speech, a special form of verb which functions as another part of speech, depending on the ending and use in the sentence; sometimes referred to as a secondary verb.

 Gerund (jėr′ənd) is a verb form ending in *ing* that may be used as a noun; *e.g.*, *swinging* is fun.

 Infinitive (in-fin′ə-tiv) is a verb form preceded by the word *to* which may be used as an adjective (there is money *to spend*), noun (*to fight* is your right), or adverb (he went home *to rest*).

 Participle (pär′tə-si-pəl) is a verb form used as an adjective; (*e.g.*, the *swaying* branch broke; the *broken* foot hurts).

Passavant's bar or **cushion** or **pad** [P. G. Passavant, Ger. physician, 1815–1893] Bulging of the posterior pharyngeal wall produced by the contraction of the overlapping superior and middle constrictors of the pharynx; in cleft palate individuals, this characteristic may aid in reducing nasal resonance.

pass-band filter Band-pass *filter.*

passive bilingualism See under bilingualism.

passive voice See voice.

past perfect progressive tense See progressive *tense.*

past perfect tense See under tense.

pathologic, pathological (path-ə-loj′ik, -i-kəl) **1.** Diseased; resulting from disease. **2.** Relating to pathology.

pathologist (pə-thol′ə-jist) Physician specializing in one or more of the subspecialties of pathology; practice is primarily in the laboratory, serving as a consultant to colleagues in the clinical specialties, performing postmortem studies, and engaging in research.

pathology (pə-thol′ə-jē) [G. *pathos*, suffering + *logos*, discourse, study] Medical science and specialty concerned with the nature of disease and the structural and functional changes that result from disease processes.

Patterned Elicitation Syntax Screening Test (PESST) See *Language Tests and Procedures* in appendices.

patterning 1. Imitating a sample or model. **2.** Form of drill which uses an entire utterance or specific linguistic structure as an aid in speech or language training; *e.g.*, *this is a* boy; *this is a* dog; *this is a* cat. See also modeling.

pavlovian conditioning See classical *conditioning.*

PBK Word Lists See under *Audiometric Tests and Procedures* in appendices.

PB max Highest speech discrimination score for PB words.

PB words Phonetically balanced words.

PDD Pervasive developmental disorder.

PE Pharyngoesophageal (junction or segment).

Peabody Picture Vocabulary Test See *Language Tests and Procedures* in appendices.

peak acoustic gain See under gain.

peak clipping Method of limiting maximum acoustic output of an amplifier, such as a hearing aid, by cutting off the highest intensities whenever they exceed a predetermined maximum output level; results in the elimination of excessive loudness and may give speech a monotonous quality.

Pearson product-moment coefficient of correlation See product moment, under coefficient of correlation.

pectoralis major muscle See *Muscles of Respiration* table, under respiration.

pectoralis minor muscle See *Muscles of Respiration* table, under respiration.

pedagogical grammar See under grammar.

pediatric (pē-dē-at′rik) Relating to pediatrics.

pediatric audiology See under audiology.

pediatrician (pē′dē-a-tri′shan) Physician specializing in pediatrics, especially in the diseases of children.

pediatrics (pē-dē-at′riks) [G. *pais (paid-)*, child + *iatrikos*, relating to medicine] Medical science and specialty concerned with the health, development, and diseases of children.

Pediatric Speech Intelligibility Test (PSI) See *Auditory Tests and Procedures* in appendices.

pedolalia (ped-ō-lā′lē-ə) [G. *pais (paid-)*, child + *lalia*, talking] Infantile perseveration.

PEG Percutaneous endoscopic gastrostomy.

peptic esophagitis See under esophagitis.

perceived noise level (PNdB) Level in dB assigned to a noise by a calculation procedure based on an approximation of subjective evaluations.

percentage (pėr-sen′tij) **1.** Rate per hundred, or proportion in a hundred parts. **2.** Proportion of what is under consideration; a part considered in its quantitative relation to the whole.

percentile (pėr-sen′tīl) Any of one hundred points measured within the range of a plotted variable, each of which denotes that percentage of the total cases lying below it in value; *e.g.*, one, two, three, etc. percent of the cases are in the first, second, third, etc., percentile.

percentile rank Type of converted score that expresses an individual's score relative to his group in percentile points; indicates the percentage of individuals tested who have scored equal to or lower than a specific score; *e.g.*, a percentile rank of 90 (corresponding to a score of 80) means that 90% of the individuals who took the test had a score of 80 or less than 80.

perception (pėr-sep′shən) [L. conception] **1.** Meaningful awareness and affective appreciation of a stimulus, ob-

ject, or situation, which are the result of a complex pattern of stimulation plus the effect of experience and attitude; in contrast to sensation, which is dependent on specific sense organ stimulation. **2.** Process by which people select, organize, and interpret sensory stimulation into a meaningful and coherent picture of the world around them; involves detection, discrimination, identification, and recognition. See also cognition.

    auditory p. 1. Identification, interpretation, or organization of sensory data received through the ear. **2.** Mental awareness of sound. See also *Auditory Tests and Procedures* in appendices.

    cross-modality p. Neurologic process of transferring sensory data received through one input modality to another system within the brain. Syn: intermodal or intersensory transfer; transducing; supramodal perception.

    haptic p. Awareness and interpretation of sensory data received through the tactile and kinesthetic modalities.

    kinesthetic p. Comprehension and awareness of sensory data obtained through body movements and muscle feeling; *e.g.*, positions taken by different parts of the body; bodily feelings of muscular contraction, tension, and relaxation. See also proprioception.

    proprioceptive p. Awareness of sensation of muscles, tendons, and joints.

    supramodal p. Cross-modality *perception.*

    tactile p. Awareness and comprehension of sensory data received through the sense of touch.

    visual p. Awareness and comprehension of visual stimuli.

perceptive hearing loss See sensorineural deafness.

perceptual analysis In acoustics, the description of sound after it has been received and interpreted in terms of pitch, loudness, and quality.

perceptual consistency Ability to accurately perceive the permanent attributes of objects, such as shape, position, and size, in spite of the variability of the impression these objects make on the senses of the observer. See also cognitive development.

perceptual disorder Disturbance involving the interpretation of sensory stimulation.

perceptual distortion Term used by some authorities to refer to peripheral problems related to hearing or vision impairment.

perceptual disturbance Aphasic-like fluctuations in the ability to receive, manipulate, and express language symbols. See also aphasia.

perceptual immaturity Delayed development of perceptual skills; intelligence is presumed to be within normal limits.

perceptually handicapped Denoting individuals who have difficulty in learning because of a disturbance in their perception of sensory stimuli.

perceptual-motor Denoting the interaction of the channels of perception (auditory, visual, kinesthetic, tactile) with motor activity.

perceptual-motor match Process of comparing and integrating sensory data received through the motor system and the sensory data received through perception.

perceptual retardation Intellectual deficiency which affects language performance.

percutaneous endoscopic gastrostomy (PEG) A minor surgical procedure which allows an individual to receive nutrition in a nonoral manner; using a local anesthetic and an endoscope, a tube is percutaneously inserted into the abdomen leading into the stomach or the jejunum. See also feeding.

perfect tense See tense.

performance In linguistics: **1.** Overt expression of competence in the linguistic activities of listening, speaking, reading, and writing. **2.** Linguistic behavior; encoding or decoding speech. **3.** Speaker's actual use of language.

Performance Assessment of Syntax Elicited and Spontaneous (PASES) See *Language Tests and Procedures* in appendices.

performance-intensity function Graph that demonstrates the percentage of words correctly identified during discrimination testing as a function of the intensity level of presentation. Syn: articulation-gain function.

performance objective Statement of desired behavior that specifically identifies and describes in observable, measurable terms what is to be achieved; written in terms of expected outcomes for the learner. Syn: behavioral, instructional, or operational objective.

Elements of performance objective are the factors necessary for the execution of an objective. These include (a) *participant*, the person performing; (b) *actual behavior*, the action; (c) *product*, the result of performance; (d) *conditions*, requirements necessary for correct performance; and (e) *measurement standard*, assessment of the performance (may be objective or subjective).

performance test Test in which the role of language is minimized; the task requires overt motor response other than verbal.

performative Verb that signifies an active process; *e.g.*, marry, promise.

performative pragmatic structures See under pragmatic structures.

perimeter earmold Skeleton *earmold*.

perinatal (păr-i-nā′təl) [G. *peri*, around + L. *natus*, born] Pertaining to or occurring in the period shortly before or after birth.

period (pēr′ē-əd) [G. *periodos*, a way round, cycle] In acoustics: **1.** Length of time for a sound wave to complete one cycle (one complete back and forth movement of a displaced air particle); determines whether a sound will be perceived as a tone or a noise. **2.** Time interval involved in the regular repetition of a cycle of sound. For type of period, see specific term.

periodic (pēr-ē-od'ik) Recurring at intervals of time, whether regular or irregular.

periodicity (pēr-ē-ə-dis'i-tē) [Fr. *périodicité*] Regular recurrence of a wave form in mathematical relationship to the fundamental (harmonics); makes sounds musical.

periodic wave See under wave.

peripheral (pèr-if'èr-əl) Relating to or situated at the periphery.

peripheral dysarthria See under dysarthria.

peripheral masking See under masking.

peripheral nervous system See under nervous system.

periphery (pèr-if'èr-ē) [G. *periphereia*] Outer or external boundary or surface of a part or body, as distinguished from its central or internal regions.

peristalsis A mostly involuntary muscular contraction throughout the entire digestive tract, carrying the bolus (of food) through the system for nutritional extraction.

perlocution (pèr-lō-kyu'shən) [L. *per-*, through + *locutio*, speaking] Effect on a listener which a speaker achieves, such as boredom, discouragement, inspiration, etc. *Cf.* illocution; locution.

permanent teeth See teeth.

permanent threshold shift (PTS) See under threshold shift.

permutation (pèr-myu-tā'shən) [L. *per-*, through + *mutatus*, changed] **1.** Thorough change in character or condition; transformation. **2.** Act or process of changing the lineal order of an ordered set of objects. **3.** In linguistics, a transformation which converts one phrase structure into another; it is accomplished by such operations as substitutions or displacements.

perpetuating factors See etiology.

perseveration (pèr-sev-èr-ā'shən) [L. *perservatus*, persisted] **1.** Tendency to continue an activity, motor or mental, once it has been started and to be unable to modify or stop the activity even though it is acknowledged to have become inappropriate. **2.** Automatic and often involuntary continuation of behavior. **3.** In speech, a prolongation into a succeeding period of life of some habit or function; usually limited to a given age, such as baby talk continued into adulthood. **4.** In stuttering, the continued act of stuttering associated with the stutterer's failure to shift readily from a mental set preceding his difficulty.

perseveration theory See under breakdown theory, under stuttering theories.

person See under deixis.

personality (pèr-sən-al'i-tē) [L. *personalitas*] Totality of one's character traits, attitudes, and habits.

personification See under figure of speech.

person who stutters Term used by some authorities in place of the word "stutterer."

perstimulatory fatigue Auditory adaptation.

pervasive developmental disorders (PDD) Disorders characterized by severe and pervasive impairment in several areas of development: reciprocal social interaction skills, communication skills, or the presence of stereotyped behavior, interests, and activities. The qualitative impairments that define these conditions are distinctly deviant relative to the individual's developmental level or mental age. These disorders contain Autistic Disorder, Rett's Disorder, Childhood Disintegrative Disorder, Asperger's Disorder, and Pervasive Developmental Disorder Not Otherwise Specified. These disorders are usually evident in the first years of life and are often associated with some degree of Mental

Retardation. The Pervasive Developmental Disorders are sometimes observed with a diverse group of other general medical conditions (*e.g.*, chromosomal abnormalities, congenital infections, structural abnormalities of the central nervous system). Although terms like "psychosis" and "childhood schizophrenia" were once used to refer to individuals with these conditions, there is considerable evidence to suggest that the Pervasive Developmental Disorders are distinct from Schizophrenia (however, an individual with Pervasive Developmental Disorder may occasionally later develop Schizophrenia) [DSM-IV]. Syn: autistic spectrum disorder. See also autism or autistic disorder.

pervasive developmental disorders not otherwise specified (including atypical autism) (PDDNOS) This category should be used when there is a severe and pervasive impairment in the development of reciprocal social interaction or verbal and nonverbal communication skills, or when stereotyped behavior, interests, and activities are present, but the criteria are not met for Pervasive Developmental Disorder, Schizophrenia, Schizotypal Personality Disorder, or Avoidant Personality Disorder. For example, this category includes "atypical autism"—presentations that do not meet the criteria for Autistic Disorder because of late age at onset, atypical symptomatology, or subthreshold symptomatology, or all of these [DSM-IV]. See also autism or autistic disorder.

PET Positron emission tomography.

petit mal (pe-tē′məl) [Fr. small sickness] Type of epileptic seizure activity characterized by a loss of consciousness for only brief periods of time, resulting in staring and loss of continuity in what one was doing or saying, but not falling or convulsing.

PE tube Pressure equalization tube.

PFAGH *P*enalty, *f*rustration, *a*nxiety, *g*uilt, and *h*ostility associated with stuttering [Van Riper].

PGSR Psychogalvanic skin response.

PGSRA Psychogalvanic skin response audiometry.

phantom speech See under speech.

pharyng-, pharyngo- Combining form relating to the pharynx.

pharyngeal (fə-rin′jē-al -rin′jəl) Relating to the pharynx.

pharyngeal flap Surgical procedure to aid in achieving velopharyngeal closure; a flap of skin is used to close most of the opening between the velum and the nasopharynx.

pharyngeal raphe See under raphe.

pharyngeal reflex See under reflex.

pharyngeal resonance See cul de sac under voice disorders of resonance.

pharyngeal speech See under alaryngeal *speech*.

pharyngeal tonsil See under tonsil.

pharynges (fə-rin′jēz) Plural of pharynx.

pharyngitis (făr-in-jī′tis) [pharyng- + G. *-itis*, inflammation] Inflammation of the pharynx.

pharyngoesophageal (PE) junction or **segment** Sphincter-like muscle located between the laryngopharynx and the esophagus; considered to be composed of the cricopharyngeal part of the inferior pharyngeal constrictor muscle, although some authorities include fibers from the inferior pharyngeal constrictor muscle and the superior esophageal sphincter. See also neoglottis.

pharyngopalatine arch See fauces.

pharyngopalatinus muscle See *Muscles of the Palate* table, under palate.

pharyngoplasty (fə-riŋ′gō-plas-tē, -rin′-jō-) [pharyngo- + G. *plassō*, to form] Plastic surgery of the pharynx.

pharyngostomy See under feeding, nonoral.

pharynx, pl. pharynges (făr′iŋks, fə-rin′-jēz) [G. pharynx] **1.** Irregular tubular space, considered to be part of the respiratory and alimentary tracts, which

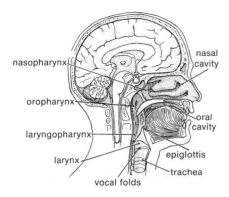

nasopharynx

oropharynx

laryngopharynx

larynx

vocal folds

nasal cavity

oral cavity

epiglottis

trachea

Pharynx

Lateral view of the head showing the nasopharynx, oropharynx, and laryngopharynx in relation to other structures.

extends from the nasal cavities to the esophagus and which is also continuous with the larynx, mouth, and eustachian tubes; in its lower two thirds it is capable of considerable change of dimension from front to back and from side to side, a factor that contributes to the act of swallowing and influences vocal resonance. It is considered to be the principal resonator of the human voice. It is divided into three sections: **laryngopharynx** (hypopharynx), extending from the level of the hyoid bone to the level of the inferior border of the cricoid cartilage where it is continuous with the esophagus; **nasopharynx,** located above the level of the soft palate and opening anteriorly into the nasal cavity; and **oropharynx,** extending from the level of the soft palate to the level of the hyoid bone and opening through the fauces into the oral cavity. **2.** Commonly referred to as the throat.

    Muscles of the pharynx alter the size and shape of the pharyngeal cavity as part of the act of swallowing. See *Muscles of the Pharynx* table.

phase (fāz) In acoustics, the time relationship between two or more pure tones occurring simultaneously.

MUSCLES OF THE PHARYNX				
Muscle	*Origin*	*Insertion*	*Innervation*	*Function*
Inferior pharyngeal constrictor	Oblique line of thyroid cartilage; side of cricoid cartilage	Median raphe of posterior wall of pharynx	Spinal accessory nerve (cranial nerve XI) via pharyngeal plexus; laryngeal branches of vagus nerve (cranial nerve X)	Constricts pharynx
Middle pharyngeal constrictor	Stylohyoid ligament and lesser cornu of hyoid bone	Median raphe of pharynx	Spinal accessory nerve (cranial nerve XI) via pharyngeal plexus	Constricts pharynx
Superior pharyngeal constrictor	Medial pterygoid lamina, pterygomandibular raphe, and mylohyoid line of mandible	Pharyngeal tubercle of occiput and median raphe of pharynx	Spinal accessory nerve (cranial nerve XI) via pharyngeal plexus	Constricts pharynx
Salpingo-pharyngeus	Cartilaginous end of eustachian tube orifice	Posterior part of pharyngopalatinus	Pharyngeal plexus	Narrows fauces and opens eustachian tube
Stylopharyngeus	Root of styloid process	Lateral wall of pharynx and thyroid cartilage	Glossopharyngeal nerve (cranial nerve IX)	Raises pharynx and larynx

In phase refers to two tones of the same frequency and intensity produced so that their periods of compression and rarefaction agree exactly; these combine into a tone with twice the amplitude of either one alone.

Opposite phase or **out of phase** refers to two sound pressure waves which tend to cancel each other at certain points, resulting in zero amplitude (no sound).

phases of stuttering See stuttering phases.

philtrum, pl. **philtra** (fil′trəm, -trə) [L. fr. G. *philtron*] Depression on the surface of the upper lip immediately below the nasal septum.

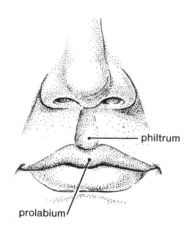

Philtrum

phobia (fō′bē-ə) [G. *phobos*, fear] Excessive and objectively unwarranted dread or fear of some particular object or situation.

phon (fon) In acoustics: **1.** Unit for measuring the loudness level of a sound in comparison with a 1000-Hz tone; the loudness level in phons is numerically equal to the sound pressure level of the 1000-Hz tone, while the sound pressure level at other frequencies will vary for the same number of phons. **2.** Unit of subjective loudness based on the observer's own value judgment;

phon and decibel values differ except at a reference of 1000 Hz where they are identical.

phon- [G. *phonē*, sound, voice] Combining form relating to sound, speech, or voice sounds.

phonagnosia See under agnosia.

phonasthenia (fō-nəs-thē′nē-ə) [phon- + G. *aisthenia*, weakness] Voice fatigue. See under voice disorders of phonation.

phonation (fō-nā′shən) [G. *phonē*, voice] **1.** Physiologic process whereby the energy of moving air in the vocal tract is transformed into acoustic energy within the larynx. **2.** Production of voiced sound by means of vocal fold vibration.

    dysrhythmic p. A type of phonation which occurs only within words. Disturbances or distortions of the so-called normal rhythm or flow of speech, and may or may not be accompanied by tension; may be attributable to a prolonged sound, an accent or timing which is notably unusual, an improper stress, or a break in pitch or voicing.

    hypervalvular p. **1.** Use of excessive tension in the larynx during vocal fold approximation; the closed portion of the vibratory cycle is given an increased amount of time. **2.** Nasal resonance of vowel sounds during speech. See also hypernasality, under voice disorders of resonance.

    reverse p. Vocalizing on inhalation.

    ventricular p. See under voice disorders of phonation.

phonation break Aphonic episode.

phone (fōn) [G. *phonē*, voice sound] Single speech sound represented by a single symbol in a phonetic system; *e.g.*, /ʃ/ = sh.

phoneme (fō′nēm) [G. *phōnēma*, voice] **1.** Group or family of closely related speech sounds, all of which have the same distinctive acoustic characteristics in spite of their differences; each phoneme corresponds roughly to one of the symbols in the phonetic alphabet; *e.g.*, p = /p/. **2.** Shortest arbitrary unit of sound in a given language that can be recognized as being distinct from other sounds in the language. **3.** Class of sounds which are phonetically similar and show certain characteristic patterns of distribution (free variation or complementary distribution) in the language or dialect under consideration. See also consonant; distinctive features; vowel.

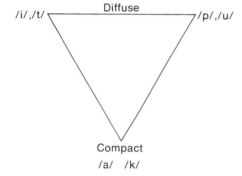

Compact and Diffuse Phonemes

acute p. Sound produced with a concentration of energy in the upper frequencies of the spectrum; *e.g.*, /i/ in s*ea*t.

back p. Phoneme produced in the back of the oral cavity; *e.g.*, /j/, /tʃ/, /ʤ/, /ʃ/, /ʒ/, /k/, /g/, /ŋ/, /h/, /u/, /ʊ/, /o/, /ɔ/, /a/.

compact p. Sound produced with a high concentration of energy in a relatively narrow, central region of the spectrum; *e.g.*, /a/ in f*a*ther; /k/ in *k*eep.

diffuse p. Sound produced in a relatively wide region of the spectrum; *e.g.*, /i/ in *ea*t; /u/ in n*ew*.

front p. Phoneme produced in the front of the oral cavity; *e.g.*, /p/, /b/, /m/, /w/, /f/, /v/, /θ/, /ð/, /t /, /d/, /n/, /s/, /z/, /r/, /l/, /i/, /ɪ/, /e/, /ɛ/, /æ/.

grave p. Sound showing a concentration of energy in the lower fre-

quencies of the spectrum; *e.g.*, /u/ in bl*ew*.

lax p., lenis p. Sound articulated with little muscular tension; *e.g.*, /ɛ/ in b*e*d. See also lax or lenis *consonant.*

segmental p.'s Manner in which the phones of speech are sorted; *e.g.*, into sound groups such as consonants and vowels.

suprasegmental p.'s Features such as pitch, stress, intonation, and juncture which affect more than a single consonant or vowel; often add meaning to an utterance; *e.g.*, He bought that. He bought *that*! Syn: prosodeme.

tense p. Sound produced with great muscular tension; *e.g.*, /i/ in s*ea*t; /u/ in f*oo*d.

phonemic (fō-nēm′ik) Relating to phonemes.

phonemic analysis Sound analysis.

phonemic articulation error See under articulation error.

phonemic regression Loss of the ability to understand speech in spite of relatively good peripheral hearing; a phenomenon often seen in elderly individuals.

phonemics (fō-nēm′iks) [G. *phonē*, voice sound] Study of the sound system of a language.

phonemic synthesis Auditory synthesis.

phonemic transcription See under transcription.

phonetic (fō-net′ik) [G. *phōnētikos*] Relating to speech or to the voice.

Phonetically Balanced Kindergarten Word Lists See *Auditory Tests and Procedures* in appendices.

phonetically balanced words (PB words)- Monosyllabic words, equal in stress, used in audiometric evaluations to determine speech discrimination abilities; *e.g.*, dad; hunt; twins.

phonetic alphabet See International Phonetic *Alphabet.*

phonetic analysis See under phonological analysis.

phonetic articulation error See under articulation error.

phonetic assembly The ability of a reader to decode a word by associating its letters with an internal phonologic system.

phonetic context Environment in which a sound occurs; may affect its production; *e.g.*, /r/ is surrounded by the vowels /ɛ/ and /ə/ in carrot. See also assimilation.

phonetic features Distinctive and nondistinctive elements of a sound. See also distinctive features.

phonetician (fo-nə-tish′ən) One who specializes in phonetics and uses knowledge of phonetics to understand the systemic classification of speech sounds of the various languages of the world.

phonetic inventory One's repertoire of speech sounds.

phonetic placement Method of correcting articulation problems which emphasizes the correct positioning of the articulators prior to the production of the specific speech sounds; *e.g.*, /θ/ = tongue between the teeth and blow.

phonetic power Distance a speech sound will "carry" and still be identifiable, as determined by its energy; *e.g.*, /b/ will be heard at a greater distance than /p/.

phonetics (fō-net′iks) **1.** Science concerned with the production and perception of speech sounds; involves the description and classification of speech sounds relative to a set of standardized sounds, such as the cardinal vowels and the phonetic alphabet. **2.** Study of the sounds of language in terms of their physical and articulatory characteristics.

    acoustic p. Study of speech sounds as they are perceived by the ear of the listener, and of the sound waves produced when they are uttered; uses electrical or mechanical equipment to register speech as sound waves and provides objective information about sounds.

    applied p. Use of findings in phonetic research for the development of acceptable and effective speech.

    articulatory p. Study of the sounds in a language in terms of the articulatory movements required to produce them. Syn: physiologic phonetics.

    auditory p. Study of hearing, perception, and processing of speech by the brain.

    descriptive p. Study and explanation of speech sound peculiarities of a particular language or dialect.

    evolutionary p. Study of speech sound changes of a language over a period of time. Syn: historical phonetics.

    experimental p. Use of objective laboratory techniques in the analysis of spoken language.

    general p. Study of the speech mechanism and of the sound-producing possibilities of man.

    historical p. Evolutionary *phonetics.*

    impressionistic p. Study of a language according to the manner in which sound waves strike the ear of the listener or speaker.

    linguistic p. Phonology.

    normative p. Entire set of rules which determines appropriate pronunciation of a language.

    physiologic p. Articulatory *phonetics.*

phonetics of juncture Assimilation.

phonetic transcription See under transcription.

phonetic variations Differences in the pronunciation of a phoneme. See also allophone.

phoniatrics (fō-nē-at′riks) [phon- + G. *iatrikos*, relating to medicine] Science concerned with the pathologic phenomena of pronunciation, whether they be articulatory in nature or are caused by disorders of the central nervous system.

phoniatrist Term used primarily in Europe and South America for speech and language pathologist.

phonics (fon'iks) [G. phonē, sound, voice] **1.** Method of teaching reading and pronunciation by learning the phonetic value of letters and groups of letters. **2.** Establishment of the sounds (phonemes) of a language with the equivalent written forms (graphemes). **3.** Study of the relationship of the English speech sounds to the letters of the English alphabet.

vocal p. Auditory synthesis.

phono- [G. *phonē*, sound, voice] Combining form relating to sound, speech, or voice sounds.

phonogram (fō'nə-gram) [phono- + G. *gramma*, mark, character] Speech sound represented by a sign or character; a phonetic symbol.

phonological (fō-nə-loj'i-kəl) **1.** Relating to phonemics, phonetics, or both together. **2.** See under linguistic components.

phonological analysis Analysis system used to explain children's sound changes when attempting to produce adultlike utterances.

a. of homonymy Assessment of the extent of homonymy in a child's speech, as when a child produces the same phonetic form for two or more adult words; *e.g.*, *bat* for *bath* and *blanket.*

distinctive feature a. Articulation errors analyzed in terms of distinctive features.

phonetic a. Determination of the child's phonetic inventory for word initial, word medial, and word final positions, and a numerical count which can be used as a gross measure of development. Syn: traditional analysis.

phonological processes a. Calculation of the percentage of occurrence of common phonological processes, as well as those that are less frequent.

place-voice-manner a. Examination of the relationship among the error sounds according to place of articulation, manner of articulation, and voicing.

substitution a. Recording of the substitutions a child uses for adult segments that are syllable initial, syllable final, and ambisyllabic, and also a measure of the extent of substitutions.

traditional a. Phonetic *analysis.*

Phonological Awareness Test See *Articulation Tests and Phonological Analysis Procedures* in appendices.

phonological conditioning Predictable differences in the sequences of phonemes determined by their environment; may recur with the same meaning; may also be found in regular third-person singular verbs; *e.g.*, cats, /-s/ occurs in voiceless environments where there is no friction; dogs, /-z/ occurs in voiced environments where there is no friction; roses, /-ɪz/ occurs in voiced or voiceless environments where there is friction.

phonological process analysis 1. Attempts to describe misarticulations and to provide an explanation for why these errors occur; emphasizes the linguistic components of speech production. **2.** Attempts to identify, describe, and explain phonological processes. See also *Articulation Tests and Phonological Analysis Procedures* in appendices.

phonological processes 1. Rules or statements that account for errors of substitution, omission, or addition; describe the difference between sounds actually produced and sounds present in the adult standard form. **2.** Techniques used by children to simplify speech when attempting to produce adult words.

assimilation p. p. Tendency to create internal symmetry within words; process whereby a child changes one or more phonemes to match production features of other sounds or characteristics of an utterance. Syn: harmony processes. See also assimilation.

Devoicing of final consonants is the process whereby a child anticipates the silence following a word and substitutes a voiceless consonant for the final voiced consonant; *e.g.*, bed = bɛt, big = bɪk.

Labial assimilation is the substitution of a labial consonant for a nonlabial consonant to make production similar to another labial consonant in a word; *e.g.*, top = bop.

Nasal assimilation is the substitution of a nasal consonant for a nonnasal consonant in a word containing a nasal; *e.g.*, Santa = nænə.

Nasalization of vowels is **1.** A tendency of vowels to take on the nasality of a following nasal consonant that has been deleted; *e.g.*, friend = frɛ. **2.** The addition of nasality to vowels that are not adjacent to nasal consonants; *e.g.*, house = haʊ.

Prevocalic voicing of consonants is inappropriate voicing of word initial voiceless consonants; *e.g.*, pen = bɛn.

Progressive vowel assimilation is assimilation of an unstressed vowel to a preceding stressed vowel; *e.g.*, apple = ʔabə.

Velar assimilation is the tendency of apical consonants to assimilate to a following velar consonant; *e.g.*, duck = gək, tongue = gəŋ.

breaking p. p. Long vowels become diphthongs; *e.g.*, fast = faeɪst, pass = paeɪs.

coalescence p. p. 1. Replacement of two contiguous consonants by a single consonant which shares features of the two original ones; *e.g.*, smoke = fok, in which the stridency of /s/ and the labialness of /m/ are combined in /f/. **2.** Combination of pho-

nemes from two syllables into one syllable; *e.g.*, pacifier = pæf.

developmental p. p. Processes that are frequently produced; characteristic of normal speech development in children.

diminutive p. p. Addition of /i/ on the end of nouns; *e.g.*, doggi, mommi.

epenthesis p. p. Addition of a vowel sound, usually to separate a group of consonants; *e.g.*, tree = tʌri, film = fɪləm.

idiosyncratic p. p. 1. Processes which are not characteristic of normal or disordered phonology but which are "unique" to the individual. **2.** Deficient pattern that does not fit into any major process classification; *e.g.*, atypical cluster reduction, initial consonant deletion, glottal replacement, fricatives substituted for stops, stops substituted for glides.

metathesis p. p. Transposition of sounds or syllables in a word; some authorities use "migration" when only one phoneme is moved to another place in a word; *e.g.*, mask = mæks; refrigerator = frɪ-ri-dʒɝ-tə-e. Syn: transposition.

substitution p. p. Replacement of one sound by another without being influenced by neighboring sounds. Syn: feature contrasts processes.

Affrication (af-ri-kā′shən) is the replacement of a fricative with an affricate; *e.g.*, zipper = tsɪpə, sun = tsʌn. Syn: stopping of fricatives.

Apicalization (ā′pi-kəl-ə-zā′shən) is the substitution of an apical consonant for a labial; *e.g.*, bow = do.

Backing is the substitution of a velar for any consonant other than a velar; *e.g.*, tub = tʌg. Syn: backing to velars.

Deaffrication (dē′af-rə-kā′shən) is **1.** Deletion of the stop feature of an affricate, with retention of the continuant or fricative feature; *e.g.*, matches = mæʃɪz. **2.** Changing of an affricate target phoneme to a continuant or a stop; *e.g.*, chair = teɚ.

Denasalization (də-nā′zəl-i-zā′-shən) is the replacement of a nasal consonant with an oral one; *e.g.*, no = dow, home = hʌb.

Gliding of fricatives is the substitution of a glide /w/ or /j/ for a fricative; *e.g.*, soap = jop, fish = wɪs.

Gliding of liquids is the substitution of a glide /w/ or /j/ for a liquid sound; *e.g.*, rock = wak, lap = jæp.

Labialization (lā′bē-əl-i-zā′shən) occurs when a labial consonant is substituted for a lingual consonant; *e.g.*, thick = fɪk.

Neutralization (nu′trə-li-zā′shən) occurs when several different phonemes are replaced by one sound; *e.g.*, replacing all prevocalic fricatives and affricates with /j/.

Palatal fronting is the replacement of palatal consonants with nonpalatal consonants; *e.g.*, mash = mæs. Syn: depalatization.

Palatization (pal′ə-ti-zā′shən) occurs when a sound is produced as a palatal rather than as a nonpalatal; *e.g.*, soup = ʃup.

Stopping is the replacement of fricatives, and occasionally other sounds, with a stop consonant; *e.g.*, seat = tit, soup = dup.

Velar fronting is the tendency to replace velar consonants with alveolar ones; *e.g.*, cot = tot.

Vowelization is the replacement of a syllabic consonant with a vowel; *e.g.*, apple = æo, flower = fawo, star = stau.

Vowel neutralization is the reduction of vowels to /ə/ or /a/; *e.g.*, fish = fəʃ.

syllable structure p. p. 1. Changes in the makeup of the structure of syllables. **2.** Simplification of the structure of syllables.

Cluster reduction is **1.** The reduction of a consonant cluster to a single consonant; *e.g.*, spoon = pun.

2. When one or more consonants is deleted from a sequence of consonants; may simplify by adding a /ə/ between members of a cluster; *e.g.*, blue = bəlu.

Deletion of final consonant is the reduction of consonant-vowel-consonant (CVC) words or syllables to a consonant-vowel (CV) form; *e.g.*, pig = pɪ. Syn: consonant-vowel preference; postvocalic obstruent singleton omissions; open syllable.

Deletion of initial consonant occurs when the speaker deletes the initial consonant of a syllable or word; uncharacteristic of normal speech development; *e.g.*, house = aus. Syn: prevocalic singleton; obstruent omission.

Deletion of unstressed syllables is the dropping of an unstressed syllable; *e.g.*, telephone = təfon.

Glottal replacement is the replacement of a deleted consonant with a glottal stop; *e.g.*, kitchen = kɪʔən.

Reduction is the deletion of a phoneme or a syllable; *e.g.*, that = æt, before = fore.

Reduplication is the assimilation of consonant and vowel; *e.g.*, kitty = tɪtɪ. Syn: syllable duplication; doubling.

Stridency deletion occurs when the stridency of a consonant is deleted by either substitution of a nonstrident consonant (fish = pɪf) or omission of the strident consonant (soup = up).

Syllable reduction is the deletion of a syllable from a word; *e.g.*, before = fore, telephone—tɛfon. Syn: syllable, weak syllable, or unstressed syllable deletion.

phonological rules 1. Rules relating the surface structure of a sentence to its representation as a sequence of phonemes, a matrix of feature values, or a phonetic transcription. **2.** Rules relating a sequence of linguistic units to a sequence of articulatory, acoustic, or neural events. **3.** Rules specifying the pronunciation of an utterance.

phonology (fō-nol′ə-jē) [phono- + G. *logos*, discourse, study] **1.** Study of the sound system of a language, including pauses and stress. **2.** Science of the phonemes of a language and the rules governing their combination; interprets surface structure (pronunciation). **3.** Branch of linguistics concerned with how the sounds within a language function to signify meaning, *i.e.*, each language's sound pattern. Syn: linguistic phonetics. See also linguistic component.

phonophobia (fō-nə-fō′bē-ə) [phono- + G. *phobos*, fear] Sense of discomfort caused by sounds above the threshold of hearing.

phonosurgery Surgical techniques that have as their aim the improvement of voice; *e.g.*, surgical removal of vocal folds or polyps.

phonotactics (fō-nə-tak′tiks) [phono- + G. *taktikos*, fit for arranging] Study of the ways in which phonemes are combined and ordered in the syllables and words of a particular language or dialect.

Photo Articulation Test (PAT) See *Articulation Tests and Phonological Analysis Procedures* in appendices.

photoglottography (fō′tō-glot-og′rə-fē) Method of indirectly measuring the glottal opening by measuring the amount of light transmitted through the glottis. Syn: transillumination.

phrase (frāz) Small group of words forming part of a sentence; does not contain a subject and a verb, and may act as any part of speech or as any sentence element.

phrase structure grammar See under grammar.

phylogenesis or **phylogeny** (fī-lə-jen′ə-sis, fī-loj′ə-nē) [G. *phylon*, tribe + *genesis*, origin] Origin and development of a species, as distinguished from ontogenesis or ontogeny.

physiogenic (fiz′ē-ō-jen′ik) [G. *physis*, nature + *genesis*, origin] Originating from physiologic causes. *Cf.* psychogenic.

physiologic, physiological (fiz′ē-ō-loj′ik, -i-kəl) **1.** Pertaining to physiology or to the functioning of a structure. **2.** Denoting normal as opposed to pathologic.

physiologic phonetics Articulatory *phonetics.*

physiology (fiz-ē-ol′ə-jē) [L. or G. *physiologica*] Science concerned with the normal functions or vital processes in living things.

Piaget's cognitive development stages See cognitive development stages. See also *General Outline of Language Development From Birth to 11 Years* in appendices.

PIC Symbols A symbol set consisting of drawings intended for use on communication boards. The drawings are white on a black background. See also augmentative and alternative communication.

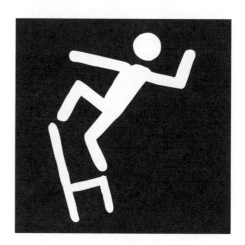

PIC Symbols
Fall

PICSYMS Acronym for picture symbols. A graphic symbol set intended for use on communication boards. The symbols—line drawings—are both ideographic and pictographic. See also augmentative and alternative communication.

PICSYM Symbols
Toast

pictographs (pik′tō-grafs) Symbols that look like the things they represent.

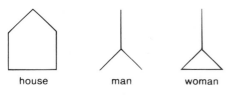

house   man   woman

Pictographs

Pictorial Test of Intelligence See *Psychological Measures and Tests* in appendices.

Picture Articulation and Language Screening Test See *Articulation Tests and Phonological Analysis Procedures* in appendices.

Picture Sound Discrimination Test See *Auditory Tests and Procedures* in appendices.

pidgin (pij′ən) [uncertain] Simplified speech used for communication between individuals with different languages; usually a corrupted form of one language with features of both languages.

pidgin sign English (PSE) Signed English (siglish). See under sign systems.

Pierre Robin syndrome [P. Robin, Fr. pediatrician, 1867–1950] Complex of disorders, characterized by micrognathia, glossoptosis, high-arched or cleft palate, and absence of gag reflex, with as-

sociated aural, ocular, skeletal, and cardiovascular anomalies.

pink noise See under noise.

pinna, pl. **pinnae** (pin′ə, -ē) [L. sing. feather, pl. wing] Auricle. See under external *ear*.

pitch [L. *pix*] **1.** Acuteness or gravity of a tone, dependent on the frequency of the vibrations producing it and their intensity and overtone structure. The greater the number of vibrations per unit of time, the higher the pitch and the more acute the tone; conversely, the less the number of vibrations, the lower the pitch and the more grave the tone. **2.** That attribute of auditory sensation in terms of its perception by the listener in which sounds may be ordered on a scale extending from low to high; measurable through discriminatory responses. **3.** Subjective quality primarily associated with frequency.

    basal p. Lowest pitch on which an utterance can be sustained.

    habitual p. 1. Fundamental frequency most often used in the act of producing spontaneous speech; should not be considered a fixed static value since it will vary in different settings. **2.** Central tendency of the pitches used by an individual. Syn: modal frequency or tone.

    natural or **optimal p.** Frequency at which the greatest vocal carrying power is achieved by the least expenditure of vocal effort; the frequency at which the movements of the vocal folds are best facilitated by factors of resonance, often found in two or three notes near the bottom of an individual's lowest possible pitch production. Optimal frequencies are approximately 125 Hz for adult males and 225 Hz for adult females.

pitch break See under voice disorders of phonation.

pitch range Distance between one's highest and lowest pitch; usually determined by instructing the individual to sing the lowest note possible and then the highest note possible. Most normal voices are capable of a pitch range of approximately two octaves.

pitch shift Change in pitch level occurring between phonations.

pivot See under parts of speech.

pivot grammar See under grammar.

pivot word See under word.

place See under deixis.

placebo effect An improvement in a condition due to a psychologically based belief in a "treatment effect" which does not exist.

place of articulation See consonant, place of articulation.

place theory See under hearing theories.

plane [L. *planus*, flat] Any flat, smooth surface, especially any assumed or conventional surface, through an axis or two points, whether dividing a body or tangent to it.

    coronal p. Frontal *plane*.

    frontal p. Any vertical plane passing from side to side and dividing a body or structure into anterior and posterior parts. Syn: coronal plane.

    horizontal p. See transverse *plane*.

    median sagittal p. Vertical plane which divides a body or structure into perfect halves in the midline.

    sagittal p. Any vertical plane which divides a body or structure into right and left parts.

    transverse p. Any plane cutting the long axis of a body or structure at right angles; such a plane of the human body is a horizontal plane.

    vertical p. See frontal *plane*.

planigraphy (plə-nig′rə-fē) [L. *planum*, plane + G. *graphe*, a writing] Tomography.

plateau (pla-tō′) [Fr.] In audiometry, the theoretical point in masking where the level of the noise in the nontest ear may be raised or lowered about 15 dB without affecting the threshold of the signal in the test ear; the levels between undermasking and overmasking at which the true threshold of the test ear may be seen.

plateau method Hood technique. See under masking techniques.

play audiometry Behavioral *audiometry*.

play therapy **1.** Method of examination and treatment in which a child is observed as he plays freely with a selected inventory; the role of the clinician or therapist is usually passive. **2.** Use of play activities in psychotherapy or speech therapy with children; based

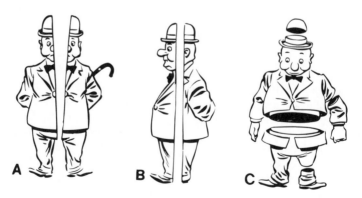

Planes of the Body

A, median sagittal plane; B, frontal (coronal) plane; C, transverse plane. From Basmajian, JV. *Primary Anatomy,* 7th ed. Baltimore: Williams & Wilkins, 1976.

on the premise that play is the child's natural medium of self-expression.

plosive See under consonant, manner of formation.

plosive-injection method See injection method, under speech, methods of esophageal speech.

plus juncture Open *juncture.*

PNdB Perceived noise level (in decibels).

pneumatic (nu-mat'ik) [G. *pneumatikos*] Relating to air or a gas, an air-filled structure, or respiration.

pneumatic artificial larynx See under artificial larynx.

pneumo- [G. *pneuma*, air, breath; *pneumōn*, lung] Combining form relating to air or gas, to breathing, or to the lung.

pneumogram (nu'mō-gram) [pneumo- + G. *gramma*, something written] Recording of measurements made by a pneumograph.

pneumograph (nu'mō-graf) [pneumo- + G. *graphē*, a writing] Device for measuring thoracic and abdominal movements during inhalation and exhalation.

pneumotachogram (nu-mō-tak'ō-gram) [pneumo- + G. *tachys*, swift + *gramma*, something written] Recording of measurements made by a pneumotachograph.

pneumotachograph (nu'mō-tak'ə-graf) [pneumo- + G. *tachys*, swift + *graphē*, a writing] Instrument used to measure airflow; airflow from the nose and mouth may be measured independently and simultaneously over a period of time; does not provide measurement of intraoral pressure. It functions on the principle that the volume of air passing through a straight tube is proportional to the difference in pressure between two points in that tube.

PNS Peripheral nervous system.

point of articulation See consonant.

poles Natural frequencies of the vocal tract; in vowel spectra, the poles are the areas of greatest sound intensity.

poly- [G. *polys*, much, many] Prefix denoting multiplicity; corresponds to Latin prefix *multi-*.

polyglot (pol'ē-glot) [G. *polyglōttos*, many-tongued] **1.** An individual who speaks, reads, and writes several languages. **2.** Denoting one who experiences a confusion of language, usually the result of foreign language influences.

polygraph (pol'ē-graf) [poly- + G. *graphē*, a writing] Instrument used for simultaneous recordings of physiologic functions such as respiration, pulse, heartbeat, and galvanic skin response; when used as a "lie detector," recorded changes in the subject's physiologic functions are presumed to be indicative of his emotional responses to questions, and thus indicators of his veracity.

polymorphemic utterances (pol'ē-môr-fēm'ik) Verbalizations containing more than one morpheme.

polyp See under laryngeal anomaly.

polypoid (pol'i-poid) [polyp + G. *eidos*, resemblance] Resembling a polyp in gross features.

polypoid degeneration of the true folds See under laryngeal anomalies.

polypoid vocal nodules See vocal nodules, under laryngeal anomaly.

polysyllabic word See under word.

polytomography (pol-ē-tə-mog'rə-fē) [poly- + G. *tomos*, cutting (section) + *graphe*, a writing] Tomography.

pons See under brainstem, under brain.

population (pop-yu-lā'shən) [L. *populus*, people, nation] In statistics, a group or set, such as persons, objects, events, operations, scores, or values, subject to study or from which a sample is to be drawn.

Porch Index of Communicative Abilities (PICA) See *Language Tests and Procedures* in appendices.

Porch Index of Communicative Abilities in Children (PICAC) See *Language Tests and Procedures* in appendices.

portmanteau word (pôrt-man'tō) [Fr.

portemanteau, suitcase opening into two halves] Telescoped *word.*

positive See under comparison.

positive correlation See under correlation.

positive emotion Sympathetic responses to stimulus circumstances; includes hope, pleasure, and positive regard.

positive reinforcer See under reinforcer.

positive response See under response.

positron emission tomography (PET) In radiology, a functional method of evaluating the brain to measure cerebral function.

possessive case See case.

possessor-possession See semantic relations.

post- [L. *post,* behind] Prefix denoting after, behind, posterior.

postcentral gyrus See under gyrus.

postcentral sulcus See under sulcus.

postconsonantal vowel See under vowel.

postdeterminer See determiner.

posterior (pōs-tēr′ē-ėr) [L. *posterus,* following] Denoting behind or after, or the back part of, an anatomical structure; opposite of anterior.

posterior vertical canal See semicircular canals, under inner *ear.*

postlingual deafness See under deafness.

postnatal (pōst-nā′təl) [post- + L. *natus,* born] Occurring after birth.

postponements (pōst-pōn′mənts) In stuttering, devices used by the stutterer to delay uttering a word which he knows he will have difficulty producing; may include pauses, repetitions of previously spoken words, or the use of a different word. In some instances, the stutterer appears to "forget" certain words. Syn: stallers.

posttraumatic amnesia (PTA) See under amnesia.

postvocalic (pōst-vō-ka′lik) Denoting a consonant position following the vowel and closing the syllable. See under consonant position.

postvocalic obstruent singleton omissions Deletion of final consonant. See under

syllabic structure, under phonological processes.

potential (pō-ten′shəl) [L. *potentia,* power, potency] Capability of being or performing.

    action p. Changes in electric potential at the surface of a nerve or muscle which occur at the moment of their excitation.

    electrical p. Electromotive *force.*

potential energy See under energy.

potentiometer (pō-ten-shē-om′ə-tėr) Instrument designed to measure electromotive force or difference of potential.

power Amount of energy used or generated in a given unit of time; in electricity, expressed in watts.

power CROS See contralateral routing of signals (CROS), under hearing aid.

pragmatic [G. *pragmatikos,* practical] **1.** Pertaining to pragmatics. **2.** Functional; useful. See also under linguistic component.

pragmatic aphasia See under aphasia.

pragmatics In oral language: **1.** Language development in the context and environment in which it is generated. It includes such factors as intention in communication; sensorimotor actions preceding, accompanying, and following the utterance; knowledge shared in the communicative dyad; and the elements in the environment surrounding the message. **2.** Set of rules governing the use of language in context. Context is treated as an integral part of language structure rather than as a cause of language, and meanings are seen as the result of the creative combination of utterance and social settings; thus meanings and context become virtually inseparable. **3.** Study of linguistic acts and the contexts in which they are performed. **4.** Study of speaker-listener intentions and relations, and all elements in the environment surrounding the message. See also pragmatic structures.

pragmatic structures Rules of use of oral language.

conversational postulates Assumptions about the nature of human conversation in general, especially as these assumptions are used to convey subtle messages to the listener.

performative Information about the identity of speaker and listener and the speaker's goal in using the sentence.

presupposition Information that is not contained in the sentence but must be known and understood if that sentence is to make sense.

pragmatic text See under text.

praxis (prak'sis) **1.** The ability to plan and execute a skilled movement. **2.** The performance of an action.

pre- [L. *prae*, before] Prefix denoting before, anterior. *Cf.* pro-.

prearticle Any word which precedes articles, demonstratives, or genitives, including the zero morpheme; *e.g.*, all, only, both, just.

precentral gyrus See under gyrus.

precentral sulcus See under sulcus.

precipitating factor See etiology.

precision fluency shaping In stuttering, a program using easy breathing, easy onsets, and then monitoring the beginning sounds and syllables of words; involves beginning the sounds and syllables gently and elongating their production for as long as one or two seconds. Syn: gentle onsets, stretched syllables.

precision therapy 1. Teaching method utilizing measurement procedures, such as charting graphs, as opposed to extrinsic rewards or reinforcements; entails recording the acceleration or change in frequency of wanted behaviors or the deceleration of unwanted behaviors, rather than simply recording level of performance. **2.** Eclectic approach to articulation therapy that results from combining the principles of behavior modification, programming, and traditional therapy into a systematic framework which permits an efficient use of time in reaching criterion levels; the components include gathering and analyzing baseline data, determining long-term and short-term objectives, arranging antecedent and consequent events to ensure a high correct and low error response rate per minute, recording responses, graphing progress, and setting criteria for each learned behavior.

preconsonantal vowel See under vowel.

predeterminer See determiner.

predicate (pred'i-kət) In traditional grammar, the part of the sentence comprising what is said about the subject; may be composed of only the verb **(simple predicate)** or the verb along with its complements and modifiers **(complete predicate);** *e.g.*, He *ran* (simple predicate). He *ran through the house* (complete predicate).

predicate adjective See complement.

predicate noun or **nominative** See complement.

predicate objective See complement.

predicate truncation Ellipsis.

predictive validity See criterion-related validity.

predispose (prē'dis-pōz) To give a tendency or bias to; to incline beforehand.

predisposing factor See etiology.

prefix Word or syllable placed before the root of another word to form a new word; *e.g.*, *un*stable. See also affix; morpheme.

prelingual deafness See under deafness.

prelinguistic language See under language.

premaxilla (prē-mak-sil'ə) [pre- + L. *maxilla*, jawbone] **1.** The intermaxillary bone. **2.** Separate element derived from the median nasal processes in the embryo which later fuses with the maxilla.

premolar teeth Bicuspid *teeth.*

prenatal (prē-nā'təl) [pre- + L. *natus*, born] Preceding birth.

preoperational thought period See Period II, under cognitive development stages.

prepalate (prē-pal'it) [pre- + L. *palatum*,

palate] Upper lip and gum ridge; those parts of the oral structure anterior to the incisive foramen. Syn: primary palate.

preparatory set 1. In stuttering, the covert rehearsal behavior of the stutterer used in preparation for the difficulty anticipated. **2.** In stuttering, the stutterer seems to preset his mouth, tongue, or jaw for the first sound of the word to be spoken; tension is present with the posture. Syn: trigger posture. **3.** In pragmatics, the semantic conditions of a speech act specifying assumed, shared, or unshared meaning.

preposition (pre-pə-zi′shən) **1.** See under parts of speech. **2.** In pragmatics, a referred intended notion, much like a basic topic conveyed to a hearer.

prepsychosis (prē-sī-kō′sis) [pre- + G. *psychosis*, an animating] Childhood *schizophrenia.*

presbycusis, presbyacusis (prez-bē-ku′ sis, -ə-ku′sis) [G. *presbys*, old man + *akousis*, hearing] **1.** Progressive loss of auditory acuity as a result of the aging process; atrophy of the cochlear mechanism causes a loss of hearing for frequencies from 2000 Hz to 8000 Hz. See also sociocusis (2). **2.** A term used when referring solely to the biologic aging of the auditory mechanism. Any hearing dysfunction resulting strictly from the aging process; *e.g.*, vascular alterations, genetic makeup, cellular aging. **3.** A term used by some to refer to hearing losses associated with the elderly. It may be the result of a number of factors which act over a person's life to produce a hearing impairment; *e.g.*, noise exposure, toxic drugs. According to Schuknecht, the effects of aging on the auditory system can be classified as:

Sensory Limited to the lower few millimeters of the basal turn of cochlea; flattening and atrophy of the organ of Corti; loss of hair cells and supporting cells resulting in an abrupt high-frequency sensorineural

hearing loss beginning in middle age and progressing slowly.

Neural Loss of neurons in auditory pathway and cochlea; decrease in the number of functional neural units available resulting in no great effect on hearing sensitivity until late in life; poor word discrimination; minimal decrease in sensitivity.

Strial (metabolic) Atrophy of the stria vascularis; reduction in the microphonic potential; reduced cellular function and bioelectrical/biochemical balance of the cochlea resulting in a flat audiogram which progresses slowly with age.

Cochlear conductive (mechanical) Problem involving motion mechanics of the cochlear duct; atrophic alterations in the spiral ligament, mass and stiffness changes in the basilar membrane; modification of middle ear mechanics resulting in a descending threshold curve with steep slope; reduced word discrimination. (From Katz, S., *Handbook of Clinical Audiology*, 4th ed. Baltimore: Williams & Wilkins, 1994, p. 709).

Preschool Language Assessment Instrument (PLAI) See *Language Tests and Procedures* in appendices.

Preschool Language Scale—Fourth Edition See *Language Tests and Procedures* in appendices.

Preschool Language Screening Test See *Language Tests and Procedures* in appendices.

Preschool Speech and Language Screening Test See *Language Tests and Procedures* in appendices.

prescription (prē-skrip′-shən) [L. *praescription*] In speech, any written formula for the preparation and administration of any program for the habilitation or rehabilitation of a communication disorder.

prescriptive grammar See under grammar.

present perfect tense See under tense.

present perfect progressive tense See progressive *tense*.

pressure equalization tube Grommet.

pressure pattern Rise and fall of air pressure as consonants leave the mouth of the speaker and are sensed by the ear of the listener.

presupposition See under pragmatic structures.

presyntactic devices (prē-sin-tak′tik) Methods used by young children to extend the length of what was essentially a one-word utterance; *e.g.*, carcar (reduplication).

prevocalic (prē-vō-ka′lik) Denoting a consonant position preceding the vowel phoneme and initiating the syllable. See under consonant position.

prevocalic singleton Deletion of initial consonant. See under syllabic structure, under phonological processes.

prevocalic voicing of consonants See under assimilatory *phonological processes*.

prevocational deafness See under deafness.

primary autism See under autism.

primary characteristics of stuttering See stuttering.

primary gain Reduction of anxiety as a result of the conversion of emotional concerns into obvious organic manifestations, as in hysterical aphonia.

primary palate Prepalate.

primary progressive aphasia See under aphasia.

primary reinforcement See under reinforcement.

primary reinforcer See under reinforcer.

primary stress See under stress.

primary stuttering See under stuttering stages.

primary stuttering theories See anticipatory and struggle behavior theories, under stuttering theories.

principal clause Main *clause*.

pro- [L. and G. *pro*, before] Prefix denoting before or forward. *Cf.* pre-.

probability curve Normal *distribution*.

probe [L. *probo*, to test] **1.** To make either an exploratory or thorough investigation. **2.** In articulation, the use of a language sample to measure an individual's success in producing the target phoneme in conversational speech without reinforcement. **3.** Slender surgical instrument used for examining a cavity. **4.** Pointed metal tip for making electrical contact with a circuit element being checked.

probe tube microphone Small microphone which can be inserted into a nostril; used to study hypernasality by comparing sound pressure levels obtained with it to those obtained with a separate microphone usually placed a few inches in front of and at the level of the mouth.

Procedures for the Phonological Analysis of Children's Language See *Articulation Tests and Phonological Analysis Procedures* in appendices.

process (pro′ses) [L. *processus*] In anatomy, a projection or outgrowth. For various processes, see specific term. See also crus.

production (prō-dək′shən) [L. *productus*, lead forth] In speech, an utterance, spontaneous or imitated; the language which one speaks, as opposed to that which he understands. See also performance.

product moment (r) See under coefficient of correlation.

profound hearing impairment or **loss** See under hearing impairment degrees.

progeria Premature senility or old age.

prognathic (prog-na′thik) [pro- + G. *gnathos*, jaw] Having a marked projection of the jaw. *Cf.* retrognathic.

prognosis (prog-nō′sis) [G. *prognosis*] **1.** Prediction of judgment concerning the course, duration, termination, and recovery from a disease or disorder. **2.** Prediction of the outcome of a proposed course of treatment; its effectiveness and duration, and the client's progress.

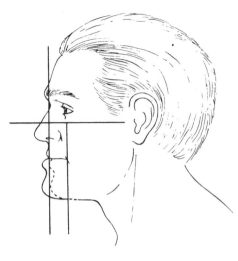

Prognathic

From *Stedman's Medical Dictionary*, 25th ed. Baltimore: Williams & Wilkins, 1990.

Prognostic Value of Imitative and Auditory Discrimination Tests See *Auditory Tests and Procedures* in appendices.

program [G. *programma*, written public notice] Set of sequentially ordered step procedures for modifying behavior which progress in a specified sequence from a previously established baseline to a predetermined goal; some steps may be optional. The program determines what response or responses will be dealt with at different times; whether those responses will be reinforced, extinguished, or punished; the type, amount, and duration of the stimuli; the schedule of presentation; and any other details necessary to achieve conditioning. See also criteria.

programmed therapy Commercial or individually constructed remediation techniques which use behavior modification principles and utilize a series of steps or goals. See also precision therapy.

programming Initiation and execution of a program. For types of programming, see specific term.

progressive assimilation See under assimilation.

progressive relaxation Technique for teaching an awareness of the state of tension in muscle groups throughout the body and an ability to bring about decreased tension when under stress; sometimes used in stuttering and voice therapy.

progressive tense See under tense.

progressive vowel assimilation See under assimilatory *phonological processes.*

projection (prō-jek′shən) [L. *projectio,* to throw before] Ascribing to others the ideas, feelings, or attitudes which the individual himself has but which he does not desire to recognize or face.

projective technique Testing method in which the subject is required to ascribe his own thoughts and feelings to a stimulus of relatively high ambiguity; designed to determine personal characteristics.

prolabium (prō-lā′bē-əm) [pro- + L. *labium,* lip] **1.** Central prominence of the lip. **2.** The small elevation at the labial termination of the philtrum.

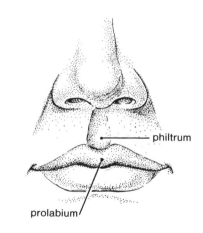

Prolabium

prolongation (prō-lon-gā′shən) In stuttering, the lengthening of a speech sound or maintaining the posture of the lips, tongue, or other parts of the speech mechanism in an attempt to modify the stuttering pattern.

prompt A type of cue; in speech, usually verbal.

prompting Assisting the listener to understand what the speaker has said by restating the utterance in a different form; *e.g.*, "What do you want?" "You want what?"

pronoun See under parts of speech.

pronunciation (prō-nən-sē-ā′shən) [L. *pronuntiation,* delivery (of a speech)] Act of speaking using the conventional sound patterns of a language.

properant (prop′ėr-ənt) [fr. *proportionally operant*] Measure of the acceptability of an individual's articulation in ongoing speech.

proposition (pro-pə-zi′shən) **1.** In case grammar, a tenseless set of relationships involving nouns and verbs; a list of sentence types, each of which is defined as a verb (V), plus some combination of cases. See also sentence (1). **2.** In pragmatics, an internal activity of speakers rather than an object located in sentences.

propositional speech See under speech.

proprioception (prō′prē-ō-sep′shən) [L. *proprius,* one's own + *receptus,* received] **1.** Term used to include kinesthesia (awareness of bodily movement and position) and taction (sense of touch or contact); speech is presumably monitored through auditory and proprioceptive feedback. **2.** Sensory data from muscles, joints, or tendons. See also perception.

proprioceptive (prō′prē-ō-sep′tiv) Relating to proprioception.

proprioceptive feedback See under feedback.

proprioceptive perception See under perception.

prosodeme (pros′ə-dēm) [See prosody] Suprasegmental *phoneme.*

prosody (pros′ə-dē) [G. *prosōidia,* modulation of voice] **1.** Physical attributes of speech that signal linguistic qualities such as stress and intonation; in-

cludes the fundamental frequency of the voice, the intensity of the voice, and the duration of the individual speech sounds. **2.** Melody of speech determined primarily by modifications of pitch, quality, strength, and duration; perceived primarily as stress and intonational patterns.

prosopagnosia See under agnosia

prosthesis, pl. **prostheses** (pros′thə-sis, pros-thē′sis, -sēz) [G. an addition] Artificial substitute for a missing part of the body; *e.g.*, artificial larynx, denture, palatal lift.

prosthetic (pros-thet′ik) Relating to a prosthesis or the use of a prosthesis.

prosthetic management of cleft palate See cleft palate.

prosthodontist (pros-thə-don′tist) [G. *prosthesis + odous (odont-),* tooth] Dentist who specializes in providing prosthetic appliances for oral structures, such as a palatal lift or obturator.

protolanguage See under language.

protoword See under word.

protrusion lisp Frontal *lisp.*

proxemics (proks-ē′miks) [L. *proximus,* nearest, next] **1.** Study of the role and function of spatial positioning in interpersonal communication. **2.** Awareness of four areas of territory: intimate, social, personal, and public.

proximal (proks′i-məl) [L. *proximus, nearest, next*] Nearest the center or point of origin; opposite of distal.

PSE Pidgin sign English.

pseud-, pseudo- [G. *pseudēs,* false] Prefix denoting a resemblance, often deceptive.

pseudobinaural hearing aid Y-cord *hearing aid.*

pseudobulbar paralysis See under paralysis.

pseudoglottis (su-dō-glot′is) [pseudo- + G. *glōttis,* aperture of larynx] Neoglottis.

pseudohypacusis, pseudohypoacusis (su-dō-hīp-ə-ku′sis, -hī-pō-ə-ku′sis) [pseudo- + G. *hypo,* under + *akousis,* hearing] Infrequently used term for functional *deafness.*

pseudolaryngeal paralysis See under paralysis.

pseudostuttering (su-dō-stət′ĕr-iŋ) Deliberately faked stuttering; used as a therapy technique to aid in reducing the client's fear of stuttering.

psych- See psycho-.

psychiatric (sī-kē-at′rik) Relating to psychiatry.

psychiatrist (sī-kī′ə-trist) Physician who specializes in psychiatry.

psychiatry (sī-kī′ə-trē) [psych- + G. *iatreia,* medical treatment] Medical specialty concerned with the diagnosis and treatment of mental illness.

psycho- [G. *psychē,* soul, mind] Combining form relating to the mind.

psychoacoustics (sī′kō-ə-ku′stiks) [psycho- + G. *akousis,* hearing] **1.** Combined disciplines of psychology and acoustics concerned with the study of man's response to sound. **2.** Study of the relationship between acoustic characteristics and human auditory perception of these characteristics. See also psychophysics.

psychoanalysis (sī′kō-ə-nal′i-sis) [psycho- + G. *analysis,* a breaking up] Clinical method of psychotherapy, originated by Sigmund Freud, which utilizes special techniques to bring repressed factors from unconsciousness to consciousness to reveal the mental processes responsible for the condition being treated and to suggest further therapeutic measures; sometimes used in the treatment of stutterers.

psychodrama (sī-kō-drä′mə) [psycho- + G. *drama,* action (of a play)] Form of psychotherapy in which patients act out their problems through roles in spontaneous performances; sometimes used with stutterers in an attempt to enable them to improve their speech and related behavior in those situations in which they have the most speech difficulty.

psychodynamic (sī-kō-dī-nam′ik) [psy-

cho- + G. *dynamis,* force] Relating to mental or emotional forces or processes, especially those developing in early childhood, and their effects on behavior.

psychogalvanic skin resistance Galvanic skin *response.*

psychogalvanic skin response (PGSR) Galvanic skin *response.*

psychogalvanic skin response audiometry (PGSRA) Electrodermal audiometry. See under electrophysiologic *audiometry.*

psychogenic (sī-kō-jen′ik) [psycho- + G. *genesis,* origin] Originating in the mind or in mental or emotional conflict. *Cf.* physiogenic.

psychogenic deafness See under deafness.

psycholinguistic (sī-kō-liŋ-gwis′tik) Relating to psycholinguistics.

psycholinguistics (sī-kō-liŋ-gwis′tiks) [psycho- + L. *lingua,* tongue] **1.** Field of study that blends the disciplines of psychology and linguistics to analyze all areas of human behavior and culture with all areas of human language function. **2.** Study of the relationship between grammatical complexity and psychological complexity; also attempts to distinguish between what people know about their language and how they make use of it.

psychologic, psychological (sī-kō-loj′-ik, -i-kəl) Relating to psychology or to the mind and its processes.

psychological measures and tests See appendices.

psychologist (sī-kol′ə-jist) One who is licensed to practice psychology as a profession, certified to teach psychology as a discipline, or whose scientific specialty is psychology.

psychology (sī-kol′ə-jē) [psycho- + G. *logos,* study] Professional specialty or discipline concerned with mental processes and behavior.

   abnormal p. Branch of psychology that examines behavior disorders, inadequate behavior abilities, and individuals exhibiting such behaviors.

clinical p. Branch of psychology concerned with the diagnosis and treatment of emotional and behavioral disorders.

experimental p. Study of the mind and mental processes by the use of experimental methods; concerned with the study of conditioning, learning, perception, motivation, emotion, language, and thinking.

gestalt p. [Ger. shape] Theory which emphasizes the wholeness and organized structures of every experience; it maintains that psychologic processes and behavior cannot be described adequately by analyzing the elements of experience alone, and emphasizes sudden learning by insight rather than by trial and error or by association.

psychometry (sī-kom′ə-trē) [psycho- + G. *metron*, measure] The broad field of psychological and mental testing.

psychomotor (sī-kō-mō′tėr) [psycho- + L. *motor*, a movement] **1.** Pertaining to muscular movements resulting from compulsive mental processes. **2.** Relating to the mental origin of voluntary movement.

psychomotor seizure State in which consciousness is altered but not lost, the individual often acting in a peculiar way with no subsequent memory of what transpired; not attributable to known organic origins.

psychoneurological (sī′kō-nu-rō-loj′i-kəl) Characterized by both psychic and organic neural components, and manifested by disturbances in behavior.

psychoneurosis (sī′kō-nu-rō′sis) [psycho- + G. *neuron*, nerve + -*osis*, condition] Mental disorder which is of psychogenic origin and which manifests itself in deviant behavior.

psychopathology (sī′kō-pə-thol′ə-jē) [psycho- + G. *pathos*, suffering + *logos*, study, discourse] **1.** Science concerned with the pathology of the mind. **2.** Science concerned with mental and behavioral disorders; includes psychiatry and abnormal psychology.

psychophysics (sī-kō-fiz′iks) [psycho- + G. *physikos*, natural, physical] Study of the relationship between the objective world and subjective awareness; study of the relation between stimulus and response.

psychosis, pl. **psychoses** (sī-kō′sis,-sēz) [G. an animating] Mental disorder characterized by disintegration of the personality and its break with reality to the degree of interfering with the capacity to cope with the demands of everyday life. *Cf.* neurosis.

childhood p. Childhood *schizophrenia.*

infantile p. Disorder of early childhood manifested by impaired contact with reality, absence of meaningful verbal communication, withdrawal from social interactions, and unevenness between mental and emotional functioning, as well as a disparity among motor, verbal, social, and adaptive behavior. See also childhood *schizophrenia;* autism.

symbiotic p. Emotional disorder believed to be caused by the failure of the child to make a separation or a differentiation of his ego from that of his mother; characterized by difficulty with pronouns and references to himself in the third person, repetition of phrases out of context, and frequently echolalia.

psychosomatic (sī′kō-sə-mat′ik) [psycho- + G. *soma*, body] Denoting especially a physical disorder attributable to emotional or other psychogenic causes, as in conversion *(q.v.).*

psychotherapy (sī-kō-thār′ə-pē) [psycho- + G. *therapeia*, treatment] Treatment of behavioral, emotional, personality, or psychiatric disorders by any of a variety of psychological methods, with emphasis on communication with the patient in contrast to chemical or physical measures; sometimes used in stuttering therapy.

PTA Posttraumatic amnesia.

PTS Permanent threshold shift.

puberphonia (pyu-bėr-fō'nē-ə) [L. *puber*, grown-up + G. *phōnē*, voice] Adolescent *voice*.

pull out In stuttering, a deliberate attempt by the stutterer to modify the stuttering block before it is completed. Syn: in-block correction.

pulmonary (pùl'mə-nā-rē) [L. *pulmonarius* fr. *pulmo*, lung] Relating to the lungs.

pulmonary pressure Intrapulmonary pressure.

pulsated voice Glottal fry. See under voice disorders of phonation.

pulsation (pəl-sā'shən) [See pulse] See beat.

pulse [L. *pulsus*, a beat or stroke] **1.** In audiology, rhythmical presentation of short bursts of a pure tone. **2.** In speech, a type of sound generation in which there is abrupt release of closures in the vocal tract or larynx.

    alternating p. Series of short bursts of pure tones which vary in amplitude in regular cycles.

    glottal p. Release of a series of pulses of air pressure when the vocal folds vibrate.

punishment Consequent event which immediately follows a behavior and decreases the frequency of that behavior.

pure agraphia See under pure *aphasias*.

pure alexia See under pure *aphasias*.

pure aphasias See under aphasia.

pure aphemia See under pure *aphasias*.

pure tone See under tone.

pure tone air-conduction threshold See under threshold.

pure-tone audiometer See under audiometer.

pure-tone audiometry See under audiometry.

pure tone average In audiometry, the average of the hearing threshold levels at frequencies of 500, 1000, and 2000 Hz for each ear as obtained on a pure tone hearing test.

pure tone bone-conduction threshold See under threshold.

pure vowel See under vowel.

pure wave Sinusoidal wave.

pure word blindness See pure alexia under pure *aphasias*.

pure word deafness See under pure *aphasias*.

purulent (pyur'ə-lənt) [L. *purulentia*, a festering] Suppurative.

purulent otitis media Suppurative *otitis media*.

push back Surgical procedure used to correct cleft palate; the velum is separated from the posterior surface of the palatine bone and shifted posteriorly, along with flaps of tissue raised from the oral surface of the soft palate.

PWS Person who stutters.

pyramidal system or **tract** Two groups of nerve fibers arising in the sensorimotor areas of the cerebral cortex and descending into the spinal cord; responsible for skillful, discrete, spatially oriented movements. Syn: direct motor system.

Q Coulomb.

quadratus lumborum muscle See *Muscles of Respiration* table, under respiration.

quadriplegia (kwäd-rə-ple'jē-ə) [L. *quattuor*, four + G. *plēgē*, stroke] Paralysis involving all four extremities. *Cf.* diplegia; hemiplegia; monoplegia; paraplegia; triplegia.

qualifier Word or word group limiting or modifying the meaning of another word or word group; *e.g.*, the *short* boy. See also adjective and adverb, under parts of speech.

quality **1.** Essential attribute, distinguishing feature, or characteristic; degree of excellence. **2.** Subjective impression of the patterns of frequencies and relative intensities of the voice. **3.** Identifying characteristic of a vowel sound, determined chiefly by the resonance of the vocal chambers producing it. See also timbre.

quantifier Word expressing amounts when used to modify another word; *e.g.*, five, twenty, a few, more. See also adjective, under parts of speech.

quantity **1.** Characteristic of a phenomenon which permits it to be measured or counted; results in variations in degree rather than in kind. **2.** In speech, the frequency, intensity, and duration of a speech sound. **3.** Amount of time the vocal organs stay in their required positions for the production of a particular sound.

  objective q. Variations of the length of speech sounds as measured by instrumental examination.

    Absolute quantity is the exact amount of time that a sound has endured; *e.g.*, /t/ in a specific production may last 4/100 of a second.

    Relative quantity is a comparison of the duration of one sound with that of another; *e.g.*, /a/ in a given position is always shorter in duration than /i/ in a given position.

  subjective q. In linguistics, the length of a sound as felt or heard during its production; *e.g.*, the vowels in *beat* and *bit* are perceived as different and give two different meanings to the *b-t* frame.

quartile One of the three points that divide a serially ranked distribution into four parts, each of which contains one fourth of the scores.

question (kwes'chən) [L. *quaestion*, to ask] Request for information demonstrated by the use of *wh-* words, verb reversals requiring a yes-no response, or tags; usually indicated by rising intonation and punctuated by /?/.

  tag q. Interrogative form following a declarative sentence and derived from that sentence; usually involves elliptical constructions. Semantically, it is a request for conformation; *e.g.*, You can go, can't you? You can't go, can you?

  wh- question Syntactic construction that begins with *who, what, which, when, where, whose, why,* and *how; e.g., Who* is that? *How* is included on the basis of its distribution in spite of the fact that it does not technically qualify by its spelling.

  yes-no q. Type of interrogative construction which requires affirmative or negative responses; the usual subject-verb order is inverted; *e.g.*, Is that a cat?

255

r Product moment.

R or **r** Roentgen.

℞ Prescription therapy.

radical mastoidectomy See under mastoidectomy.

radiogram (rā′dē-ō-gram) [L. *radius*, ray + G. *gramma*, a writing] Radiograph.

radiograph (rā′dē-ō-graf) [see radiography] Photographic film or plate depicting images of internal structures of the body which is produced by the actions of x-rays on a specially sensitized film. Syn: x-ray (2); radiogram; roentgenogram.

radiography (rā-dē-og′rə-fē) [L. *radius*, ray + G. *graphē*, a writing] Technique of x-ray exposure of human anatomy for display on a film; the most common and frequent type of x-ray, *e.g.*, of the chest, neck, skull. Syn: roentgenography. *Cf.* cineradiography; fluoroscopy; tomography. See also x-ray.

radiologic, radiological (ra-dē-ō-loj′ik, -i-kəl) Relating to radiology.

radiologist (rā-dē-ol′ə-jist) Physician specializing in the diagnostic and therapeutic use of x-rays and other forms of radiant energy.

radiology (rā-dē-ol′ə-jē) [L. *radius*, ray + G. *logos*, study, discourse] Medical specialty and science concerned with the use of radiant energy, including x-rays, in the diagnosis and treatment of disease and in the evaluation of physical abnormalities and pathologic conditions.

Rainville technique See under masking techniques.

Ramsay Hunt syndrome [J. Ramsay Hunt, U.S. neurologist, 1872–1937] Herpes zoster virus infection of the ganglion of the facial nerve (cranial nerve VII) with lesions involving the external ear, mastoid process, and oral mucosa; results in intense pain in the affected areas, paralysis of the nerve with attendant manifestations, tinnitus, hearing loss, and vertigo. Syn: Hunt's syndrome.

ramus, pl. **rami** (rā′məs, -mī) [L.] A branch; in anatomical nomenclature, a general term used to designate a smaller structure given off by a larger one or one into which a larger structure divides, such as a blood vessel or nerve.

random Occurring by chance.

random activity or **movement 1.** Behavior made without purpose or foresight, not determined by instinct or habit, and not obviously elicited by any specific cue in the situation. **2.** Movement which is not guided or directed toward any goal or biological purpose; *e.g.*, movements of an infant.

random noise See under noise.

random sample See under sample.

range Interval or distance between two extreme values (inclusive of the extremes) in a series of data, stimuli, sensibilities, movements, variations from the mean, and so forth. For various ranges, see specific terms.

range of frequencies See band *frequency.*

range of motion (ROM) or **movement** or **excursion** Those limits within which a motion may occur.

rank order See under coefficient of correlation.

raphe (raf′ē) [G. *raphē*, suture, seam] Seam or ridge indicating the line of junction of two symmetrical halves.

  lingual r. Median lingual *sulcus.*

  median longitudinal r. Median lingual *sulcus.*

  palatine r. Narrow ridge of mucosa in the median line of the palate.

  pharyngeal r. Fibrous band in the median line of the posterior wall of the pharynx.

Rapidly Alternating Speech Perception

Test (RASP) See *Audiometric Tests and Procedures* in appendices.

rare clefts Atypical *clefts*.

rarefaction (răr-ə-fak′shən) [L. *rarus*, thin + *factus*, made] **1.** Process or act of making less dense. **2.** In acoustics, a separating of particles in a sound wave resulting in a less compact condition; the second half of the cycle of a sound wave. See also wave (2).

rate [L. *ratum*, a computation, reckoning] **1.** Expression of the speed or frequency with which a certain event or circumstance occurs in relation to a certain period of time, a specific population, or some other fixed standard. For various rates, see specific terms. **2.** In speech, the speed with which phonemes, syllables, and words are uttered; reflects phonetic duration of silence as well as sound; may be freely responsive to the nature of the communicative situation and to the psychological condition of the speaker. See also speech sound flow.

rate control In stuttering, a technique in which the stutterer, in an attempt to avoid a stuttering block, speaks more slowly, often in a monotone with each syllable given equal stress.

rate of decay Decay period or rate.

rate of maturation Sequential development of certain skills during infancy and early childhood which usually occur within certain time periods; *e.g.*, sitting, crawling, standing, walking, speaking, social interactions.

ratio (rā′shē-ō) [L. *ratio*, a reckoning] Value obtained by dividing one number by another, indicating their relative proportions; *e.g.*, IQ equals mental age divided by chronological age.

rationalist theory of language Nativist theory. See under language theories.

rationalization (ra′shən-əl-i-zā′shən) Process of justifying one's behavior by presenting plausible or socially acceptable reasons in place of the real reasons.

raw score Record of test performance

presented in terms of the original test units; the number of items "passed."

re- Prefix from Latin meaning again, backward, contrary.

reactance (rē-ak′tens) That part of the impedance (opposition to alternating-current flow) of an alternating-current circuit that is due to the capacitance or inductance or both; computed by formula and expressed in ohms.

  inductive r. Measure, in ohms, of the resistance to electrical current flow in an induction coil.

reaction (rē-ak′shən) Partial or total response made to any kind or degree of stimulation.

  conversion r. Transformation of an emotion into a physical manifestation, as in conversion hysteria.

  dissociative r. Attempt to escape from excessive tension and anxiety by separating some parts of a personality function from the other parts.

  escape r. 1. Response that tends to remove an organism from contact with an undesirable stimulus. **2.** In stuttering, the behavioral reaction of the stutterer on escape from a moment of stuttering.

  manic r. Psychotic excitements characterized by overactivity and delusional elation or self-assertion, but without disorganization.

  obsessive compulsive r. Useless but irresistible repetitious acts, words, or thoughts whose aim is to reduce tensions and anxiety by (a) indulging in something forbidden; (b) denying such indulgence or guarding against it; or (c) punishing oneself for having had the impulse to indulge.

  paranoid r. Attempt to escape from tension and anxiety through the process of denial and projection which may result in systemized delusions.

reaction time Minimum time between a stimulus and a response.

real-ear gain See under gain.

Real Ear Measurement See *Audiometric Tests and Procedures* in appendices.

reasoning Problem solving by means of general principles.

reauditorization (rē′ôd-i-tôr-i-zā′shən) [re- + L. *auditus*, heard] Verbal mediation.

rebus (rē′bəs) [L. by things, fr. *res*, thing] Puzzle representing a word, phrase, or sentence by letters, numerals, pictures, etc., often with pictures of objects whose names have the same sound as the words represented; used as an alternative method of teaching reading. See also aided *augmentative communication*.

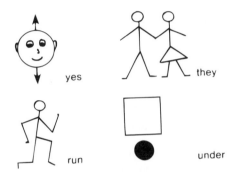

yes they run under

Rebus

recall 1. Memory. 2. Process of remembering something in the past in an attempt to recapture its essence.

receiver (rē-sē′vėr) [L. *recipio*, to receive] In a hearing aid, the earphone or bone-conduction vibrator which provides the inverse function of a microphone by converting electrical impulses from the amplifier to an acoustic output (sound pressure waves); composed of a magnet, coil, and diaphragm. See also hearing aid.

   air-conduction r. Device which receives the amplified electronic signal of the hearing aid circuit and converts it to sound pressure waves which activate the eardrum.

   bone-conduction r. Vibrator or oscillator designed to transmit sound pressure waves through the bones of the skull.

reception (rē-sep′shən) [L. *recipio*, to receive] In speech and language, the admission of language (oral or other) via single or multi-modality avenues (auditory, visual, etc.); does not necessarily imply comprehension.

receptive aphasia See under aphasia.

Receptive-Expressive Emergent Language Scale (REEL)—Second Edition See *Language Tests and Procedures* in appendices.

Receptive-Expressive Observation Scale (REO) See *Language Tests and Procedures* in appendices.

receptive language See under language.

Receptive One-Word Picture Vocabulary Test (ROWPVT)—2000 See *Language Tests and Procedures* in appendices.

receptor (rē-sep′tėr) [L. one who receives] Any one of the various sensory nerve endings in the skin, viscera, and sense organs.

reciprocal assimilation See under assimilation.

reconditioning (rē-kən-dish′ən-iŋ) Reestablishing a conditioned response after extinction has begun by further repetition of the stimulus with reinforcement.

recruitment (rē-krut′ment) [Fr. *recrutement* fr. L. *recretus*, grown again] 1. Phenomenon, sometimes accompanying a sensorineural impairment of hearing, in which a relatively slight increase in the intensity of a sound results in a disproportionate increase in the sensation of loudness; may be indicative of a lesion of the organ of Corti; *e.g.*, the actual decibel intensity may have increased only 20 dB, while it is perceived as having increased from 0 dB to 60 dB. 2. Pathologic condition in which the intensity function is so disturbed that the individual is extremely sensitive to small increases in the loudness of sound. 3. Activity that requires additional motor neurons and thus causes greater activity in response to increased duration of the stimulus applied to a given receptor or afferent nerve. See also decruitment.

complete r. Sensation of loudness of a tone in the affected ear equals the sensation of loudness in the better ear at higher intensity levels.

hyperrecruitment Sensation of intensity of a tone in the affected ear exceeds the sensation of loudness in the better ear at higher intensity levels. Syn: overrecruitment.

incomplete r. Sensation of loudness of a tone in the affected ear approaches, but does not equal, the sensation of loudness in the better ear at high-intensity levels. Syn: partial recruitment.

overrecruitment Hyperrecruitment (see above).

partial r. Incomplete *recruitment*.

rectus abdominis muscle See *Muscles of Respiration* table, under respiration.

recurrent laryngeal nerve paralysis See laryngeal motor *paralysis* and its subentries.

reduced screening audiometry See under screening *audiometry*.

reduction (rē-dək′shən) [L. *reductio*, to lead back] **1.** Act or process of decreasing or lessening. **2.** In phonetics, a method of facilitating pronunciation by suppressing certain consonants in heavy clusters or decreasing double consonants belonging to different words or morphemes; *e.g.*, can't, hasn't, didn't. See also under syllabic structure, under phonological processes. **3.** Altering of unstressed vowels to /ə/; *e.g.*, tɛləgram = tɛləgram. **4.** Processes whereby a full form is abbreviated to a shorter form; *e.g.*, *influenza* to *flu*. **5.** In transformational grammar, a rule which allows a lengthy utterance to be shortened without loss of meaning; *e.g.*, *I can cook and I sew* to *I can cook and sew.*

reduction of clusters See under syllabic structure, under phonological processes.

redundancy (rē-dən′dan-sē) [L. *redun-*

dantia, an excess] **1.** That part of a message which can be eliminated without the loss of essential information. **2.** Information repeated.

reduplicated babbling See under babbling.

reduplication See under syllabic structure, under phonological processes.

REEL Receptive-Expressive Emergent Language Scale.

reference (ref′ėr-əns) [L. *referre*, bring back] Semantic meaning of a word or expression; *e.g.*, pig = animal. Syn: referential function. See also denotation.

reference zero level See audiometric zero.

referent (ref′ėr-ənt) [see reference] Object, event, abstraction, or person indicated by a symbol, verbal or otherwise.

referential function Reference.

referential semantics See under semantics.

reflected wave See under wave.

reflection (rē-flek′shən) [L. *reflexio*, a bending back] In acoustics, the return of sound pressure waves toward their source. See also reflected *wave.*

reflex [L. *reflexus*, bent back] **1.** A reaction; an involuntary movement excited in response to a stimulus applied to the periphery and transmitted to the nervous centers in the brain or spinal cord. **2.** Simple mechanical act which appears not to involve volition or choice.

acoustic r. 1. Contraction of the intra-aural muscles (tensor tympani, and stapedius) in response to sound; one of three measurements utilized in acoustic immittance. **2.** Any reflex occurring in response to a sound. Syn: auditory, cochlear, or intra-aural reflex; middle ear muscle reflex.

acoustic contralateral r. Measurement of reflex-related change in acoustic immittance in one ear, with acoustic stimulation of the opposite ear.

acoustic ipsilateral r. Measurement of reflex-related change in acoustic immittance in the ear that is acoustically stimulated.

acousticopalpebral r. Auropalpebral *reflex.*

acoustic stapedial r. Contraction of the stapedial muscle elicited by high-intensity acoustic stimulation; in the normal ear, a contralateral reflex is elicited at 70–95 dB sensation level while the ipsilateral reflex is elicited at 3–16 dB lower (67–79 dB) sensation levels.

audito-oculogyric r. Turning of the two eyes toward the source of a sudden sound.

auditory r. Acoustic *reflex.*

auropalpebral r. (ARP) Wink or twitch at the corner of the eye as a result of a sudden sound near the ear. Syn: acousticopalpebral, cochleoorbicular, or cochleopalpebral reflex.

Babinski r. [J. F. Babinski, Fr. neurologist, 1857–1932] Extension of the great toe with fanning of the other toes on stimulation of the sole of the foot; may be indicative of a lesion involving the pyramidal tract.

cochlear r. Acoustic *reflex.*

cochleoorbicular r. Auropalpebral *reflex.*

cochleopalpebral r. (CPR) Auropalpebral *reflex.*

flexion r. Withdrawal of an extremity from an irritating or painful stimulus; *e.g.*, bending of the ankle, knee, and hip when the foot is painfully stimulated.

gag r. Pharyngeal *reflex.*

intra-aural r. Acoustic *reflex.*

laryngeal r. Cough resulting from irritation of the larynx.

middle ear muscle r. Acoustic *reflex.*

Moro's r. [E. Moro, Ger. physician, 1874–1951] Reaction of infants to a variety of stimuli which is characterized by a sudden extension and ab-

duction of the arms, hands, and fingers from their usual fixed posture; the legs may follow the same movement pattern. It is present at birth and is strongest during the first three months of life. Syn: startle reflex.

myotatic r. Stretch *reflex.*

orienting r. (OR) Aspect of attending in which an organism's initial response to a change in its environment or to a novel stimulus is such that the organism becomes more sensitive to the situation; *e.g.*, dilation of the pupil of the eye in response to dim light.

pharyngeal r. Medial movement of the lateral walls of the oropharynx and elevation and retraction of the soft palate as a result of touching the posterior pharyngeal wall of the oropharynx; included in oral peripheral examinations to observe functioning of the velopharyngeal port mechanism. Syn: gag reflex.

rooting r. A response whereby the head turns in the direction of a stimulus in a food-seeking movement. This occurs when stroking or other tactile stimulation is given at the upper lip, at the lower lip, or at the corners of the mouth. The tongue, lips and jaw may also move in the direction of the stimulus. The rooting reflex is present at birth and disappears at 2–4 months. It is retained for a longer period by breast-fed infants than by bottle-fed infants. Syn: rooting reaction.

stapedius r. Contraction of the stapedius muscle in response to a loud sound.

startle r. Moro's *reflex.*

stretch r. Tonic contraction of the muscles in response to a stretching force, due to stimulation of muscle proprioceptors. Syn: myotatic reflex.

reflex arc Functional unit of the nervous system, as establishing a connection between receptor and effector, or between the situation with which an organism is confronted and the motor response which the organism makes; consists of two or more structural units or neurons, one afferent, conducting the nerve impulse from the receptor, and the other efferent, conducting the impulse to the effector muscle or gland. Syn: sensorimotor arc.

reflex conditioning See under classical *conditioning.*

reflex time Period between the stimulus and the beginning of the response.

reformulation (rē'fôr-myu-lā'shən) In oral language, false starts, *i.e.*, pauses, starting over, stopping, starting over; *e.g.*, "He, she, he said, she, she said, she said, 'Let's go home'."

refracted wave See under wave.

refraction (rē-frak'shən) [L. *refractio*, to break up] In acoustics, the deflection of sound waves around obstacles. See also refracted *wave.*

refractory period Time between nerve impulses during which the nerve will not respond to a stimulus of threshold intensity; during this period the ions of the nerve return to a prefiring or resting position.

regional dialect See dialect.

register (rej'i-stėr) See vocal register; voice register.

regression (rē-gresh'ən) [L. *regressus*, gone back] A return to an earlier mental, physical, or behavioral level. For types of regression, see specific terms.

regressive assimilation See under assimilation.

regular determiner See determiner.

rehabilitation (rē-hə-bil-i-tā'shən) [L. *rehabilitatus*, made fit] Restoration to normal, or to as satisfactory a status as possible, of impaired functions. *Cf.* habilitation. For types of rehabilitation, see specific terms.

rehabilitative audiology Aural rehabilitation.

reinforcement (rē-in-fôrs'ment) Procedure of following a response with a reinforcer (positive or negative); used in conditioning.

differential r. Any procedure in which one response is supported and another, usually similar to the first, is not; encourages the desired response to occur more often and the undesired response to occur less often. See also shaping.

partial r. Procedure in which only a portion of all responses is reinforced.

primary r. Use of reinforcers whose effectiveness does not depend on learning, such as food and water.

reinforcement schedule Procedural plan used in conditioning which prescribes when the subject's response to a stimulus is to be rewarded, either in terms of time intervals or in terms of the succession of responses; *e.g.*, every third response to be rewarded.

continuous r. s. Schedule in which a reinforcer follows every desired response.

extinction r. s. (eks-tiŋk'shən) [L. *extinctio*] Progressive reduction in the strength of a conditioned response on withdrawal of the reinforcer; *e.g.*, learning which requires reinforcement will show a reduction in performance if the reinforcement is omitted.

fixed-interval r. s. Schedule of reinforcers received for the first response to occur after a specified time period has elapsed, measured from the last reinforcement.

fixed-ratio r. s. Schedule in which the subject receives a reinforcer only after emitting a specified number of responses.

intermittent r. s. Schedule in which only some occurrences of a response are followed by a reinforcer.

variable-interval r. s. Schedule in which reinforcement of a response occurs at random or semirandom periods around a specified mean time length.

variable-ratio r. s. Schedule in which

reinforcement occurs after a number of responses, the number varying randomly or semirandomly about a mean.

reinforcer (rē-in-fôrs′ėr) **1.** A reward; a satisfactory or unsatisfactory stimulus, object, or stimulus event given to the subject on his performance of a specified or predetermined behavior. **2.** Consequence which increases or decreases the frequency of a response. See also stimulus.

    conditioned r. Stimulus which is originally neutral but which acquires reinforcing characteristics by being paired with a reinforcing stimulus; *e.g.*, a social consequence, such as a smile, frown, praise, criticism produced by the behavior of other people, which is often paired with a primary reinforcer. Syn: Secondary reinforcer.

    delayed r. Consequence which is not administered immediately after the response.

    generalized r. Conditioned reinforcer which may be paired with several primary reinforcers; *e.g.*, mother's voice paired with food, warmth, and the removal of unpleasant stimuli.

    negative r. 1. Consequence which is unpleasant, unsatisfying, or painful to the recipient. **2.** Adverse stimulus used to decrease the probability of a response. **3.** Distasteful stimulus, removal of which is contingent on a response, with a resulting increase in the frequency of that response. Syn: noxious stimulus.

    positive r. 1. Consequence which is pleasant or satisfying to the recipient. **2.** Anything, following a response, which increases the frequency of that response; may be extrinsic, such as a token, edible item, or money, or social, in the form of praise.

    primary r. Consequence which appears to have reinforcing characteristics as a function of the biological makeup of the organism; *e.g.*, response that terminates a painful stimulus. Syn: unconditioned reinforcer.

    secondary r. Conditioned *reinforcer.*

    unconditioned r. Primary *reinforcer.*

Reissner's membrane [E. Reissner, Ger. anatomist, 1824–1878] Vestibular *membrane.*

relational words See under word.

relative quantity See under objective *quantity.*

release (rē-lēs′) **1.** Movement of the speech organs from a position of articulation to a state of rest. **2.** Act or manner of ending a sound. **3.** In stuttering, the reduction in muscle tension of the stutterer when his atypical speech behaviors are discontinued.

releasing consonant See under consonant.

reliability (rē-lī-ə-bil′ə-tē) In mental measurements, the dependability of a test as reflected in the consistency of its scores on repeated measurements of the same group.

reliability coefficient Coefficient of correlation between two forms of a test, between scores on two administrations of the same test, or between halves of a test; all three measures vary as to the aspects of reliability determined, but all are properly spoken of as reliability coefficients.

    alternate forms r. c. Correlation between results on alternate, equivalent, or parallel forms of a test; a measure of the extent to which the two forms are consistent in measuring what they purport to measure. Syn: comparable forms reliability coefficient.

    comparable forms r. c. Alternate forms *reliability coefficient.*

    odd-even method Split-half *reliability coefficient.*

    split-half r. c. Measure of estimating the reliability of a test by splitting it into comparable halves (usually the odd-numbered and even-numbered items), correlating the scores of the two halves, and applying the Spearman-Brown prophecy formula to estimate the correlation. Syn: odd-even method.

test-retest r. c. Reliability coefficient obtained by administering the same test a second time, after a short interval, and correlating the two sets of scores.

remission (rē-mish′ən) [L. *remissio,* to send back, slacken] Lessening of the severity or a temporary abatement of symptoms of a disorder or of a disease.

repetition (rep-ə-tish′ən) [L. *repetitio,* to repeat] **1.** In oral language, the ability to reproduce, from aural presentation, patterns of familiar speech sounds. **2.** In stuttering, a type of behavior which involves the repeating of a sound, syllable, word, or phrase as part of the stuttering pattern.

representative sample See under sample.

repress [L. *repressus,* pressed back] To suppress from conscious awareness those memories, thoughts, or feelings that are painful or distasteful to the self.

repressed need theory See under stuttering theories.

reserve air Expiratory reserve volume. See under respiratory volume.

residual (rē-zid′yu-əl) [L. *residuus,* remaining] **1.** Denoting that which remains of a part, substance, or function after a portion has been removed or lost. **2.** Statistical term indicating the expected error in the analysis.

residual air Residual volume. See under respiratory volume.

residual hearing The range of hearing that an individual with a hearing loss possesses; *e.g.,* 80% hearing loss = 20% residual hearing.

residual volume (RV) See under respiratory volume.

resistance (rē-zis′təns) [L. *resisto,* to withstand] **1.** Action of a body against an opposing force. **2.** In electronics, the opposition in a conductor to the passage of a current of electricity, where there is a loss of energy and a production of heat; resistance equals the voltage divided by the current. **3.** In acoustics, dissipation of energy by friction of the molecules of the sound medium; a part of acoustic impedance measured in acoustic ohms.

galvanic skin r. Galvanic skin *response.*

psychogalvanic skin r. Galvanic skin *response.*

resistor (rē-zis′tėr) [see resistance] Device used to control the flow of electricity, as in the circuit of a hearing aid.

resonance (rez′ə-nəns) [L. *resonantia,* echo] Sympathetic or forced vibration of the air in the cavities above, below, in front of, or behind the source of a sound.

nasal r. 1. Energy pattern added to the spectrum of a speech sound when the nasal tract is coupled to the vocal tract; consists of both resonances and antiresonances. **2.** Modification of the glottal tone by the nasal chambers. See also nasal, under consonant, manner of formation; nasality and its subentries; voice disorders of resonance.

vocal r. Modification of the laryngeal tone by passage through the chambers of the throat and head, so as to alter its quality; may, without actually increasing its intensity, alter the wave form, causing it to affect the ear more vigorously and thus to increase the loudness of the tone.

resonance disorders See voice disorders of resonance.

resonance-volley theory See under hearing theories.

resonant frequency Natural *frequency.*

resonator (rez′ə-nā-tėr) [L. *resonatus,* resounded] Any cavity which is responsible for the changes in the fundamental vibrations produced by the vocal folds.

subglottic r.'s The trachea and the thoracic cavities.

supraglottic r.'s The pharynx and the oral and nasal cavities.

respiration (res-pə-rā′shən) [L. *respiratio*, to breathe] **1.** Act of breathing with the lungs which consists of two actions: (a) *inspiration*, the drawing in of atmospheric air or oxygen, and (b) *expiration*, the expulsion of mixed air and gases resulting from respiratory metabolism. Syn: breathing. **2.** Energy source for speech; a physical process of pumping air, the movement of which eventually is transformed into acoustic energy. See *Muscles of Respiration* table.

abdominal-diaphragmatic r. Respiration utilizing the contraction of the diaphragm and the elasticity of the abdominal wall and viscera; considered by some authorities to be the preferred method of respiration. *Cf.* thoracic *respiration.*

bronchial r. Breathing heard over the trachea or bronchial tubes; it is high in pitch (equal in inspiration and expiration), blowing in character, and marked by a brief pause between inspiration and expiration.

clavicular r. Breathing in which the shoulders are elevated on inhalation, using the neck accessory muscles as the primary muscles of inhalation; characterized by noticeable elevation of the clavicles. This manner of breathing is unsatisfactory for good voice because it requires too much effort for too little breath.

cortical r. Conscious control of breathing usually characterized by exertion of excessive muscular force while attempting to speak, such as holding the abdominal muscles in a fixed contracted state.

laryngeal r. Widening of the glottis during inspiration and its narrowing during expiration.

nasal r. Breathing through the nasal

cavity; usually considered the "normal" manner of breathing.

opposition r. Breathing in which the thorax and diaphragm work against each other in providing breath support for the voice.

oral r. Breathing through the oral cavity; usually the result of nasal congestion or obstruction.

thoracic r. Respiration in which there is no noticeable upper thoracic elevation, as with clavicular breathing, or abdominal expansion, as with abdominal-diaphragmatic respiration; considered by some authorities to be the preferred method of respiration. *Cf.* abdominal-diaphragmatic *respiration.*

respiratory (res′pėr-ə-tôr-ē,   rə-spīr′ə-tôr-ē) Pertaining to respiration.

respiratory capacity Potential cubic contents of the lungs and airways; includes two or more respiratory volumes. Syn: lung capacity. See also respiratory volume.

functional residual c. (FRC) Amount of air contained within the lungs and airways at the resting expiratory level; includes expiratory reserve volume and residual volume (*q.v.,* under respiratory volume).

inspiratory c. (IC) Maximum amount of air that can be inspired from the resting expiratory level; the sum of tidal volume and inspiratory reserve volume (*q.v.,* under respiratory volume).

total lung c. (TLC) Amount of air contained within the lungs and airways at the end of maximum inspiration; includes all of the respiratory volumes (*q.v.*).

vital c. (VC) Greatest amount of air that can be expelled from the lungs and airways after maximum inspiration; includes all of the respiratory volumes except residual volume (*q.v.*).

respiratory disorder Abnormal breathing pattern which may manifest itself in

MUSCLES OF RESPIRATION

Muscle	Origin	Insertion	Innervation	Function
		INHALATION (QUIET)		
Diaphragm	Xiphoid process of sternum, lower 6 costal cartilages, and lumbar vertebrae	Central tendon	Phrenic nerve	Acts as main muscle of inhalation; aids in expulsive actions
Intercostalis externus (11 pairs)	Lower border of rib above	Superior border of rib below	Anterior branch of thoracic nerve	Accessory muscle of respiration
Scalenus anterior (paired)	Transverse processes of 3rd to 6th cervical vertebrae	Tubercle of 1st rib	Anterior branches of 3rd and 4th cervical nerves	Flexes vertebral column laterally; accessory muscle of respiration
Scalenus medius (paired)	Transverse processes of 2nd to 6th cervical vertebrae	Upper surface of 1st rib	Anterior branches of 3rd and 4th cervical nerves	Flexes vertebral column laterally; accessory muscle of respiration
Scalenus posterior (paired)	Tubercles of 4th to 6th cervical vertebrae	2nd rib	Anterior branches of 3rd and 4th cervical nerves	Flexes vertebral column laterally; accessory muscle of respiration
Levator costae (12 pairs)	Transverse processes of 7th cervical and upper 11 thoracic vertebrae	Medial to angle of corresponding rib below	Anterior branch of thoracic nerve	Aids in raising ribs in inspiration
		INHALATION (FORCED)		
Serratus anterior (paired)	Upper 8 or 9 ribs	Vertebral border of scapula	Long thoracic nerve	Draws scapula forward, draws inferior angle laterally
Serratus posterior inferior (paired)	Lumbodorsal fascia, spines of lowest thoracic and upper lumbar vertebrae	Last 4 ribs	Lower thoracic nerve	Accessory muscle of respiration
Serratus posterior superior (paired)	Spines of 7th cervical and upper thoracic vertebrae	2nd to 5th ribs	2nd and 3rd thoracic nerves	Accessory muscle of respiration; elevates ribs
Pectoralis major (paired)	Clavicle, sternum, first 6 ribs, and aponeurosis of external oblique muscle of abdomen	Intertubercular sulcus of humerus	Medial and lateral anterior thoracic nerves	Adducts and medially rotates humerus; flexes shoulder joint; depresses shoulder girdle
Pectoralis minor (paired)	3rd to 5th ribs	Coracoid process of scapula	Medial and lateral anterior thoracic nerves	Draws shoulder forward
Latissimus dorsi (paired)	Spines of lower 6 thoracic vertebrae, spines of lumbar vertebrae, lumbodorsal fascia, crest of ilium, lower ribs, and inferior angle of scapula	Intertubercular sulcus of humerus	Thoracodorsal nerve	Adducts and extends humerus; used to pull body up in climbing; accessory muscle of respiration

(Continued)

MUSCLES OF RESPIRATION—Continued

Muscle	Origin	Insertion	Innervation	Function
Subclavius (paired)	1st costal cartilage and 1st rib	Clavicle	Nerve to subclavius	Depresses lateral end of clavicle
Sternoclavicularis (variable)	Small separate slip of subclavius occasionally arising from sternum			
Sternocleidomastoideus (paired)	Manubrium of sternum and clavicle	Mastoid process	Accessory nerve and branches from 2nd and 3rd cervical nerves	Flexes head
		EXHALATION		
Obliquus abdominus externus (paired)	Lower 8 ribs	Xiphoid, linea alba, pubis, crest of ilium	Lower 6 thoracic nerves	Supports abdominal viscera; flexes vertebral column
Obliquus abdominus internus (paired)	Lumbodorsal fascia, iliac crest, and inguinal ligament	Lower 3 ribs, linea alba, xiphoid, pubis	Lower 6 thoracic and iliohypogastric nerves	Supports abdominal viscera; flexes vertebral column
Intercostalis internus (11 pairs)	Lower border of costal cartilage and rib above	Superior border of costal cartilage and rib below	Anterior branch of thoracic nerve	Accessory muscle of respiration
Iliocostalis dorsi	Lower 6 ribs	Upper 6 ribs	Posterior branch of thoracic nerve	Extends vertebral column and assists in lateral movements of trunk
Iliocostalis lumborum	Iliac crest, lumbar vertebrae, sacrum, and lumbodorsal vertebrae	Lower 6 ribs	Posterior branch of lumbar nerve	Extends vertebral column and assists in lateral trunk movements
Quadratus lumborum (paired)	Iliac crest, lumbodorsal fascia, and lumbar vertebrae	Transverse processes of lumbar vertebrae 1 through 4, medial half of last rib	Anterior branches of first 3 lumbar nerves	Assists in lateral movements of vertebral column
Serratus posterior inferior (paired)	Lumbodorsal fascia, spines of lowest thoracic and upper lumbar vertebrae	Last 4 ribs	Lower thoracic nerve	Accessory muscle of respiration
Subcostalis (paired)	Lower ribs	Lower ribs	Thoracic nerves	Muscle of respiration
Transversus abdominus (paired)	Costal cartilages of lower 6 ribs, lumbodorsal fascia, iliac crest, and inguinal ligament	Xiphoid, linea alba, inguinal ligament, and pubis	Anterior branches of lower 6 thoracic and iliohypogastric nerves	Supports abdominal viscera and flexes vertebral column
Transversus thoracis (paired)	Mediastinal surface of xiphoid and body of sternum	2nd to 6th costal cartilages	Thoracic nerve	Pulls ribs downward, decreasing thoracic cavity
Rectus abdominus (paired)	Pubis	Xiphoid, 5th to 7th costal cartilages	Anterior branches of lower 6 thoracic nerves	Supports abdominal viscera; flexes vertebral column

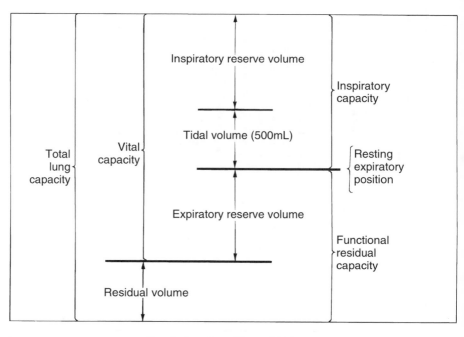

Respiratory Capacities and Volumes

any of a variety of speech characteristics. See *Respiratory Disorders* table.

respiratory frequency See under frequency.

respiratory system or **tract** Air passages from the nares into the lungs, including the nasal cavities, pharynx, larynx, trachea, and bronchi; allows passage of inhaled air into and exhaled air from the lungs, and provides adequate expiratory pressures to vibrate the vocal folds and an airstream from which

RESPIRATORY DISORDERS

Breathing Patterns	*Speech Characteristics*
Rapid rate of breathing	In infants, reduced vocalizing; in older children, prevention of the prolongation of exhalation essential to speech production
Difficulty with deep inhalation	Production of only one or two syllables on an exhalation; tension increases when longer vocalizations are attempted
Difficulty with prolonged exhalation	Problems in initiating vocalization; noticeable escape of air before initiation of vocalization; production of only a few syllables on exhalation
Antagonistic diaphragmatic-abdominal and thoracic movements	Difficulty sustaining vocalization as the result of insufficient air when antagonism occurs on inhalation
Involuntary movement in respiratory musculature	Varied loudness of voice; interruptions of vocalization
Speaking on residual air	Difficulty with adequate intensity and resonance

vowel and consonant sounds can be produced.

respiratory volume Actual space occupied by the air in the lungs and airways; expressed in milliliters. Syn: lung volume. See also respiratory capacity.

   expiratory reserve v. (ERV) Maximum volume of air that can be expelled from the lungs after normal expiration. Syn: reserve or supplemental air.

   forced expiratory v. (FEV) Maximum volume of air that can be expired in a specific time interval when starting from maximum inspiration.

   inspiratory reserve v. (IRV) Maximum volume of air that can be taken into the lungs and airways after normal inspiration, less tidal volume. Syn: complemental air.

   residual v. (RV) Volume of air remaining in the lungs and airways at the end of maximum expiration. Syn: residual air.

   tidal v. (V_T, TV) Volume of air inspired or expired during a respiratory cycle; considered the ideal breathing for speaking. Syn: tidal air.

respirometer (res-pə-rom′ə-tėr) [L. *respiro*, to breathe + G. *metron*, measure] Spirometer.

respondent conditioning Classical *conditioning*.

response (rē-spons′) [L. *responsus*, an answer] **1.** Any muscular, glandular, or psychic process that depends on stimulation; a reaction to a stimulus. **2.** In acoustics, the pattern of output of a transducer, such as a hearing aid, when measured at various frequencies after the input has been amplified. **3.** In conditioning, observable reactions, the result of stimulation, which can be counted, recorded, and manipulated.

   conditioned r. New or modified behavior that is elicited by a given stimulus after conditioning.

   covert r. Behavior that cannot be directly observed by another.

delayed r. Lapse of time occurring between a presented stimulus and a reaction to it; it may be deliberate or a result of an inability to react.

differential r. Reaction that is elicited by only one stimulus from among several similar stimuli.

false-negative r. In audiometry, the failure of a subject to respond during a hearing test when he has heard the stimulus.

false-positive r. In audiometry, response from a subject during a hearing test when no stimulus has been presented or the stimulus is below his threshold.

frequency r. Range of frequencies over which an acoustic or an electroacoustic device, such as a hearing aid, operates.

galvanic skin r. (GSR) Opposition of the skin to electrical impulse; a stimulus that excites any type of emotional response will cause the opposition of the skin to decrease, and the resulting increased flow of electrical current may be amplified and displayed on a graphic recorder. Syn: galvanic skin resistance; psychogalvanic skin resistance or response. See also *Audiometric Tests and Procedures* in appendices.

generalization r. (jen′ėr-əl-i-zā′ shən) In conditioning, the theory that, after an organism learns to emit a certain reaction to a given stimulus, a stimulus becomes effective in eliciting "similar" responses; the greater the similarity of reactions, the more frequently the stimulus will elicit the reaction. See also carryover.

latent r. Time between the beginning of a stimulus and the earliest detectable response.

maladaptive r. 1. Instrumentally conditioned response for which the reinforcement is the escape from or avoidance of stimulation. **2.** Response made at great sacrifice of energy, or perhaps even harmful to the organism, for a reinforcement of dubious or nonexistent value.

negative r. 1. Reaction which removes the organism from the source of stimulation. **2.** Reduced activity in which the subject ignores, is indifferent to, or resists the stimulus; may be overt or covert.

overt r. Behavior which can be observed by another.

paradigmatic r. Reply which is in the same grammatical class as the stimulus; *e.g.*, hot-cold (adjectives). *Cf.* syntagmatic *response.*

positive r. Increased activity in which the subject recognizes, is motivated by, and reacts to the stimulus.

psychogalvanic skin r. (PGSR) Galvanic skin *response.*

syntagmatic r. Reply which is in a different grammatical class than the stimulus; *e.g.*, big (stimulus-adjective)-boy (reply-noun). *Cf.* paradigmatic *response.*

target r. Reaction singled out as the one that will receive some predetermined consequence (positive or negative).

unconditioned r. Unlearned reaction evoked by a certain stimulus situation.

vibrotactile r. In audiometry, the response obtained during bone-conduction audiometry to stimuli that have been felt rather than actually heard; may occasionally occur during air-conduction testing. Syn: tactile exteroception.

response hierarchy Arrangement of a group of behaviors in the order of probability in which they will be elicited in a specific situation.

response magnitude Response strength.

response rate In conditioning, the number of responses given per unit of time, determined by dividing the number of responses by the number of minutes involved; correct, erroneous, or total number of responses may be recorded.

response strength Behavior described in

terms of amplitude, duration, frequency, or intensity. Syn: response magnitude.

response system Physiologic, neurologic, and psychologic processes involved in a reaction.

response time Period of time involved in producing a response to a stimulus.

restrictive modifier See under modifier.

retardation (rē-tär-dā′shən) [L. *retardatus*, delayed, hindered] Slowness or limitation of development; may be physiologic, neurologic, psychological, or any combination of these. For types of retardation, see specific terms.

retrieval (rē-trēv′əl) Ability to recall from memory the desired or correct symbol (auditory, visual, tactile, etc.). See also memory; word retrieval.

retro- [L. back, backward] Prefix denoting backward, behind.

retroactive amnesia See under amnesia.

retroauricular (re-trō-ôr-ik′u-lėr) Behind the ear.

retrocochlear (re-trō-kō′klē-ėr) Behind the cochlea.

retrocochlear deafness See under deafness.

retroflex See under consonant, manner of formation.

retroflex vowel See under vowel.

retrognathic (re-trō-na′thik) [retro- + G. *gnathos*, jaw] Having an underdeveloped maxilla, mandible, or both. *Cf.* prognathic.

reverberation (rē-vėr-bėr-ā′shən) [L. *reverbratus*, struck back] In acoustics, the persistence of sound in an enclosed space as a result of multiple reflections after the source of the sound has ceased.

reverberation room Chamber with minimal sound absorption capacity; sound will be reflected many times therein. Syn: echo chamber. *Cf.* anechoic chamber.

reverberation time 1. Rate of sound decay; the length of time required for sound pressure waves to decay to

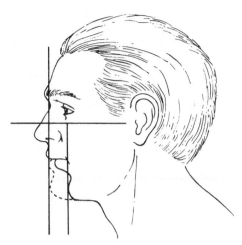

Retrognathic
From *Stedman's Medical Dictionary,* 25th ed.
Baltimore: Williams & Wilkins, 1990.

some fixed fraction of their original value in a chamber after the initial sound source has ceased. **2.** Time required for the sound field to decay to inaudibility.

reverse phonation See under phonation.

reverse swallowing Tongue thrust.

reversibility Ability to follow a line of reasoning back to where it began [Piaget].

Revised Token Test See *Language Tests and Procedures* in appendices.

reward See reinforcer (1). See also consequence (2).

rheobase (rē′ō-bās) [G. *rheos*, stream + *basis*, base] Minimum voltage of an electric current required to stimulate a nerve or muscle.

rhin-, rhino- [G. *rhis*, nose] Combining form pertaining to the nose.

rhinitis (rī-nī′tis) [rhin- + G. *-itis*, inflammation] Inflammation of the mucous membranes of the nose.

rhinolalia (rī-nō-lā′lē-ə) [rhino- + G. *lalia*, speaking] Nasality.

    r. aperta Hypernasality. See under voice disorders of resonance.

    r. clausa Hyponasality. See under voice disorders of resonance.

rhinophonia (rī-nō-fō′nē-ə) [rhino- + G. *phonē*, sound, voice] Nasality.

rhotacized vowel See under vowel.

rhotic See under consonant, manner of formation. Syn: retroflex.

rhythm (rɪTH′em) [G. *rhythmos*] In speech: **1.** Cadence or melody of oral language; the pattern of speech flow. It is established by patterns of stress and rate. See also speech sound flow. **2.** That aspect of oral language concerned with the periodic recurrence in time of similar patterns of pitch, loudness, duration, or quality. **3.** In stuttering, a therapy technique to help the stutterer speak fluently by altering the rhythm of speech through such means as singing or speaking in a singsong manner, speaking with a regularly recurring rhythm such as to the beat of a metronome, or timing the speech and syllable gestures to an arm swing. See specific terms.

ridge (rij) Linear elevation on a surface. For various ridges, see specific terms.

rigidity (ri-jid′i-tē) Muscular resistance to passive motion from simultaneous agonist and antagonist muscle group contractions. See also under cerebral palsy symptomatology.

rima glottidis Glottis.

Rinne Test See *Audiometric Tests and Procedures* in appendices.

Robbins Speech Sound Discrimination and Verbal Imagery Type Tests See *Auditory Tests and Procedures* in appendices.

Rochester method [Rochester School for the Deaf, Rochester, N.Y.] Method of teaching the deaf in which oralism is supplemented by fingerspelling. See also simultaneous method, under aural rehabilitation.

roentgen (R, r) (rent′gən) [W. K. Roentgen, Ger. physicist, 1845–1923] International unit of x-ray radiation.

roentgenogram (rent′gen-ə-gram) Radiograph.

roentgenography (rent-gən-og′rə-fē) Radiography.

roentgen ray X-ray (1).

ROM Range of motion.

root of the tongue See tongue.

root word Base *word*.

Ross Information Processing Assessment—Geriatric See *Language Tests and Procedures* in appendices.

Ross Information Processing Assessment—Primary See *Language Tests and Procedures* in appendices.

Ross Information Processing Assessment—Second Edition See *Language Tests and Procedures* in appendices.

Rotation Test See *Audiometric Tests and Procedures* in appendices.

rote See under memory.

rough hoarseness See hoarseness, under voice disorders of phonation.

round See under distinctive feature.

rounded vowel See under vowel.

rounding See lip rounding.

round window See under middle *ear*.

rubella (ru-bel'ə) [L. fem. reddish, dim. *ruber*, red] Viral disease characterized by reddish eruptions on the skin and enlargement of the lymph nodes, but with little fever or other constitutional disturbances; if contracted within the first three to four months of pregnancy, it may produce in the fetus varying combinations of deafness, blindness, mental deficiency, cleft palate, cerebral palsy, or other anomalies. Syn: German or three-day measles.

Rudmose audiometer See under audiometer.

ruga, pl. **rugae** (ru'gə, -gē) [L. a wrinkle] Crease or furrow, such as found on the surface of the middle anterior portion of the upper alveolar or rugal ridge.

rule [Fr. *reule* fr. L. *regula*, guide or pattern] Prescribed guide for conduct or action; a law or regulation; a standard of judgment. *Cf.* criteria.

running speech Connected *speech*.

RV Residual volume.

saccule (sak′yul) [L. *sacculus*, small sac or pouch] Smaller of the two vestibular sacs. See vestibule, under inner *ear.*

saddle curve See under audiogram configuration.

sagittal (saj′i-təl) [L. *sagitta*, arrow] In an anterior to posterior direction (and in the line of an arrow shot from a bow).

sagittal plane See under plane.

salience (sā′lē-əns) In speech, the psychological prominence a speaker assigns, in his own mind, to a speech unit.

salpingopharyngeus muscle See *Muscles of the Pharynx* table, under pharynx.

SAL test Sensorineural acuity level technique. See under masking techniques.

sample Part of the population which is taken as representative of the whole population, so that certain conclusions based on this group will be valid for the whole population.

    random s. Any sample of a limited number of cases from a large group or population for testing and statistical treatment, based on the assumption that the sample may be taken as representative, for a particular purpose, of the whole group.

    representative s. Any sample which includes the characteristics of the entire population from which the sample was drawn.

sarcoma (sär-kō′mə) [G. *sarkōma*, fleshy excrescence] Malignant tumor composed of cells derived from nonepithelial tissues, primarily connective tissue.

SAT Speech awareness threshold.

saturation output Maximum acoustic *output.*

saturation sound pressure level In hearing, the maximum output of a hearing aid regardless of the input level.

saucer curve See under audiogram configuration.

sawtooth noise See under noise.

scala, pl. **scalae** (skā′lə, -lē) [L. stairway] One of the three spiral cavities of the cochlea.

    s. media See cochlea, under inner *ear.*

    s. tympani See cochlea, under inner *ear.*

    s. vestibuli See cochlea, under inner *ear.*

scalenus anterior muscle See *Muscles of Respiration* table, under respiration.

scalenus medius muscle See *Muscles of Respiration* table, under respiration.

scalenus posterior muscle See *Muscles of Respiration* table, under respiration.

Scales of Cognitive Ability for Traumatic Brain Injury (SCATBI) See *Language Tests and Procedures* in appendices.

scanning communication board See under communication board.

scanning speech See under speech.

SCATBI Scales of Cognitive Ability for Traumatic Brain Injury.

schema, pl. **schemata** (skē′mə, skē-mä′tə) [G. *schēma*, shape, form] **1.** Number of ideas or concepts combined into a coherent plan; a model that displays the essential or important relations between concepts. **2.** In the plural only, the cognitive structures by which individuals intellectually adapt to and organize their environment [Piaget].

Schiefelbush-Lindsey Test of Sound Discrimination See *Auditory Tests and Procedures* in appendices.

schizophrenia (skit-sō-frē′nē-ə, skiz-ō-) [G. *schizō*, to split or cleave + *phrēn*, mind] Group of psychoses characterized by fundamental disturbances in reality relationships, by a conceptual world determined excessively by feeling, and by marked affective, intellectual, and overt behavioral disturbances.

childhood s. Disorder of childhood characterized by lack of contact with reality, little or no communication with others, and lack of integration and uniformity in ego development; speech, when present, is related to early instinctual processes, and words do not serve reality and have no conventional significance. Syn: childhood *psychosis;* prepsychosis. See also autism.

Schmidt's syndrome [J. F. M. Schmidt, Ger. laryngologist, 1838–1907] Unilateral paralysis of the vocal folds, soft palate, and sternocleidomastoideus and trapezius muscles (partial or total), with attendant speech and swallowing disorders; due to lesions of the vagus and spinal accessory nerves (cranial nerves X and XI); a variant of Jackson's and of Mackenzie's syndrome, *q.v.*

school language See under language.

schwa (ə) (schwä') Neutral *vowel.*

Schwabach Test See *Audiometric Tests and Procedures* in appendices.

schwannoma (shwä-nō'mə) [T. Schwann, Ger. histologist, 1810–1882 + G. *-oma,* tumor] Neurilemoma.

scientific grammar See under grammar.

scintigraphy A nuclear medicine test in which the patient swallows measured amounts of a radioactive substance. The procedure enables visualization of the food being swallowed, but not of the anatomy and physiology of the oropharyngeal region during deglutition.

score Evaluation, usually expressed numerically, of achievement, rank, or condition in a particular set of circumstances. For types of scores, see specific terms.

screening Any gross measure utilized to separate those who may require specific help in a specific area, such as language, hearing, articulation, fluency, and voice, from those who obviously do not need help.

screening audiometry See under audiometry.

Screening Deep Test of Articulation See *Articulation Tests and Phonological Analysis Procedures* in appendices.

Screening Kit of Language Development (SKOLD) See *Language Tests and Procedures* in appendices.

screening test See under articulation test.

Screening Test for Auditory Comprehension of Language See *Language Tests and Procedures* in appendices.

Screening Test for Auditory Perception See *Auditory Tests and Procedures* in appendices.

Screening Test for Developmental Apraxia of Speech—Second Edition See *Articulation Tests and Phonological Analysis Procedures* in appendices.

Screening Test for Identifying Central Auditory Disorders (SCAN) See *Auditory Tests and Procedures* in appendices.

Screening Test of Adolescent Language See *Language Tests and Procedures* in appendices.

SD Speech discrimination.

SDS Speech discrimination score.

SDT Speech detectability threshold.

secondary articulation See assimilation (2 and 3).

secondary autism See under autism.

secondary characteristics of stuttering Associated behaviors in stuttering. See stuttering.

secondary gain Neurotic profit.

secondary palate Palate.

secondary reinforcer Conditioned *reinforcer.*

secondary stress See under stress.

secondary stuttering See under stuttering stages.

secondary verb Term sometimes used for verbal.

second cranial nerve See *Cranial Nerves* table, under cranial nerves.

second deciduous molar or **second premolar teeth** Bicuspid *teeth.*

Secord Contextual Articulation Test See *Articulation Tests and Phonological Procedures* in appendices.

secretory otitis media Serous otitis media.

SEE₁ Seeing Essential English.

SEE₂ Signing Exact English.

Seeing Essential English (SEE₁) See under sign systems.

segmental analysis Analysis of speech sounds in which sounds are studied either in isolation or when separated arbitrarily from other sounds in continuous speech.

segmental phoneme See under phoneme.

seizure (sē′zhėr) An attack or sudden occurrence of a disease or of certain symptoms, such as convulsions. For types of seizures, see specific terms.

selective listening Auditory figure-ground *discrimination.*

self-concept Individual's evaluation of himself.

self-esteem Concept or description indicative of an individual's self-concept.

self-role concept 1. In stuttering, the stutterer's self-concept that he cannot meet demands for verbal fluency. **2.** Dilemma resulting from what one expects from himself and that which is expected from one by others.

self-talk 1. Subvocal *speech.* **2.** See also inner *language.*

semanteme (sə-man′tēm) Base *word.*

semantic (sə-man′tik) **1.** Of, pertaining to, or arising from the meanings of words or other symbols. **2.** Pertaining to semantics.

semantic aphasia See under aphasia.

semantic constraints Limitations in the selection of words or structures imposed by meaning or context.

semantic feature Distinguishing element of meaning in a lexical item; *e.g., man/ woman* has the semantic features of being animate, human, and male/female.

semantic implication Causes, effects, and concomitant conditions implied

by the content and structure of sentences.

semantic relations Linguistic structures usually exhibited by children 12 to 24 months of age; semantic concepts and cause-effect relations are demonstrated by (a) **action-locative,** verb plus locative, as in *come here;* (b) **action-object,** verb plus noun, as in *eat lunch;* (c) **agent-action,** noun plus verb, as in *boys play;* (d) **agent-object,** noun plus noun, as in *Billy home;* (e) **demonstrative-entity,** demonstrative plus noun, as in *that ball;* (f) **attribute-entity,** adjective plus noun, as in *big dog;* (g) **entity-locative,** noun plus locative, as in *puppy there;* (h) **possessor-possession,** possessor plus noun, as in *my house.*

semantic rule In transformational grammar, an operation on syntactic structures to describe the way in which an utterance is used and understood.

semantics (sə-man′tiks) [G. *sēmantikos,* having meaning] **1.** Study of meaning in language, includes the relations between language, thought, and behavior. **2.** Study of meanings of speech forms, especially of the development and changes in meanings of words and word groups. **3.** Study of the development of the meanings of words; its goal is to account for the knowledge a native speaker has which enables him to judge some sentences as meaningful, some as ambiguous, and some as anomalous. See also linguistic component.

> **behavioral s. 1.** Theory that the meaning of a word or expression is the set of responses it produces in the listener. **2.** Reaction of a particular listener, reader, or observer to a specific word or expression; *e.g., dirty* as soiled or as smutty.
>
> **extension s.** Theory that a term denotes a concrete referent which never changes; *e.g.,* George Washington, the first president of the United

States. See also referential *semantics*.

general s. Educational discipline intended to improve people's responses to their environment and to one another by training in the more critical use of words.

generative s. Theory which replaces the mathematical syntactic objects and separate semantic component of generative transformational grammar with a single set of abstract logical structures containing all of the semantic relations holding among the lexical items in a sentence.

intention s. Belief that something must possess sets of properties to be referred to by a specific term; *e.g.*, *house* as one's home, as the White House as a business setting. See also behavioral *semantics*.

referential s. Theory that words are symbols which by themselves have little meaning until associated with a particular object or class; *e.g.*, *cat* refers to a particular class of animals; *red* refers to a specific class of colors.

semantic theory of stuttering Diagnosogenic theory. See under anticipatory and struggle behavior theory, under stuttering theories.

sememics (sə-mēm′iks) Semology.

semiaural hearing protection device See under hearing protection device.

semiautonomous systems concept of brain function Theory which suggests that a given modality functions semi-independently or in a supplementary way with another modality system; all the modality systems may, at times, function together as a unit.

semicircular canals. See under inner *ear*.

semiology (sēm-i-ôl′ə-jē) [G. *sēmeion*, sign + *logos*, study, discourse] Science and study of signs and language.

semitone (sem′i-tōn) In music, an interval approximately equal to half of a major tone on the musical scale.

semivowel 1. See under consonant, manner of formation. **2.** See under vowel.

semology (sēm-ôl′ə-jē) [G. *sema*, sign + *logos*, study, discourse] Awareness and understanding of linguistic information; it is related to semantics as phonemics is to phonetics. Syn: sememics.

Semon's law or **symptom, Semon-Rosenbach law** [F. Semon, Eng. laryngologist, 1849–1921] Theory that impairment of the mobility of the vocal folds in malignant disease of the larynx occurs first in the abductor muscles and may or may not progress to the adductor muscles.

senescence (sə-nes′əns) [L. *senesco*, to grow old] Act of aging, of growing old; a process that may involve psychological, social, and physical changes which may include sensory limitations and slowness of response, decline in intellectual efficiency, recent memory impairment, confusion, disorientation in time and place, reduction of activities and interests, impaired affect, diminished involvement with the environment, use of highly personal associations in verbal communications, increased inversion and suspiciousness of close emotional relationships, and increased resistance to change.

senile (sē′nīl) [L. senilis] Relating to or characteristic of old age (senility).

senility (sə-nil′ə-tē) Old age, the cognitive and physiologic expressions of the sum of the physical and mental changes occurring in advanced life. See also senescence.

sensation (sen-sā′shən) [L. *sensatio*, perception, feeling] Conscious awareness of the action of a stimulus, such as pain, heat, odor, noise, or taste, on a sensory organ or receptor.

sensation level (SL) In audiology, a description of loudness in terms of decibels above the threshold of hearing; *e.g.*, for an individual with a 50-dB hearing threshold, a signal presented at 70 dB would be 20 dB SL above threshold.

sensation unit (SU) In audiology, the smallest change of intensity that can be detected by the normal ear; approximately equal to one decibel.

sense [L. *sensus*, felt, perceived] Awareness of a stimulus through one or more of the five receptor pathways (sight, sound, smell, taste, and touch).

sensitivity (sen-sə-tiv′ə-tē) [fr. L. *sensus*, felt, perceived] Ability of an organism or sense organ to respond to a stimulus.

sensitivity prediction from the acoustic reflex (SPAR) Procedure in which the middle-ear muscle reflex threshold for pure tones is compared to those for wide-band noise and low- and high-frequency filtered wide-band noise to approximate the degree of hearing loss.

sensorimotor (sen′sôr-ē-mō′tėr) Denoting the combination of the input of sensations and the output of motor activity; motor activity reflects what is happening to the sensory organs.

sensorimotor act Act primarily dependent on the combined functioning of the sensory and motor mechanisms. See also reflex arc.

sensorimotor arc Reflex arc.

sensorimotor intelligence period See Period I, under cognitive development stages.

sensorineural (sen′sôr-ē-nu′rəl) Pertaining to or conveying sensation to nerves or nervous tissue.

sensorineural acuity level technique See under masking techniques.

sensorineural deafness See under deafness.

sensor operation Return of information to the speaker on all aspects of the output of a speech signal via various sensory channels. See also feedback.

sensory aphasia See under aphasia.

sensory impairment Abnormal functioning of one or more of the five receptive pathways (vision, auditory, olfactory, tactile, and taste).

sensory integration (SI) The brain's ability to interpret and organize information from the senses—vision, hearing, taste, smell, touch, balance, gravity position, and movement. Problems in sensory integration may result in learning problems, hyperactivity, distractibility, poor coordination, poor balance, and behavior problems, and may contribute to difficulties at school, at home, at work, and in play.

sensory nerve See under nerve.

sensory paralysis See laryngeal sensory *paralysis.*

sensory receptor See receptor.

sensory scale Numerical relations between magnitudes (loudness, pitch) of a specified attribute which bear a reasonable relation to the experience of the observer; the basic method in the development of such a scale is fractionalization judgments; *e.g.*, in tuning a guitar, adjusting one tone until it is in harmonic balance with the others (half as high, half as low).

sentence 1. Basic unit for expressing a complete idea. It consists of (a) in traditional grammar, a subject and predicate; (b) in transformational grammar, a noun phrase and verb phrase; or (c) in case grammar, a modality and proposition. **2.** Combination of morphemes arranged grammatically and syntactically to constitute a complete unit of meaning. **3.** Any utterance which contains at least two structurally related morphemes. See also sentence classification.

sentence classification Any unit of meaning organized according to structure.

In traditional grammar:

complex sentence Sentence containing a main clause and one or more subordinate clauses; *e.g.*, "The visiting students arrived at the airport where they were met by their teacher."

compound sentence Sentence containing two or more main clauses but no subordinate clause; *e.g.*,

"The visiting students arrived at the airport and they were met by their teacher."

compound-complex sentence Sentence containing two or more main clauses and at least one subordinate clause; *e.g.*, "The visiting students, who landed at the airport, were met by their teacher, and she took them to the university."

simple sentence Sentence containing one main clause and no subordinate clause; *e.g.*, "The visiting students were met at the airport by their teacher."

In transformational grammar:

constituent or **embedded sentences** Sentences in which two kernels are combined one within the other; may result in sentences that are compound or have modification, appositives, subordination, or parallel structure. The process allows for all adjective modifiers and subordinate clauses in English; e.g., Fred bought a car. + Fred did not have enough money. = Although Fred did not have enough money, he bought a car.

derived sentence Nonkernel sentence which is formed from a kernel sentence through various operations; *e.g.*, "When will mom go?"

kernel sentence Basic sentence pattern from which all other sentences originate; *e.g.*, "Betty sat." "The boy hit the ball."

matrix sentence The main clause; in traditional grammar, the independent clause; *e.g.*, "The students arrived at the airport."

sentence constituents Units of words into which a sentence can be divided; *e.g.*, clauses, phrases, words. For immediate sentence constituents, see sentence (1).

sentence derivation See derivation of a sentence.

sentence types In traditional and transformational grammars, sentences organized according to the purpose of the sentence.

declarative sentence Sentence that makes a statement; *e.g.*, "I am going home."

exclamatory sentence Sentence that expresses a strong feeling; *e.g.*, "It is hot!"

imperative sentence Sentence that gives a command or makes a request; *e.g.*, "Ring the bell." "Please be on time."

interrogative sentence Sentence that asks a question; *e.g.*, "Where have you been?" See also question.

sequence (sē′kwens) [L. *sequor*, to follow] **1.** Order of succession; a continuous or connected series of things or events. See also speech sound flow. **2.** In speech, the temporal arrangement of phonemes in proper order for pronunciation.

Sequenced Inventory of Communication Development (SICD)—Revised Edition See *Language Tests and Procedures* in appendices.

sequencing rules In linguistics, an aspect of syntax which governs the order in which words may be combined into phrases and sentences.

sequential memory See under memory.

serial content speech See under speech.

serial list learning See under learning.

seriatim speech (sēr-ē-ā′təm) Serial content *speech.*

seriation (sēr-ē-ā′shən) [L. *series*, connection] Ability to mentally arrange elements in a series according to value, size, or other criterion.

serous fluid Thin watery fluid secreted by a serous membrane.

serous otitis media (SOM) See under otitis.

serratus anterior muscle See *Muscles of Respiration* table, under respiration.

serratus posterior inferior muscle See *Muscles of Respiration* table, under respiration.

serratus posterior superior muscle See

Muscles of Respiration table, under respiration.

servomechanistic theory (sėr'vō-me-kə-nis'tik) [L. *servus*, servant + *mechaniscus*, mechanic] In speech, a theory that a control system composed of different sensory modalities is part of the receptive mechanism, and is considered to be error-sensitive and self-adjusting.

servosystem (sėr'vō-sis-təm) [L. *servus*, servant + G. *systēma*, an organized whole] In speech, an application of a concept of cybernetics to the speaking process; if performance does not match the intent of the speaker, then future output is corrected on the basis of negative feedback until the desired performance is achieved.

sessile vocal nodules See under vocal nodules, under laryngeal anomaly.

set 1. Collection which may contain an infinite number of units; *e.g.*, in linguistics, the English language is a collection of the infinite number of possible English sentences. **2.** Attitude or predisposition to perceive or to respond in some manner.

seventh cranial nerve See *Cranial Nerves* table, under cranial nerves.

severe hearing impairment or **loss** See under hearing-impairment degrees.

SFOAE Stimulus-frequency otoacoustic emissions. See under otoacoustic emissions.

shadow curve See under curve.

shadowing Echolalia.

shadowing method Hood technique. See under masking techniques.

shaping Technique for obtaining responses that are not in the subject's repertoire. First, the desired response is specified, and then responses which resemble that response (even remotely) are reinforced. Once the frequency of these responses has been increased, the subject must emit a response even more like the desired one; at this point, the technique is a special form of differential reinforcement. The criterion for reinforcement is continuously shifted in the direction of the desired response until that response is emitted, reinforced, and acquired.

sharply falling curve See under audiogram configurations.

shell earmold See under earmold.

shimmer 1. In voice, denotes the cycle-to-cycle variations in amplitude of glottal pulses that occur when an individual attempts to sustain phonation at a constant frequency and intensity; contributes to the perception of roughness. See also jitter. **2.** Rhythmic variations in intensity (dB) of a sound. Syn: amplitude shimmer.

SHM Simple harmonic motion.

Short Increment Sensitivity Index (SISI) See *Audiometric Tests and Procedures* in appendices.

Short-Term Auditory Retrieval and Storage Test (STARS) See *Auditory Tests and Procedures* in appendices.

short-term memory See under memory.

shower collar Collar-like device often used by a laryngectomee while showering to avoid water intake to the lungs through the stoma in his neck.

shunt 1. To bypass or to divert. **2.** Diversion of accumulations of fluid to an adsorbing or excreting system by surgical reconstruction or by a mechanical device as for the relief of hydrocephalus.

shunting Stereotyped motor activities of an individual who has persistent spinal and tonic reflexes.

SI Sensory integration.

sibilant See under consonant, manner of formation.

sibling [A.S. *sib*, relation + *-ling*, diminutive] One of two or more persons having one common parent.

sigh voice A therapy technique often used with stuttering and voice clients in which word are uttered while making a deep audible expiration of the breath. Voice is released on the outgoing breath stream with a breathy voice quality.

siglish [contraction of signed English] Signed English. See under sign systems.

sigmatism (sig′mə-tiz-əm) [G. *sigma*, Letter S] Lisp.

sign (sīn) [L. *signum*, mark] **1.** American sign language. See under sign systems. **2.** Any abnormality indicative of a disease or disorder; an objective symptom. *Cf.* symptom. For various signs, see specific terms.

signal-to-noise ratio (S/N) 1. Mathematical ratio of a signal to a noise. **2.** In audiometry, the relationship between the intensity of the speech signal and the intensity of the noise signal; the ratio should exceed 6 dB for satisfactory communication.

signed English See under sign systems.

sign or **manual English** See under sign systems.

significantly subaverage See mental retardation.

Signing Exact English (SEE₂) See under sign systems.

sign language See under language.

sign marker In sign or manual English, used to represent certain basic and common English word form changes, usually inflections and endings that change the meaning of the word, *e.g.*, look to looked.

sign systems Manual communication systems used by the deaf. See also International Standard Manual *Alphabet;* verbotonal method.

    American Indian sign language (Amer-Ind) Manual gestural communication system used by North American Indians for intertribal communication among tribal members not speaking a common language. Gestural signs are pictographic and ideographic rather than phonetic; they represent ideas and in many cases are kinetic pictorial representations of the ideas conveyed. See

also unaided *augmentative communication.*

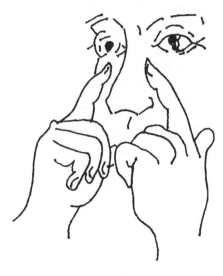

Amer-Ind Sign
cry

American Sign Language (ASL, Ameslan) Communication method used by the deaf in which gestures function as words; has its own morphology, semantics, and syntax (not based on English syntax). Syn: sign.

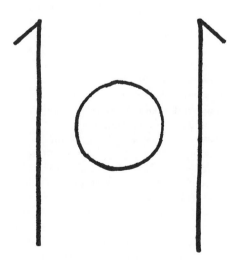

Ameslan-based Sigsymbol
sorry

cued speech In aural rehabilitation, speechreading combined with a system of manual cues that discriminate between similar visual configurations. Twelve cues are available which enable the viewer to identify phonemes if they are used in conjunction with speechreading; four hand positions are associated with four groups of visually contrastive vowels. See also simultaneous method, under aural rehabilitation.

Seeing Essential English (SEE₁) System that uses modification of American sign language to resemble English and may be utilized by all age groups. SEE₁ signs represent word forms or word parts such as roots, prefixes, or suffixes and are used in combinations to form any desired word. Complete English syntax is emphasized. Verb tense is clearly indicated and irregular verb forms have signed representation. English words are represented by the traditional American sign word plus a suffix and/or a prefix.

sign or **manual English** Method of communication used by the deaf which utilizes a rapid succession of specific gestures, including fingerspelling, and uses English syntax as a base. It differs from ASL, which does not use English syntax as a base, and from sign language, which has a semantic base.

signed English (siglish) Manual communication system used by the deaf which shares some of the characteristics of ASL and some of English; the grammar of each language is reduced. Syn: pidgin sign English.

Signing Exact English (SEE₂) System that utilizes signs which represent words rather than roots, as well as affixes as needed.

sign word In sign or manual English, used to represent the meaning of one English word, *e.g.*, mother, baby, man.

sigsymbols Contraction of SIG from man-

ual sign and SYMBOL from graphic symbol. Sigsymbols are pictographic or ideographic line drawings intended for use on communication boards. Sigsymbols are primarily intended for use with individuals learning Manual Sign to facilitate communication. See also augmentative communication.

SIL Speech interference level.

similarity disorders of aphasia See under aphasia.

simile See under figure of speech.

simple aphasia See under aphasia.

simple future progressive tense See progressive *tense.*

simple future tense See under tense.

simple harmonic motion (SHM) **1.** Symmetrical periodic to and fro motion of a body over a rest position. When the amplitudes of the body are plotted as a function of time, the resulting pattern is a sine wave. Pure tones are produced by SHM. **2.** Linear projection of uniform circular motion.

simple past progressive tense See progressive *tense.*

simple past tense See under tense.

simple predicate See predicate.

simple present progressive tense See progressive *tense.*

simple present tense See under tense.

simple sentence See under sentence classification, traditional grammar.

simple sound source Source that radiates sound uniformly in all directions under free-field conditions.

simple subject See subject (1).

simple syllabic Vowel.

simple tense See tense.

simple tone Pure tone.

simple wave Sinusoidal *wave.*

simple word Base *word.*

simplification See natural phonological processes.

simultagnosia See under agnosia.

simultaneous auditory feedback Auditory *feedback.*

simultaneous method See under aural rehabilitation.

sine wave Sinusoidal *wave.*

singer's formant See under formant.

singer's nodes or **nodules** Vocal nodules. See under laryngeal anomaly.

sinistral (sin-is'trəl) [L. *sinister*, left] Pertaining to the left side; opposite of dextral.

sinistrality (sin-is-tral'ə-tē) Preferential use of organs or members of the left side of the body. See also laterality (1).

sinus, pl. **sinuses** (sī'nəs, -səz) [L. cavity, channel, hollow] Cavity or hollow space in a bone or other tissue.

sinus of the ventricle One of three divisions of the larynx, *q.v.*

sinusoidal wave See under wave.

SISI Short Increment Sensitivity Index.

six-hertz positive spikes See under electroencephalogram.

six-hertz positive spike-waves See under electroencephalogram.

sixth cranial nerve See *Cranial Nerves* table, under cranial nerves.

sixty-cycle hum Type of noise heard as a buzz occurring naturally in electrical appliances, such as radios and televisions, at the frequency of 60 Hz; not present in battery-powered appliances. See also under noise.

skeleton earmold See under earmold.

skill Activity requiring expertise for competent performance; learning through practice in coordinating a set of developed responses to certain stimuli to perform an activity.

    minimum acceptable s. Smallest number of correctly performed responses that must be passed for approval.

skinnerian conditioning See operant *conditioning*.

ski slope curve See under audiogram configurations.

Sklar Aphasia Scale See *Language Tests and Procedures* in appendices.

skull [Early Eng. *skulle*, bowl] Bony framework of the head composed of eight cranial bones [*ethmoid, frontal, occipital, parietal* (paired), *sphenoid, and temporal* (paired)] and fourteen facial bones [*lacrimal* (paired), *nasal*

(paired), *nasal conchae* or *turbinates* (three), *mandible* or *inferior maxillary, maxilla* or *superior maxillary, palatine* (paired), *vomer*, and *zygomatic* or *malar* (paired)].

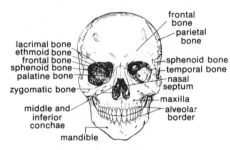

Anterior View

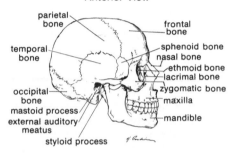

Bones of the Skull
From *Stedman's Medical Dictionary,* 24th ed. Baltimore: Williams & Wilkins, 1982.

ethmoid bone (eth'moid) [G. ēthmos, sieve + *eidos*, resembling] Irregularly shaped bone at the base of the cranium which, with the nasal bones and nasal conchae, forms the upper bony portion of the nose; it is perforated with air cells and passages for the olfactory nerves.

frontal bone Bone at the front of the cranium that consists of a vertical portion which forms the forehead and articulates with the parietal and sphenoid bones, and an orbital portion which extends backward to enter into the formation of the roofs of the orbital and nasal cavities.

inferior maxillary bone Mandible.

inferior turbinated bone Inferior nasal concha. See nasal conchae.

lacrimal bone Paired thin scalelike bones, about the size of a fingernail, that lie in the medial wall of the orbit on the ethmoid bone; the smallest and most fragile of the facial bones. Each lacrimal bone contains a groove that is part of the lacrimal canal (tear duct) from the orbit to the nasal cavity.

malar bones (ma'lẻr) [L. *mala*, cheek] Zygomatic bones (see below).

mandible (man'di-bəl) [L. *mandibula*, jaw] The lower jaw; the longest facial bone, consisting of a horseshoe-shaped body with two upturned rami which have a hinged articulation with the temporal bones. The lower teeth are rooted in sockets in the upper margin of the body. Syn: inferior maxillary bone.

maxilla (mak-sil'ə) The upper jaw; an irregularly shaped facial bone formed by midline fusion of paired bones which articulates with the frontal bone. It forms most of the palate, part of the floor of the orbits, the floor and lateral walls of the nasal cavity, and part of the wall of the nasolacrimal canal. The upper teeth are rooted in sockets on the projecting ridge on its undersurface. Syn: superior maxillary bone.

medial turbinated bone Medial nasal concha. See nasal conchae (below).

nasal bones Paired small oblong facial bones that together form the bridge of the nose.

nasal conchae, sing. **concha** (kon'-kē, -kə) [L. shells] Shell-shaped projections of thin facial bone covered by mucous membrane and forming the lateral wall of the nasal cavity. Syn: turbinated bones; turbinates.

Inferior n. c. is a bone forming the lower part of the lateral wall of the nasal cavity. Syn: inferior turbinated bone.

Medial n. c. is the lower and larger of two bony plates with upcurved margins which projects from the

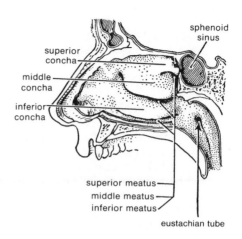

Nasal Conchae

inner wall of the ethmoidal labyrinth and separates the superior from the middle meatus of the nose. Syn: medial turbinated bone.

Sphenoidal n. c. are the paired curved plates of bone at the anterior and lower part of the body of the sphenoid bone which form part of the roof of the nasal cavity.

Superior n. c. is the upper and smaller of two bony plates with upcurved margins which projects from the inner wall of the ethmoidal labyrinth and forms the upper boundary of the superior meatus of the nose. Syn: superior turbinated bone.

Supreme n. c. is the highest of the nasal conchae which is frequently present on the posterosuperior part of the lateral nasal wall; it overlies the supreme nasal meatus. Syn: supreme turbinated bone.

occipital bone (ok-sip'ə-təl) [L. *occiput*, back of the head] Trapezoidal-shaped bone situated at the inferior posterior part of the cranium; it articulates laterally with the parietal and temporal bones and anteriorly with the sphenoid bone.

palatine bones Paired "L"-shaped facial bones, each lying between the maxilla and the pterygoid process of the sphenoid bone; the upright portion forms part of the lateral wall of the nasal cavity and part of the palate.

parietal bones Paired quadrilateral bones forming part of the superior and lateral parts of the cranium, and joining each other in the midline at the sagittal suture; they articulate anteriorly with the frontal bone, posteriorly with the occipital bone, and inferiorly with the temporal and sphenoid bones.

sphenoid bone Bone shaped like a butterfly with extended wings which forms the anterior part of the base of the cranium and forms portions of the cranial, orbital, and nasal cavities.

superior maxillary bone Maxilla (see above).

superior turbinated bone Superior nasal concha. See nasal conchae (above).

supreme turbinated bone Supreme nasal concha. See nasal conchae (above).

temporal bones Paired irregularly shaped bones forming part of the lateral surfaces and the posterior base of the cranium; they articulate with the occipital, parietal, sphenoid, and zygomatic bones, and contain the organs of hearing.

turbinates or **turbinated bones** (tẻr′bināts, -nāt-əd) [L. *turbinatus*, shaped like a top, scroll shaped] Nasal conchae (see above).

vomer (vo′mẻr) [L. plowshare] Flat trapezoidal facial bone forming the interior and posterior portion of the nasal septum and separating the right and left chambers of the nasal passage.

zygomatic bones (zī-gō-mat′ik) [G. *zygon*, yoke] The cheekbones; paired bones situated at the upper and lateral part of the face which ar-

ticulate with the maxilla and the frontal, sphenoid, and temporal bones. Syn: malar bones.

SL Sensation level.

slang 1. Commonly used informal vocabulary which disregards the principle of linguistics. **2.** Adaptations of meanings of words.

slide In stuttering, a technique used by the stutterer to control his dysfluencies; the initial sound of a word is prolonged and blended into the rest of the word, keeping the release of the initial sound as smooth and gradual as possible.

slight hearing impairment or **loss** See hearing-impairment degrees.

slit fricative See fricative, under consonant, manner of formation.

Slosson Articulation, Language Test with Phonology (SALT-P) See *Articulation Tests and Phonological Analysis Procedures* in appendices.

Slosson Intelligence Test for Children and Adults See *Psychological Measures and Tests* in appendices.

slurring Speech sounds so lightly uttered that they appear to be only partially produced. See also general oral inaccuracy, under articulation disorder.

Smit-Hand Articulation and Phonology Evaluation (SHAPE) See *Articulation Tests and Phonological Procedures* in appendices.

Smith-Johnson Nonverbal Performance Scale See *Language Tests and Procedures* in appendices.

S/N Signal-to-noise ratio.

sniff method See under speech, methods of esophageal speech.

SOAE Spontaneous otoacoustic emissions. See under otoacoustic emissions.

Social Adequacy Index (SAI) In audiology, a measure based on the results of speech audiometry (speech-reception threshold and articulation tests) which represent the degree of handicap in understanding oral language.

social babbling See under babbling.

social behavior See under behavior.

social gesture speech Nonpropositional *speech*.

social interaction Interchange of ideas among people.

social learning theory Set of concepts and principles from behavior learning theory frequently used in describing and explaining personality character- istics and social behavior.

sociocusis (sō-sē-ə-ku′sis) [L. *socius*, companion + G. *akousis*, hearing] **1.** Increase in hearing threshold resulting from noise exposures that are part of the social environment, but exclusive of occupational noise exposure, physi- ologic changes with age, and otologic disease. **2.** Progressive hearing loss due to aging, disease, or noise expo- sure. See also presbycusis.

sociolect (sō′sē-ō-lekt) Characteristics of an individual's speech patterns which may reveal his socioeconomic status and educational background.

sociolinguistics (sō′sē-ō-liŋ-gwis′tiks) **1.** Discipline utilizing the concepts of so- ciology and linguistics in the study of the functioning of language in a soci-

ety. **2.** Study of the sociological influ- ence on language learning and use; es- pecially includes such variables as dialects, bilingualism, and parent-child interactions.

soft neurological signs Mild neurologic abnormalities which are difficult to de- tect, as in Strauss syndrome, *q.v.*

soft palate Velum.

soft palate cleft See cleft palate.

soft whisper See whisper.

SOM Serous otitis media.

somesthetic (sōm-es-thet′ik) [G. *soma*, body + *aisthēsis*, sensation] Denoting conscious sensory awareness of the body.

somesthetic area See parietal lobe, under cerebrum, under brain.

somesthetic dysarthria See under dysar- thria.

SOMPA System of Multicultural Pluralis- tic Assessment.

sonant (son′ant) Sonorant. See under consonant, manner of formation.

sone (sōn) Basic unit for a loudness scale, arbitrarily defined as the loud- ness of a pure tone of 1000 Hz at 40

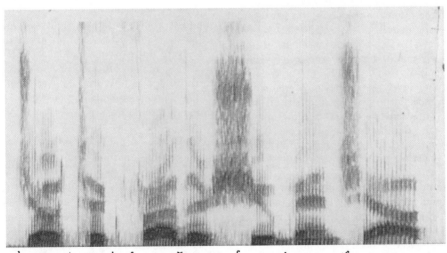

dʒ ou t ʊ k f ɑ ð ɚ z ʃ u b ɛ ntʃ a ʊ t

Sound Spectrogram

dB above the listener's threshold of audibility.

sonogram (son'ə-gram) [L. *sonus*, sound + G. *gamma*, something written] Electromechanically produced graph of a sound; often used to study the characteristics of speech formants. See also sound spectrogram.

sonorant See under consonant, manner of formation.

sonority (sə-nôr'i-tē) [L. *sonorus*, noisy sounding] Fullness or resonance in tone; loudness; volume.

sound Air wave or vibration that causes a sensory stimulation of the auditory mechanism. For sound to be created and heard, the following are essential: (a) a vibrator, (b) a force to activate the vibrator, (c) a medium to convey the wave motion originated by the vibrator, and (d) a hearing mechanism to receive the energy of the wave. For types of sound, see specific terms.

sound analysis Ability to analyze spoken syllables or words into their component sounds or phonemes. Syn: phonemic analysis.

sound blending Auditory synthesis.

sound field See under field.

sound field localization audiometry See visual reinforcement *audiometry*.

sound intensity or **level** Ratio between a sound being measured and a reference level of intensity measured in decibels. Syn: sound power density. See also noise.

sound level meter Device designed for measurement of the intensity of sound waves in air; consists of a microphone, an amplifier, a frequency-weighting circuit, and a meter calibrated in decibels with a reference of 0.0002 dyne/cm^2.

sound power density Sound intensity.

sound pressure level (SPL) Level stated in decibels which is a ratio of the measured sound pressure to a reference sound of 0.0002 dyne/cm^2.

sound pressure level range Maximum and minimum sound pressure levels that an individual can produce or detect at specific points in his frequency range.

sound quality 1. Psychological sensation of auditory stimuli resulting from the difference in overtones generated with the fundamental frequency through varying resonators. **2.** Patterning of sounds by which a speaker or instrumental generator is recognized; a function of the blends of various overtones; identified physically on waveforms and modes of vibration.

sound quantity In audiometry, the duration of sounds.

sound spectrogram [L. *spectrum*, image + G. *gramma*, something written] Photograph of the pressure waves of a particular sound.

sound spectrograph [L. *spectrum*, image + G. *graphē*, a writing] Electronic instrument for graphically recording the changing intensity levels of the frequency components in a complex sound wave. See also electrical measurement of speech production.

sound spectrum Analysis of a specific type of noise, such as masking noise or factory noise; the spectrum depicts the frequencies present in the sound and the relative intensity of each frequency component.

sound-symbol association Ability to learn an association between an event received through one modality (auditory) and another event received through a different modality (visual). See also cross-modality *perception*.

sound or **sound pressure wave** See under wave.

spacial balance Improved perception of auditory orientation obtained through binaural listening.

spasm (spa'zəm) [G. *spasmos*] **1.** Convulsive, involuntary contraction of a muscle or a group of muscles. **2.** In stuttering, an involuntary, sudden, and temporary interruption during speech of the normal movements of the speech musculature. See also block.

spasmodic croup See under croup.

spasmodic dysphonia See under voice disorders of phonation.

spastic Relating to spasm or spasticity.

spastic dysarthria See dysarthria.

spastic dysphonia See spasmodic dysphonia.

spasticity (spas-tis′i-tē) [G. *spastikos*, drawing in] Hypertonicity of a muscle characterized by hyperactivity of the stretch reflex. See under cerebral palsy symptomatology.

spastic paralysis See under paralysis.

speaker's nodes or **nodules** Vocal nodules. See under laryngeal anomaly.

spectrogram See sound spectrogram.

spectrograph See sound spectrograph.

spectrum, pl. **spectra, spectrums** (spek′ trəm, -trə, -trəmz) [L. an image] **1.** Plot showing the frequencies and amplitudes of the individual components of a wave; also used to denote a range of frequencies that possess a common characteristic, such as the audio-frequency spectrum. **2.** Array of the components of an emission or wave separated and arranged in the order of some varying characteristic, such as wavelength, mass, or energy.

speech [A.S. *spaec*] **1.** Medium of oral communication that uses a linguistic code (language); through this medium one can express thoughts and feelings and understand those of others who use the same code. **2.** Communication through vocal symbols. **3.** Motor act of respiration, phonation, articulation, and resonation.

  accelerated s. Extremely rapid speech which results in changes in pitch and intensity.

  alaryngeal s. Speech without a larynx.

    buccal s. Alaryngeal speech in which the air supply for phonation originates from an air chamber created in the buccal cavity, with the cheek and upper jaw forming a neoglottis; the tongue is allowed to remain free to serve as an articulatory organ.

    esophageal s. Alaryngeal speech in which the air supply for phonation originates in the upper portion of the esophagus, with the pharyngoesophageal segment functioning as a neoglottis. Syn: esophageal voice. For methods of esophageal speech, see speech, methods of esophageal speech.

    pharyngeal s. Alaryngeal speech produced by use of the pharyngeal and glossopharyngeal muscles at the site of the pharyngeal wall and velum; the neoglottis may be the tongue and palate or the tongue against the pharyngeal wall or upper alveolar ridge; the tongue is often restricted in movement for articulation because of its involvement in voice production. Air supply is from the pharyngeal and oral cavities.

  automatic s. Linguistic material often repeated with little awareness as to its meaning; may include such utterances as consecutive numbers, days of the week, expletives, verses, prayers, songs, and various kinds of common expressions. See also automatic *language* (1).

  buccal s. See under alaryngeal *speech* (above).

  cold-running s. In audiology, connected speech which is informative in content and delivery, rather than emotional; may be used to establish the speech reception threshold of hearing.

  compressed s. Speech which is altered by a mechanical technique which "squeezes" it into smaller than normal bandwidths, as in the telephone.

  connected s. Oral discourse; consists of a sequence of words which may or may not convey meaning. Syn: running speech.

  dactyl s. Fingerspelling.

  deaf s. Type of speech common to individuals with severe hearing losses; characteristics may include (a) slow, labored speech; (b) expenditure of an excessive amount of breath for phrasing; (c) substitutions and distortions of vowels and consonants; (d) dysprosody; (e) excessive nasal emissions; (f) improper releasing or arresting of consonants; and (g) production of inappropriate extraneous syllables.

delayed s. Broad classification with implication that a child has not acquired speech at the expected time or with the expected accuracy; also usually implies multiple articulation errors in addition to language errors.

demand s. A form of communicative pressure, especially prevalent in the early childhood years, where the young talker is pressured into giving specific answers to difficult and demanding questions; *e.g.*, "Why were you late to school?" or "Explain why you do not have your homework done."

deviant s. Speech defect.

displaced s. Ability to speak with varying degrees of abstractness; the direct referent for the topic need not be present; *e.g.*, talking about beautiful roses while in a barren desert.

echo s. Echolalia.

egocentric s. Egocentric *language.*

esophageal s. See under alaryngeal *speech* (above).

infantile s. Infantile perseveration.

inner s. Inner *language.*

intelligible s. That aspect of oral speech-language output that allows a listener to understand what a speaker is saying.

mimic s. Echolalia.

narrative s. Discourse by an individual without interruption by another; a technique often used to obtain a language sample.

nonpropositional s. Form of linguistic content in which individual words and their specific symbolic significance are relatively unimportant;

e.g., "How are you?" "Pleased to meet you." Syn: social gesture speech.

phantom s. Pantomime speech; talking and moving the lips and tongue but without making any sound.

pharyngeal s. See under alaryngeal *speech* (above).

propositional s. 1. Use of linguistic symbols to communicate a specific idea or to elicit a specific response. **2.** Communication of meanings, as contrasted with the expression of feelings.

running s. Connected *speech.*

scanning s. Alteration of prosodic features resulting in an overly even emphasis on words; unnatural prolongation and too even stress on the syllables within a word; lengthening of the intervals between syllables.

serial content s. Recitation of a series of words which have been learned and memorized in a given order, such as the alphabet, numbers, poetry. Syn: seriatim speech.

seriatim s. Serial content *speech.*

social gesture s. Nonpropositional *speech.*

spontaneous s. Verbalizations which occur with no prompting.

subvocal s. Barely audible commentary by an individual describing what he is doing, perceiving, or feeling. Syn: self-talk.

tremulous s. See under voice disorders of phonation.

unintelligible s. Verbalizations that cannot be understood by the listener.

visible s. 1. System of symbols indicating the position of the various speech organs used in producing vocal sounds; used to assist in the teaching of the deaf to speak [A.M. Bell]. **2.** Combined use of speech and fingerspelling. See also Rochester method.

speech, methods of esophageal speech Any of several procedures used to produce alaryngeal speech by means of an airflow originating in the upper portion of the esophagus, with the pharyngoesophageal segment functioning as a neoglottis.

breathing method Inhalation method (see below).

inhalation method Use of air pressure changes above or below the pharyngoesophageal segment coordinated with lung pressure. Syn: breathing method; suction.

injection method Use of air, compressed between the tongue, hard and soft palates, and pharynx, which is pushed back into the lower portion of the pharynx. It involves two techniques which may work independently or together: (a) **consonant-injection method, plosive-injection method,** or **glossopharyngeal press,** in which the throat is relaxed and the air in the oropharyngeal cavity is compressed from consonant positions /p/, /t/, or /k/ back and down into the esophagus, and (b) **tongue press,** in which the tongue pumps air into the esophagus in rapid swallowing motions.

sniff method Use of air pressure in the laryngopharynx which is built up by "sniffing" and contracting the nares.

suction Inhalation method (see above).

swallow method Use of air which has been inhaled through the mouth and then swallowed with the lips closed.

speech acts See illocution.

speech and hearing science Study, analysis, and measurement of all components of the processes involved in the production and reception of speech.

speech and language characteristics of cleft palate See cleft palate.

speech and language clinician Speech and language pathologist.

speech and language pathologist An individual with a degree or certification in speech and language pathology who is qualified to diagnose speech, language, and voice disorders and to prescribe and implement therapeutic measures. Syn: communicologist; language clinician, pathologist, or therapist; logopedist; speech and language clinician; speech correctionist, pathologist, or therapist; voice clinician, pathologist, or therapist.

speech and language pathology Study of speech, language, and voice disorders for the purposes of diagnosis and treatment. Syn: communicology; logopedics; speech correction or pathology.

speech apraxia See under apraxia.

speech aspects Features of speech (articulatory, auditory, linguistic, and phonatory) usually necessary for oral communications.

speech audiometer See under audiometer.

speech audiometry See under audiometry.

speech awareness See under speech *audiometry.*

speech awareness threshold (SAT) Speech detection *threshold.*

speech community Group of individuals who communicate with one another directly or indirectly through a common language.

dialect s.c. Group of individuals who use a language which is not typical of that spoken by the dominant dialect group in that particular geographic region; the language used by this subset of the community may differ from the dominant one in terms of its phonological, semantic, or syntactic components.

speech conservation Speech and language intervention designed for newly deafened individuals to minimize disintegration of speech, language, and voice.

speech correction Speech and language pathology.

speech correctionist Speech and language pathologist.

speech defect Speech disorder (1).

speech detection Speech awareness. See under speech *audiometry*.

speech detection or **detectability threshold (SDT)** See under threshold.

speech discrimination (SD) 1. See under discrimination. **2.** See under speech *audiometry*.

Speech Discrimination in Noise See *Audiometric Tests and Procedures* in appendices.

speech disorder 1. Any deviation of speech outside the range of acceptable variation in a given environment. Speech may be considered defective if it is characterized by any of the following to a significant degree: (a) is not easily audible; (b) is not readily intelligible; (c) is vocally or visually unpleasant; (d) deviates in respect to specific sound production; (e) is labored in production; (f) lacks conventional rhythm or stress; (g) is linguistically deficient; or (h) is inappropriate to the speaker in terms of age, sex, or physical development. Syn: deviant speech; speech defect or impairment. **2.** Interruptions in the production of voice, phoneme, or rhythm. See also communicative disorder, language disorder.

speech distortion See distortion, under articulation disorder.

speech education Broad area concerned with the training of an individual to speak and listen more effectively.

speech frequencies See under frequency.

speech impairment Speech disorder (1).

speech impediment Obsolete term for speech impairment.

speech improvement Technique used to enrich poor or average speech.

speech initiation time Voice-onset time (VOT).

speech innateness theory See nativist theory, under language theories.

speech interference level (SIL) Noise interference level.

speech mechanism Structures involved in the production of speech; includes (a) *articulators* (lips, tongue, velum, pharynx, and lower jaw), which serve to interrupt or modify the voiced or unvoiced airstream into meaningful sounds; (b) *larynx*, which creates sound energy (phonation); (c) *resonators*, cavities (pharyngeal, laryngeal, oral, and nasal) whose changes in size and shape alter the fundamental vibrations produced by the vocal folds; and (d) *respiratory system* (lungs and air passages), which furnishes the air necessary for the production of sounds.

speech-motor function Assessment of articulatory skills in combination with the movements of the speech mechanism.

speech noise See under noise.

speech pathologist Speech and language pathologist.

speech pathology Speech and language pathology.

speech perception Identification of phonemes, the vowels and consonants of language, largely from acoustic cues and the recognition of phonemes in combination as a word.

speech processor A device used to convert a microphone or other input (e.g. telephone, TV, etc.) into patterns of electrical stimulation.

speechreading See under aural rehabilitation.

speechreading aphasia See under aphasia.

speech reception (SR) See under speech *audiometry*.

speech reception in noise See under threshold.

speech reception threshold (SRT) See under threshold.

speech rehabilitation Process of attempting to restore a previously functioning speech system through an appropriate form of training.

speech science See speech and hearing science.

speech sound development See *Speech Sound Development* in appendices.

speech sound discrimination See under discrimination.

speech sound flow Components that

allow the natural movement of speech; includes (a) *duration*, length of time any phonetic element occurs; (b) *fluency*, smoothness with which sounds are articulated; (c) *rate*, speed with which phonetic elements are articulated with each other; (d) *rhythm*, pattern of speech flow; and (e) *sequence*, appropriate linguistic order of sounds.

Speech Sound Memory Test See *Auditory Tests and Procedures* in appendices.

speech therapist Speech and language pathologist.

speech training units See auditory training units.

Speech With Alternating Masking Index (SWAMI) See *Audiometric Tests and Procedures* in appendices.

speed quotient Ratio of the duration of the opening phase of the glottis to that of the closing phase.

sphenoid, sphenoidal (sfē'noid, noi'dəl) [G. *sphēnoeidēs*, wedge-shaped] Wedge-shaped; relating to the sphenoid bone.

sphenoidal nasal conchae See nasal conchae, under skull.

sphenoidal turbinated bones Sphenoidal nasal conchae. See nasal conchae, under skull.

sphenoid bone See under skull.

spinal accessory nerve See *Cranial Nerves* table, under cranial nerves.

spiral effect In stuttering, the perpetuation of stuttering due to the stutterer's fear, frustration, or embarrassment concerning stuttering.

spirant Fricative. See under consonant, manner of formation.

spirometer (spi-rom'ə-tėr) [L. *spiro*, to breathe + G. *metron*, measurement] Instrument used to measure and record air capacity of the lungs; breathing functions associated with speech production also can be measured. Syn: respirometer.

SPL Sound pressure level.

split-half reliability coefficient See under *reliability coefficient.*

split word See under word.

spondee See under word.

spontaneous imitation See imitation (2).

spontaneous otoacoustic emissions (SOAE) See under otoacoustic emissions.

spontaneous recovery 1. In aphasia, the return, complete or incomplete, of impaired abilities, such as speech, intellectual functions, motor functions; may occur with or without therapeutic intervention, usually within a period of three months. **2.** In stuttering, the remission of stuttering without formal therapy. **3.** In stuttering, the return of stuttering frequency or severity to a previous level after a sufficient interval of time following adaptation.

spontaneous speech See under speech.

square brackets In phonetic transcription, [ ] used to indicate that the symbols within represent speech sounds and not spelling, and are to be pronounced as speech sounds rather than by the letter names. See phonetic *transcription.*

SR Speech reception.

SRT Speech reception threshold.

stabilization (stā'bil-i-zā'shən) [L. *stabilitas*, firm, steady] In conditioning, process of making a response permanent.

staffing Multidisciplinary team approach in which members of the team utilize their respective expertise in matters relevant to diagnosis and treatment of a disorder or disease, educational processes, and so forth.

stages of stuttering See stuttering stages.

stage whisper Forced *whisper.*

Staggered Spondaic Word Test (SSW) See *Audiometric Tests and Procedures* in appendices.

stallers Postponements.

stammering Disorder of fluency, rhythm, and rate; often refers to involuntary speech stoppages. In the United

States, this term is not specifically differentiated from stuttering.

standard deviation See under deviation.

standard earmold See under earmold.

standardization (stan′där-di-zā′shən) Process of administering a test to a group of students to determine uniform or standard procedures and methods of interpretation.

standardized test 1. Test composed of empirically selected materials; must have definite directions for use, adequately determined norms, and data on reliability and validity. **2.** Test that has undergone standardization procedures; an individual's performance can be compared to other individuals who are the same chronological age. Syn: norm-referenced tests.

standard language See under language.

standard reference In audiology, a value expressed as a number which serves as a base for a scale of comparison with regard to intensity, frequency, sound pressure, etc.; *e.g.*, 0.0002 dyne/cm^2 is the standard reference level for sound pressure.

standard score 1. Derived score which uses as its unit the standard deviation of the population on which the test was standardized. **2.** A **z** score (the difference between the obtained score and the mean, divided by the standard deviation).

standard speech sound Accepted manner in which native speakers of a language produce a specific sound or combination of sounds; judged to be nonstandard only when the native speakers declare it to be so. See also standard *word*.

standard word See under word.

standing wave See under wave.

Stanford-Binet Intelligence Scale See *Psychological Measures and Tests* in appendices.

stanine (stā′nĭn) Statistical measure representing one-ninth of the range of the standard scores of a distribution.

stapedectomy (stā-pē-dek′tə-mē) [L. *sta-*

pes, stirrup + G. *ektomē*, excision] Surgical removal of the stapes followed by its replacement with a synthetic prosthesis between the incus and oval window; used for correction of lesions caused by otosclerosis.

stapedial acoustic reflex See under acoustic *reflex*.

stapedius reflex See under reflex.

stapes, pl. **stapes** (stā′pēz) [L. stirrup] Third and smallest bone of the ossicular chain in the middle ear. Syn: stirrup. See under middle *ear*.

stapes mobilization Surgical technique used to restore movement to the footplate of a stapes which has become fixated in the oval window because of otosclerosis.

starter In stuttering, any means, such as eye blinking, arm swinging, or excessive use of "uh, uh," that the stutterer uses as a means of breaking a block to initiate the word he intends to say. See also associated behavior in stuttering, under stuttering.

startle reflex Moro's *reflex*.

startle technique See under behavioral *audiometry*.

static acoustic impedance See under impedance. See also under acoustic impedance.

statistics Mathematical discipline concerned with the analysis of numerical data. Statistical methods are designed to summarize such data, assess their reliability and validity, determine the nature and magnitude of relationships among sets of data, and guide in attempts to generalize from observed events to new events.

steep drop curve Ski slope curve. See under audiogram configurations.

Stenger Test See *Audiometric Tests and Procedures* in appendices.

stenosis, pl. **stenoses** (ste-nō′sis, -sēz) [G. *stenōsis*, a narrowing] Narrowing of any canal; a stricture; *e.g.*, a narrowing of the external auditory canal.

Stephens Oral Language Screening Test

See *Language Tests and Procedures* in appendices.

stereognosis (stēr′ē-og-nō′sis) [G. *stereos*, solid + *gnōsis*, knowledge] Perception of an object or form through the sense of touch.

   oral s. Ability to discriminate and identify the types and locations of various objects and sensations in the mouth; in speech, this ability is tested on the surface of the lips and tongue. Syn: oral form recognition; oral sensory discrimination.

stereotyped stress See under stress.

sternoclavicularis muscle See *Muscles of Respiration* table, under respiration.

sternocleidomastoideus muscle See *Muscles of Respiration* table, under respiration.

sternohyoid muscle See *Muscles of the Larynx* table, under larynx.

sternothyroid muscle See *Muscles of the Larynx* table, under larynx.

stimulability (stim′yu-lə-bil′i-tē) Degree to which a misarticulated sound can be produced correctly by imitation.

stimulus, pl. **stimuli** (stim′yu-ləs, -lī) [L. a goad] Anything in an organism's environment, external or internal, that is capable of eliciting a response by the organism.

   conditioned s. Originally ineffective (neutral) cue for a given response which by conditioning has become capable of eliciting that response.

   neutral s. Cue which the individual will neither approach nor avoid; in conditioning procedures, the individual will not respond in any specific way to such a cue. It may be converted to a conditioned stimulus.

   novel s. Stimulus which is radically different from others presented.

   noxious s. Negative *reinforcer.*

   unconditioned s. Any cue that evokes an unconditioned response.

stimulus-frequency otoacoustic emissions (SFOAE) See under otoacoustic emissions.

stimulus generalization Process by which a response that is instrumentally or classically conditioned to occur in the presence of a certain stimulus will also occur in the presence of similar stimuli (which were not presented during conditioning) to the degree that they are similar to the original stimulus.

stimulus substitution See classical *conditioning.*

stirrup [so called because of fancied resemblance] Stapes. See under middle *ear.*

stoma, pl. **stoma, stomata** (stō′mə, stō′mə-tə) [G. a mouth] **1.** A small opening, such as the mouth. **2.** Artificial opening between cavities or canals, or between such and the surface of the body, such as the opening made into the trachea between the thyroid glands during a laryngectomy. Syn: tracheostoma.

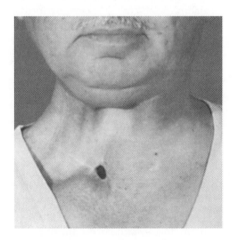

Stoma

stoma blast Sound produced by the forced or excessive expiration of air through the stoma by a laryngectomee.

stoma button Small plastic tube inserted into the stoma by a laryngectomee to maintain or enlarge the stoma.

stomata (stō′mə-tə) Plural of stoma.

stop See under consonant, manner of formation.

stopping See under substitution, under phonological processes.

stopping of fricatives Affrication. See under substitution, under phonological processes.

Strauss syndrome [A. A. Strauss] Collection of behavioral characteristics describing the child who has difficulty in learning; may include inhibited, perseverative, distractible, or hyperactive behavior. See also attention deficit/hyperactivity disorder.

stress [L. *strictus*, tight] **1.** Amount of force or strength of movement in the production of one syllable as compared with another; usually results in the syllable sounding longer and louder than other syllables in the same word. **2.** Variations in intensity by which one syllable is produced with greater intensity than are others. **3.** A condition of emotional tension.

   iambic s. (ī-am′bik) Stress pattern of two syllables in which the first is unstressed and the second is stressed, usually a consonant-vowel-consonant-vowel (CVCV) combination; used as a stimulus in articulatory training.

   primary s. Emphasis placed on the most prominently pronounced syllable in a word; symbol (′) or (´); *e.g.*, go, g̈.

   secondary s. Emphasis placed on syllables more strongly accented than neighboring unstressed syllables, but less prominently stressed than the syllable with the primary stress; symbol (ˌ) or (ˋ); *e.g.*, ′pen man ˌship, pén man shı̂p.

   stereotyped s. Regular, predictably occurring stress that contributes little to the reinforcement of meaning.

   tertiary s. Recognition given unstressed syllables which are not weakened to the point where the vowel becomes a murmur or schwa symbol (ə) or no symbol; *e.g.*, ′ma kiṅg, m̈a king.

   trochaic s. (trō-kā′ik) Stress pattern in which an accented syllable is followed by an unaccented syllable, usually vowel-consonant-vowel-consonant (VCVC) combination; used as a stimulus in articulatory training.

   weak s. Minimal amount of emphasis given a syllable in a word; such syllables are short, often low in pitch, and indefinite in quality. Conventionally, the absence of a symbol indicates weak stress, but the following symbols have been used for this purpose: u, ə, ɚ, m̩, n̩, l̩, ʊ.

stress patterns Recognizable patterns of stress in the language being spoken which reinforce the meaning of what is being said.

stretched syllables Precision fluency shaping.

stretch reflex See under reflex.

stridency deletion See under syllabic structure, under phonological processes.

strident 1. See under voice disorders of phonation. **2.** See under distinctive features.

strident lisp See under lisp.

stridor See under voice disorders of phonation.

stroboscope (strō′bə-skōp) [G. *strobos*, twisting around + *skopeō*, to view] Instrument which furnishes an intermittent light of adjustable pulse frequency; can be used to illuminate the vibrating vocal folds.

stroke 1. Cerebral vascular accident. **2.** A sudden attack or onset, as of a disorder or disease. For such usages, see specific term.

structural linguistics See under linguistics.

structure (strək′chėr) [L. *structura*, something built] In linguistics, the relationships between the morphemes of a sentence.

   base s. Deep *structure.*

   deep s. Specific rules whereby individual word meanings are combined to form the meaning of a sentence;

related to the semantic system of a language before transformations have occurred. Syn: base or underlying structure.

intermediate s. In transformational grammar, the constructions formed between the deep structure and the surface structure of a sentence.

surface s. 1. Specific rules whereby the pronunciation of the sentence, including stress and intonation, is determined. **2.** Actual form of the sentences as revealed through the speaking process; includes syntactical and phonological contributions to the deep structure.

underlying s. Deep *structure*.

Structured Photographic Expressive Language Test II See *Language Tests and Procedures* in appendices.

structure word Function *word*.

Studebaker technique See under masking techniques.

stutterer Person who experiences difficulty with normal fluency and time patterning of speech.

stuttering 1. Disturbance in the normal fluency and time patterning of speech. *Primary characteristics* include one or more of the following: (a) audible or silent blocking; (b) sound and syllable repetitions; (c) sound prolongations; (d) interjections; (e) broken words; (f) circumlocutions; or (g) words produced with an excess of tension. *Associated behaviors* or *secondary characteristics* include the habitual use of speech musculature or of other body parts which a stutterer uses along with the primary characteristics; thought to be initiated to release, conceal, or modify the dysfluency. The disturbance may be at the level of neuromuscular, respiratory, phonatory, or articulatory mechanisms. Dysfluencies are so numerous that they exceed the normal number or degree for the individual's age, sex, or speaking situation. **2.** Involuntary repetition and prolongation of speech sounds and syllables, and fluency interruptions that the individual struggles to end. See also *Stuttering—Children's Referral Checklist* in appendices.

Adaptation effect is the tendency for stuttering to decrease with repeated reading or speaking of the same sounds, words, sentences, or paragraphs.

Consistency effect is the tendency for stuttering to occur on the same sounds or words; most noticeable in repeated readings of the same material.

exteriorized s. Stuttering blocks that are readily apparent to the observer, because of the auditory or visual cues associated with them.

hysterical s. Rhythmic, usually temporary, stuttering which may result from extreme excitement, shock, or psychogenic causes.

implicit s. Interiorized *stuttering*.

incipient s. Primary *stuttering stage*.

interiorized s. Form of behavior by the stutterer in which he is able to conceal the overt manifestations of his stuttering, but at the price of constant vigilance, avoidance, and anxiety. Syn: implicit stuttering.

laryngeal s. Spastic dysphonia. See under voice disorders of phonation.

primary s. See under stuttering stages.

secondary s. See under stuttering stages.

transitional s. See under stuttering stages.

voluntary s. May refer to attempts made by the stutterer to imitate or duplicate as closely as possible, or with specific predetermined modifications, his usual, habitual, pattern of stuttering. It may also take the form of easy prolongations or relatively spontaneous and effortless repetitions of sounds, syllables, or the word itself. This style of talking may be used as a deliberate replacement for the usual stuttering behavior and is intended to reduce fear of difficulty by voluntarily doing that which is dreaded. This conscious affectation of repetitions or other forms of dysfluency is also designed to eliminate other avoidance reactions.

stuttering pattern Specific behaviors a particular stutterer demonstrates in speech interference; these usually become predictable and reoccurring.

stuttering phases Various developmental sequences of dysfluencies that an individual may experience. See also stuttering stages.

> **Phase I** Episodic, repetitious dysfluency which occurs usually at the beginning of a sentence on small parts of speech and which appears in situations of communicative pressure, with little concern or awareness shown by the stutterer; often observed in children during the preschool years [Bloodstein].
>
> **Phase II** Essentially a chronic dysfluency on "major" parts of speech; although the stutterer sees himself as one with a dysfluency increasing during excitement or rapid speech, he evidences little or no concern [Bloodstein].
>
> **Phase III** Dysfluency which occurs typically in specific situations on certain sounds and words; the stutterer begins to use circumlocutions and word substitutions, but does not avoid speech situations or exhibit embarrassment; most often observed in late childhood and early adolescence [Bloodstein].
>
> **Phase IV** Dysfluency marked by fearful anticipation of words, sounds, and speech situations; the stutterer uses many circumlocutions and word substitutions, exhibits embarrassment, and begins to avoid speech situations; most typical of later adolescence and adulthood, although it may be observed earlier [Bloodstein].

stuttering stages Various developmental sequences of dysfluencies that an individual may experience. See also stuttering phases.

> **primary s. s.** Characterized by easy repetitions of first words or syllables of a sentence, unaccompanied by signs of emotion or stress [Bluemel, Van Riper]; some speech and language pathologists do not consider these behaviors as true stuttering. Syn: incipient stuttering.
>
> **secondary s. s.** Characterized by the stutterer's awareness of his dysfluencies, with attempts to consciously modify them (thus beginning the process of anticipation and fear often associated with stuttering) [Bluemel, Van Riper].
>
> **transitional s. s.** Stage that occurs between the primary and secondary stuttering stages during which surprise, frustration, struggle, and avoidance begin to accompany the effortless repetitions and prolongations of words and syllables in a sentence; generally results in progression to the secondary stuttering stage [Van Riper].

stuttering theories Major developmental theories of stuttering classified by the manner of their concern with the issues of onset of stuttering or the moment of stuttering. There are six such theories, three of which have several subtheories: (a) anticipatory and struggle behavior theory, with communication failure theory, diagnosogenic theory, and primary stuttering theory; (b) breakdown theory, with cerebral dominance and handedness theory, dysphemia and biochemical theory, and perseveration theory; (c) capacities and demands theory; (d) cybernetic theory of stuttering; (e) learning theory, with approach-avoidance theory, conditioned disintegration theory, instrumental avoidance act theory, and operant behavior theory; and (f) repressed need theory.

anticipatory and struggle behavior theory Stutterer causes interference with the way he speaks because he believes that speech is difficult or will result in a failure. Three primary subtheories differ as to etiology.

Communication failure theory states that stuttering behaviors begin as a response to tension and fragmentation in speech, brought about and sustained by continued or severe failures in communication under pressure [Bloodstein].

Diagnosogenic theory states that stuttering is caused by the misdiagnosis of normal dysfluencies in a child's speech, *i.e.*, stuttering begins "not in the child's mouth but in the listener's ear" [Johnson]. Syn: semantic theory of stuttering.

Primary stuttering theory: 1. Stuttering emerges from a child's own normal hesitations and repetitions; occurs first without effort or awareness by the child and develops when the child learns to anticipate, avoid, and fear speech or speech situations because of reactions by listeners [Van Riper]. **2.** Stuttering can originate from constitutional, neurotic, or environmental factors [Van Riper].

breakdown theory An individual possesses a constitutional predisposition toward stuttering which is precipitated by psychosocial or environmental stress elements. The precise nature of the organic predisposing factors and the extent to which heredity is an influence is not agreed on by adherents to this concept, as indicated by three primary subtheories.

Cerebral dominance and handedness theory states that one cerebral hemisphere is dominant over the other for both speech and motor activities; ambidexterity or a change in handedness is presumed to cause a disruption in the smooth flow of nerve impulses to the speech musculature and results in stuttering [Travis, Orton]. It is referred to by some as laterality theory of stuttering.

Dysphemia and biochemical theory states that stuttering is an outward symptom of an inner condition triggered by illness or emotional or environmental stress (dysphemia), and may also be the result of biochemical imbalance [West].

Perseveration theory states that an individual has an organic predisposition to motor and sensory perseveration which manifests itself in the stuttering act [Eisenson].

capacities and demands theory Dysfluencies emerge when the capacities of the child for fluency are not equal to the demands of the environment for speech performance.

cybernetic theory of stuttering Theory based on the servomechanism feedback model in which the sensor is the ear, the effector is the vocal organs and motor innervations, and the controller is the function of the brain; stuttering is seen as a breakdown in the model's efficiency at any level [Fairbanks, Mysak, Lee and Black, Sutton and Chase, Cherry].

learning theory Any one of several theories of stuttering in the context of the behavioral sciences which concentrates on defining the processes by which stuttering is originally learned and maintained, and which seeks to identify the motivational factors, stimulus variables, and reinforcing conditions.

Approach-avoidance theory: 1. Stuttering is the result of a conflict between opposing drives within the individual to speak or to refrain from speaking [Sheehan, Perkins]. **2.** The stuttering block is the involuntary outcome of other learned approach-avoidance drives and not itself a learned behavior [Sheehan, Perkins].

Conditioned disintegration theory states that stuttering is the involuntary disruption of speech resulting from negative emotional responses that are classically conditioned; secondary characteristics (escape and avoidance) are the instrumentally conditioned responses of the individual to unpleasant experiences. It is often referred to as the two-factor model of stuttering [Brutten and Shoemaker].

Instrumental avoidance act theory states that stuttering is an acquired response incorporating the phenomena of expectancy, anticipation, adaptation, or anxiety and is motivated by the learned drive of apprehension about the normal dysfluencies of speech [Wischner].

Operant behavior theory states that speech is a behavior under operant control of positive and negative reinforcements for which there is no simple cause for stuttering; stuttering is maintained on a complex schedule of reinforcement [Azrin, Flanagan, Goldiamond, Martin and Siegel, Shames and Sherrick].

neurotic theory See repressed need theory (below).

repressed need theory Stuttering as neurotic behavior, as proposed by Freudian models, in which denial of basic psychological needs results in one of many behaviors, including stuttering; this theory poses the question of a possibility of a stuttering personality [Coriat, Bluemel, Fenichel, Freud, Glauber].

styloglossus muscle See *Muscles of the Tongue* table, under tongue.

stylohyoid muscle See *Muscles of the Larynx* table, under larynx.

stylopharyngeus muscle See *Muscles of the Pharynx* table, under pharynx.

SU Sensation unit.

sub- [L. *sub*, under] Prefix denoting under, beneath, inferior, less than the normal or usual.

subclavius muscle See *Muscles of Respiration* table, under respiration.

subcortical motor aphasia See under aphasia.

subcostalis muscle See *Muscles of Respiration* table, under respiration.

subcultural language See under language.

subglottic 1. Below the vocal folds; opposite of supraglottic. **2.** One of three divisions of the larynx, *q.v.*

subglottic resonators See under resonator.

subject [L. *subjectus*, lying beneath] **1.** In traditional grammar, the person or thing in a sentence or clause about which an assertion is made. It may be a **simple subject,** consisting of one word (The *cow* mooed.), or a **complete subject,** consisting of one word and the words associated with it (The *cow in the barnyard* mooed). **2.** A person or animal used in research.

subjective [L. *subjectivus*, thrown under] Denoting opinions or feelings of an individual which are influenced by his personal bias, information, and limitations; opposite of objective (1).

subjective case See case.

subjective quantity See under quantity.

subjunctive mood See under mood.

submucous cleft palate See under cleft palate.

subordinate clause See under clause.

subsonic [sub- + L. *sonus*, sound] Infrasonic.

substandard language Nonstandard *language.*

substantive In grammar, denotes existence, as of nouns, verbs, and adjectives. See substantive universals, under linguistic universals.

substantive universals See under linguistic universals.

substitution (səb-sti-tu′shən) [L. *substitutio*, to put in place of another] **1.** In stuttering, the use of synonyms for words which the stutterer fears. **2.** See under articulation disorder. **3.** See under phonological processes.

substitutional lisp Frontal *lisp.*

substitution analysis See under phonological analysis.

subtotal cleft palate Incomplete *cleft palate.*

subtotal laryngectomy See under laryngectomy.

subvocal speech See under speech.

successive approximation See shaping.

sucking The rhythmical method of obtaining liquid in which the tongue action is primarily a raising and lowering of the body of the tongue. There is much less jaw movement than in the earlier suckling pattern. Negative pressure builds up in the mouth with the combined closure of the lips and lowering of the tongue. This works to pull liquid in the mouth. Emergence of a true sucking pattern is gradual, generally being present by 6 to 9 months.

    nonnutritive s. In infants occurs in the absence of nutrient flow and may

be used to satisfy an infant's basic sucking urge.

    nutritive s. The process of obtaining nutrition through sucking.

suckling The earliest method of sucking observed in infants. It involves a definite backward-and-forward movement of the tongue. Commonly observed in the normal infant during the first 5 to 6 months.

suction (sək'shən) Inhalation method. See under speech, methods of esophageal speech.

sudden and progressive hearing loss See under deafness, sensorineural.

sudden drop curve Ski slope curve. See under audiogram configurations.

suffix Letter or syllable added to the end of a word; may indicate tense, degree, or number. See also affix.

sulcus, pl. **sulci** (səl'kəs, -sī) [L. furrow or groove] Long, narrow, shallow furrow or groove, as on the surface of the brain bordering the gyri or in the oral cavity.

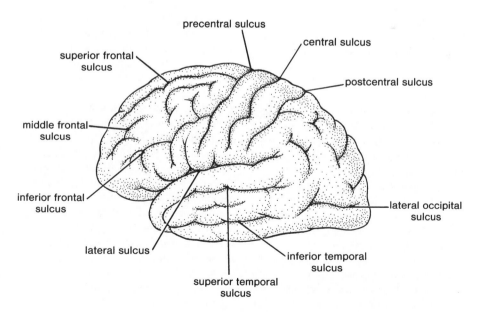

Sulci
Lateral view of the left cerebral hemisphere.

central s. Prominent fissure on the lateral aspect of each cerebral hemisphere, running from the superior margin downward and forward toward the lateral sulcus; it constitutes the boundary between the frontal and parietal lobes. Syn: fissure of Rolando.

frontal s. Three landmark grooves on the lateral aspects of the frontal lobes. The **inferior frontal sulcus** constitutes the boundary between the inferior and middle frontal gyri. The **middle frontal sulcus** divides the middle frontal gyrus into an upper and lower part. The **superior frontal sulcus** constitutes the boundary between the middle and superior frontal gyri.

lateral s. Prominent fissure on the lateral aspect of each cerebral hemisphere, running from the basal surface up toward the central sulcus and then back toward the occipital lobe; it constitutes the principal boundary of the temporal lobe, separating it from the frontal and parietal lobes. Syn: fissure of Sylvius.

median lingual s. Median furrow on the dorsal surface of the tongue, corresponding to the fibrous septum which divides it into symmetrical halves. Syn: median longitudinal raphe.

postcentral s. Sulcus of the parietal lobe immediately posterior and roughly parallel to the central sulcus, with which it forms the borders of the postcentral gyrus.

precentral s. Sulcus on the frontal lobe immediately anterior and roughly parallel to the central sulcus, with which it forms the borders of the precentral gyrus.

temporal s. Two landmark grooves on the lateral aspect of the temporal lobes. The **inferior temporal sulcus** constitutes the boundary between the inferior and middle temporal gyri. The **superior temporal sulcus** constitutes the boundary between the superior and middle temporal gyri.

terminal s. V-shaped groove, with apex pointing posteriorly, on the dorsal surface of the tongue, marking the separation between the oral and pharyngeal parts.

super- [L. *super*, above beyond] Prefix signifying in excess, above, superior, in upper part of; corresponds to Greek *hyper-*.

superior (su-pēr'ē-ėr) [L. above] Higher than or above in relation to another structure; opposite of inferior.

superior maxillary bone See under skull.

superior nasal concha See nasal conchae, under skull.

superior pharyngeal constrictor See *Muscles of the Pharynx* table, under pharynx.

superior turbinated bone Superior nasal concha. See nasal conchae, under skull.

superlative See under comparison.

supernumerary (su-pėr-nu'mėr-ar-ē) [super- + L. *numerus*, number] **1.** In phonetics, denoting an additional needless sound or syllable in a word; *e.g.*, [aɪdɪr] for *idea*. **2.** Accessory; exceeding the normal number.

supernumerary teeth See under teeth malpositions.

supplemental air Expiratory reserve volume. See under respiratory volume.

suppletion (sə-plē'shən) [L. *suppletus*, made complete] Changing of a singular form to a plural form by substituting another base; *e.g.*, is/are, man/men.

suppression (sə-pre'shən) [L. *subpressus*, pressed down] Any of a number of effects, not dependent on learning, which results in a temporary decrease in the frequency with which a response occurs; *e.g.*, a punishing consequence typically suppresses, but does not extinguish, a behavior that it follows; when the punishing consequence is removed, the behavior generally returns to its original rate of emission.

suppurative (səp'yə-rā-tiv) [L. *suppuratus*, having formed pus] Containing, forming, or discharging pus. Syn: purulent.

suppurative otitis media See under otitis.

supra- [L. above] Prefix denoting a position above that indicated by the word to which it is joined.

supraglottic (su-prə-glot'ik) **1.** Above the vocal folds; opposite of subglottic. **2.** One of three divisions of the larynx, *q.v.*

supraglottic laryngectomy See under laryngectomy.

supraglottic resonators See under resonator.

suprahyoid muscles See *Muscles of the Larynx* table, under larynx.

supramarginal gyrus See under gyrus.

supramodal perception Cross-modality *perception.*

suprasegmental (su'prə-seg-men'təl) Prosodic feature of a language, including stress, intonation, duration, and juncture.

suprasegmental analysis Analysis of speech in terms of sequence, duration, rate, rhythm, and fluency.

suprasegmental phoneme See under phoneme.

Suprathreshold Adaptation Test (STAT) See *Audiometric Tests and Procedures* in appendices.

supraversion See under teeth malpositions.

supreme nasal concha See nasal conchae, under skull.

supreme turbinated bone Supreme nasal concha. See nasal conchae, under skull.

surd Voiceless speech sound; *e.g.*, /s/, /h/, /h/, /θ/.

surface structure See under structure.

sustained bite See under mature *bite.*

SUVAG System Universal Verbotonal Audition Guberina.

swallow (swä'lō) [A.S. *swelgan*] **1.** To pass a substance through the oral cavity and pharynx, past the cricopharyngeal constriction, and into the esophagus; an act usually initiated voluntarily but almost always performed reflexively. It may be divided into four phases: (a) *oral preparatory phase*, when food is manipulated in the mouth and masticated if necessary; (b) *oral* or *voluntary phase*, when the tongue propels food posteriorly until the swallowing reflex is triggered; (c) *pharyngeal phase*, when the reflexive swallow carries the food through the pharynx; (d) *esophageal phase*, when the food is propelled through the cervical and thoracic esophagus into the stomach. **2.** A complex motor sequence involving the coordination of a large number of muscles in the mouth, pharynx, larynx, and the esophagus. Provides the mechanism by which food is transported from the environment to the alimentary tract for the survival of the individual. See also barium swallow.

swallowing disorder A swallowing disorder occurs when an impairment reduces an individual's ability to get adequate nutrition by mouth, or when it raises the danger of aspiration of foodstuffs or liquid into the lungs rather than the stomach.

SWALLOWING DISORDER SYMPTOMS

1. Excessive mouth movement during chewing and swallowing
2. Difficulty starting a swallow
3. Coughing or choking while eating or drinking
4. Coughing or choking after eating or drinking
5. Needing to swallow two or three times
6. Food remaining on tongue after swallowing
7. Pocketing of food on one side of mouth
8. Excessive drooling, especially immediately after eating
9. A large amount of extra secretions
10. Gargled-sounding voice after eating or drinking
11. Increased body temperature of unknown cause
12. Pneumonia
13. Chronic respiratory distress

---

swallow method See under speech, methods of esophageal speech.

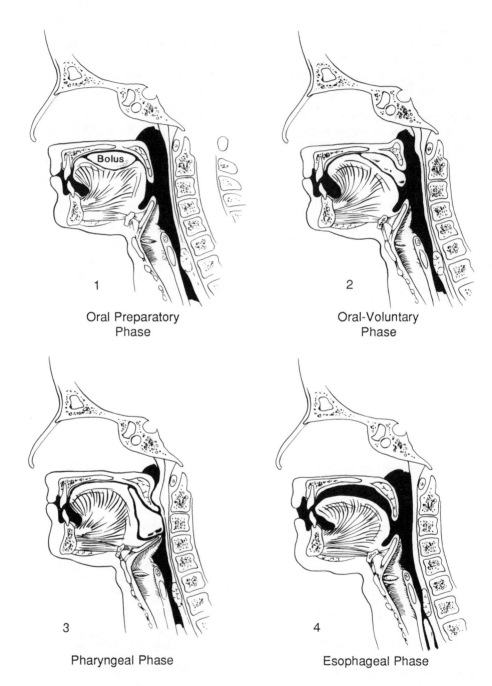

1

Oral Preparatory
Phase

2

Oral-Voluntary
Phase

3

Pharyngeal Phase

4

Esophageal Phase

Sequence of Normal Swallowing
From Cherney, LR, Chantieri, CA, Pannell, JJ. *Clinical Evaluation of Dysphagia,* Rockville, MD:
Aspen Publishers, Inc., 1986.

sweep-check test Screening *audiometry.*

Swinging Story Test See *Audiometric Tests and Procedures* in appendices.

syllabic (si-lab′ik) [G. *syllabikos*] Pertaining to or consisting of a syllable.

syllabic aphonia See under voice disorders of phonation.

syllabication, syllabification (si-la-bə-kā′shən, si-la′bə-fi-kā′shən) Process of dividing a word into syllables.

syllabic speech sound Vowel.

syllable (sil′ə-bəl) [G. *syllabē*] **1.** One of a series of pulses of sound energy; considered the basic physiologic and acoustic unit of speech. **2.** Unit of speech consisting of a vowel for a central phoneme; the vowel may stand alone or be surrounded by one or more consonants; *e.g.*, I, in, me, men.

    closed s. Vowel followed by one or more consonants: *e.g.*, on, off.

    consonant-vowel (CV) s. Syllable containing the consonant-vowel sequence; *e.g.*, see, to, toe.

    consonant-vowel-consonant (CVC) s. Syllable containing the consonant-vowel-consonant sequence; *e.g.*, sun, man.

    nonsense s. Artificial combination of letters not forming a true word; used in learning experiments to exclude possible preformed personal associations. There are three main types: (a) CV (consonant-vowel), *e.g.*, la, va; (b) VC (vowel-consonant), *e.g.*, ab, ap; (c) CVC (consonant-vowel-consonant), *e.g.*, kal, bal.

    open s. 1. Syllable which ends in a vowel; *e.g.*, to, doe. **2.** Deletion of final consonant. See under syllable structure, under phonological processes.

    paired s.′s Repetitive sounds, such as bye-bye, mama, dada.

    vowel-consonant (VC) s. Syllable that begins with a vowel and ends with a consonant; *e.g.*, at, or.

syllable deletion Syllable reduction. See under syllabic structure, under phonological processes.

syllable duplication Reduplication. See under syllabic structure, under phonological processes.

syllable reduction See under syllabic structure, under phonological processes.

syllable sequence Utterances of more than one syllable produced in their proper order; *e.g.*, re pre sent, not re sent pre.

syllable shape Syllable structure.

syllable structure Organization of phonemes in a syllable; *e.g.*, CCVC = consonant-consonant-vowel-consonant. Syn: syllable shape. See also under phonological processes.

symbiotic (sim-bē-ot′ik) [G. *symbiōsis*, state of dwelling together] Pertaining to symbiosis, the mutually advantageous association or interdependence of two individuals, such as mother and infant or husband and wife; sometimes used to denote excessive or pathologic interdependence.

symbiotic psychosis See under psychosis.

symbol (sim′bəl) [G. *symbolon*, mark or sign] **1.** Sign associated with that which it represents by an arbitrary bond agreed on by those who use the sign; *e.g.*, "dog" for a certain quadripedal animal; V_T for tidal volume. **2.** In speech, a character used to denote a speech sound; *e.g.*, /θ/ = /th/, /ʃ/ = /sh/, /ŋ/ = /ng/.

symbolism (sim′bə-liz-əm) [See symbol] **1.** Representation of one thing in terms of another; the use of a symbol. **2.** Investment of ordinary object with imaginative meanings.

symbol set system See augmentative communication system.

sympathetic vibration See under vibration.

symptom (simp′təm) [G. *symptōma*] Any change or abnormality of structure, function, or sensation experienced by the individual and indicative of disease or a disorder; a subjective sign. *Cf.* sign. For various symptoms, see specific terms.

symptomatic therapy Therapy designed to effect relief either through elimination or modification of symptoms presented, rather than of their causes.

symptomatology (simp′tə-mə-tol′ə-jē) [G. *symptōma*, symptom + *logos*, study, discourse] Systematic study of symptoms of disease.

syn- [G. *syn*, with, together] Prefix indicating together, with, joined; appears as sym- before b, p, ph, or m; corresponds to Latin *con-*.

synapse, pl. **synapses** (sin′aps, si-nap′sēz) [L. syn- + G. *haptein*, to clasp] Point of communication between one neuron and another, an effector, or a receptor at which an impulse passes from the axon of one to the dendrite of another.

synaptic (si-nap′tik) Of or associated with a synapse.

synchronic linguistics See comparative *linguistics*.

syncope (sin′kə-pē) [G. *synkopē*, a cutting short, a fainting] **1.** Deletion of a syllable in a word or deletion of an entire word in an utterance; *e.g.*, did you eat = dijeet. **2.** Fainting or a loss of consciousness resulting from a sudden drop in blood pressure or from an interruption of the heartbeat.

syncretism (sin′kre-tiz-əm) [G. *synkrētismos*, union of opposing factions against a common foe] Eclecticism.

syndrome (sin′drōm) [G. *syndromē*, a running together, a concurrence] Group of signs and symptoms which when considered together characterize a disease or lesion. For particular syndromes, see specific terms.

synecdoche See under figure of speech.

synonym See under word.

syntactic (sin-tak′tik) Of or pertaining to syntax.

syntactic aphasia See under aphasia.

syntactic rule Rule which associates the order in which the elements of a sentence can occur and indicates how the information in that sentence is organized. See also linguistic component.

syntagmatic response See under response.

syntagmatic word See under word.

syntax (sin′taks) [L. *syntaxis* fr. G. *syntaktos*, ordered, arranged together] **1.** The internal structure of language, including the order in which the elements of a language can occur and the relationships among the elements in an utterance. **2.** Rules that dictate the acceptable sequence, combination, and function of words in a sentence. **3.** The way in which words are put together in a sentence to convey meaning. See also linguistic component.

synthesis, pl. **syntheses** (sin′thə-sis, -sēz) [syn- + G. *thesis*, a placing, arranging] Combining of the elements of separate entities into a single or unified entity, as contrasted with analysis (1). For types of syntheses, see specific terms.

synthetic (sin-thet′ik) Pertaining to or produced by synthesis.

synthetic method See aural rehabilitation.

Synthetic Sentence Identification Test See *Audiometric Tests and Procedures* in appendices.

syphilis A sexually transmitted disease which may be transmitted to the fetus by intrauterine infection from the mother; may result in a sensorineural hearing loss. The degree of loss depends on the onset of the disease.

system (sis′təm) [G. *systema*, organized whole] **1.** Any organized body of knowledge or procedural plan. **2.** Any complex of anatomically and physiologically related structures; *e.g.*, speech mechanism, respiratory system, pyramidal tract. For various systems, see specific terms.

systematic method Analytic method. See aural rehabilitation.

System of Multicultural Pluralistic Assessment (SOMPA) See *Psychological Measures and Tests* in appendices.

System Universal Verbotonal Audition Guberina (SUVAG) A group of auditory training units designed by Peter Guberina in Zagreb, Croatia. These instruments are an integral part of verbotonal therapy. See also verbotonal.

s/z ratio Technique used to determine the presence or absence of vocal nodules: time (in seconds) in which a patient can sustain an /s/, divided by the time a /z/ can be sustained. The s/z ratios in excess of 1.25 usually indicate that hoarseness is accompanied by vocal nodules; those less than 0.60 strongly suggest hoarseness with normal vocal folds.

T & A Tonsillectomy and adenoidectomy.

tabulation (tab-yu-lā′shən) [L. *tabulatus*, planked, boarded] Any condensed, systematic arrangement of data by rows or columns in a table; *e.g.*, in phonemic analysis, the recording of the distribution of allophones.

tachistoscope (tə-kis′tə-skōp) [G. *tachistos*, very rapid + *skopeō*, to view] Projector with a shutter that allows a timed exposure of projected material; used in figure-ground training.

tachylalia or **tachyphemia** (tak-ə-lā′-lē-ə, -fē′mē-ə) [G. *tachys*, rapid + *lalia*, talking, or + *phemē*, speech] Excessive rate of speaking.

tactile (tak′təl) [L. *tactilis*] Relating to the sense of touch; perceived by touch.

tactile agnosia See under agnosia.

tactile exteroception Vibrotactile *response.*

tactile feedback See under feedback.

tactile kinesthetic perception See haptic *perception.*

tactile perception See under perception.

tact operant See under operant, verbal.

tag question See under question.

tainting Suffix which has acquired a given connotation and may be extended to other words; *e.g.*, *-er*, as in listen*er*, paint*er*.

tangible reinforcement operant conditioning (TROCA) See under audiometry.

Tapia syndrome [A. Tapia, Sp. otolaryngologist, 1875–1950] Ipsilateral paralysis of the larynx and tongue (with atrophy of the latter), but not of the soft palate; due to unilateral lesions of the vagus and hypoglossal nerves (cranial nerves X and XII); variant of Jackson's and of Mackenzie's syndrome, *q.v.*

target [It. *targhetta*, small shield] Goal to be achieved; *e.g.*, /p/, the sound to be corrected; *is playing*, the structure to be stabilized.

target response See under response.

task analysis Technique involving the study of a specific job to find its elements and the processes required to perform it.

tautologous (tô-tol′ə-gəs) [G. *tautos*, identical + *logos*, study, discourse] True in terms of the logic from the meanings of the words in a sentence; *e.g.*, every square is an equilateral rectangle.

TBI Traumatic brain injury.

TC Total communication.

TD Threshold of discomfort.

TDD Telecommunication device for the deaf.

technique See the specific term.

teeth, sing. **tooth** Hard conical structures in the alveoli of the upper and lower dental arches, which are used in mastication and assist in articulation; normally, there are 20 **deciduous teeth,** 10 in each jaw (four incisor, two canine, and four molar), which are replaced by 32 **permanent teeth,** 16 in each jaw (four incisor, two canine, four premolar, and six molar). Teeth play an important role as articulators by serving as markers for tongue positioning and by modifying the airstream for various speech sounds.

> **bicuspid t.** Teeth having two cusps, which are located between the first canine and first permanent molar teeth. Syn: first and second premolar or first and second deciduous molar teeth.

> **canine t.** Teeth having a single cusp, which are located between the lateral incisor and bicuspid teeth. Syn: cuspid or eye teeth.

> **central incisor t.** See incisor *teeth.*

> **cuspid t.** Canine *teeth.*

> **deciduous t.** See teeth.

> **eye t.** Canine *teeth.*

> **first deciduous molar** or **first premolar t.** Bicuspid *teeth.*

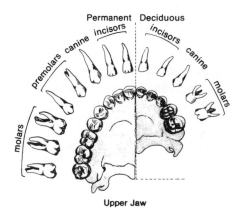

Upper Jaw

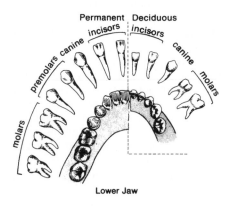

Lower Jaw

Teeth

From *Stedman's Medical Dictionary*, 24th ed.
Baltimore: Williams & Wilkins, 1982.

incisor t. Four chisel-shaped cutting teeth located in the front of the mouth: two **central incisor teeth,** one on either side of the midline or each dental arch, and two **lateral incisor teeth,** one each adjacent to the central incisor teeth on each side of each dental arch.

lateral incisor t. See incisor *teeth.*

molar t. 1. In deciduous dentition, the posterior two teeth on each side of each dental arch. **2.** In permanent dentition, the posterior three teeth on each side of each dental arch; the

most posterior ones and the last to erupt are also called wisdom teeth.

permanent t. See teeth.

premolar t. Bicuspid *teeth.*

second deciduous molar or **second premolar t.** Bicuspid *teeth.*

supernumerary t. See under teeth malpositions.

wisdom t. See molar *teeth* (2).

teeth malocclusion Misalignment of the maxillary teeth with the mandibular teeth; may contribute to poor articulation of particular sounds or to overall general oral inaccuracies. Normal occlusion is based on the relationship of the maxilla and mandible by which the anterior buccal cusp of the maxillary permanent first molar teeth fits into the buccal groove of the mandibular permanent first molar teeth; any deviation from this alignment is considered to be a malocclusion. See also teeth malpositions.

distoclusion (dis-tō-klu′zhən) [L. *distalis*, distal + *occlusus*, closed up] Malocclusion in which the lower dental arch is in a posterior relation to the upper dental arch. In Division I distoclusion, the maxillary incisor teeth protrude in a facioversion or overjet malposition and may result in an excessive overbite. In Division II distoclusion, the mandibular dental arch may assume an irregular curve, with supraversion of the mandibular incisor teeth, and the maxillary dental arch may be wider than normal; results in a closed bite [Angle's Class II].

mesioclusion (mez′ē-ō-klu′zhən) [G. *mesos*, middle + L. *occlusus*, closed up] Malocclusion in which the first permanent mandibular molar teeth are anterior in their relationship with the maxillary first molar teeth, causing the mandibular incisor teeth to protrude and creating an underbite; the maxillary dental arch is constricted, and the tongue frequently rests on the floor of the mouth; a prognathic jaw may result from an extreme version of the malocclusion [Angle's Class III].

neutroclusion (nu-trō-klu'zhən) [L. *neutralis*, neutral + *occlusus*, closed up] Normal anteroposterior relationship between the maxillary and mandibular dental arches, with possible anterior deviations of individual tooth positions, missing teeth, and tooth size discrepancies [Angle's Class I].

teeth malpositions Positioning of the teeth which may interfere with mastication and articulation or with cosmetic appearance; the teeth alone may be in improper positions, or they may be affected in conjunction with various malocclusions. See also teeth malocclusions.

    axioversion (aks'ē-ō-vėr'zhən) [L. *axis*, axle + *versus*, turned] Slanting of teeth along an improper axis.

    buccoversion (bək-ə-vėr'zhən) [L. *buccus*, cheek + *versus*, turned] Facioversion (see below).

    closed bite Supraversion (see below).

    cross-bite Condition in which the maxillary and mandibular teeth are not aligned vertically with each other; one or more teeth may be abnormally malpositioned buccally, lingually, or labially with reference to the opposing tooth or teeth.

distoversion (dis-tō-vėr'zhən) [L. *distalis*, distal + *versus*, turned] Tipping or slanting of teeth away from the middle of the dental arch.

facioversion (fā'shē-ō-vėr'zhən) [L. *facies*, face + *versus*, turned] Slanting of teeth toward the lips or cheeks (face). Syn: buccoversion; labioversion.

infraversion (in-frə-vėr'zhən) [L. *infra-*, below + *versus*, turned] Condition in which teeth have not erupted sufficiently to reach the proper line of occlusion.

jumbling Overcrowding of teeth, resulting in their being overlapped or massed together.

labioversion (lā'bē-ō-vėr'zhən) [L. *labium*, lip + *versus*, turned] Facioversion (see above).

linguoversion (liŋ-gwə-vėr'zhən) [L. *lingua*, tongue + *versus*, turned] Slanting or tipping of teeth toward the tongue or the inside of the mouth.

mesioversion (mez'ē-ō-vėr'zhən) [G. *mesos*, middle + L. *versus*, turned] Slanting or tipping of teeth toward the midline of the dental arch.

open bite Condition in which the anterior upper teeth appear to be too short to reach the midline; the posterior teeth may have grown past the midline point, and thumb sucking may also be a contributing factor.

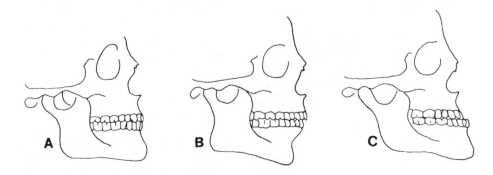

Teeth Malpositions
A, normal occlusion; B, overbite; C, underbite.

overbite Excessive supraversion.

overjet Condition in which the maxillary teeth extend past the normal line of occlusion and in the direction of the lips.

supernumerary teeth Teeth in excess of the usual number in the dental arch.

supraversion (su-prə-vėr′zhən) [L. *supra-*, above + *versus*, turned] Extension of upper teeth beyond the normal line of occlusion. Syn: closed bite.

torsiversion (tôr-si-vėr′zhən) [L. *torsio*, to twist + *versus*, turned] Rotation of teeth along their vertical axis.

transversion (tranz-vėr′zhən) [L. *trans*, through, across + *versus*, turned] Condition in which teeth are in the wrong sequential order along the dental arch, even though they may be inclined properly.

underbite Condition in which the mandibular teeth protrude and overlap the maxillary teeth; results in the appearance of the mandible jutting forward.

telecoil (tel′ə-koil) Induction coil in a hearing aid designed to pick up signals from a telephone; may also be used in loop induction auditory training units.

telecommunication device for the deaf (TDD) Telephone communication device that allows hearing-impaired or deaf individuals to send or receive messages; the sender types in messages which are then transmitted through telephone lines and received visually. Syn: text telephone (TT).

telegraphic utterance Condensed speech in which only the most essential words are used; brief expression carrying a high level of information, resembling a telegram or written lecture notes; primarily composed of nouns and verbs, with only a few adjectives and adverbs; functors (prepositions, conjunctions, articles, and auxiliary verbs) are omitted.

telephone device for the deaf A previously used term for telecommunication device for the deaf.

telephone theory Volley theory. See under hearing theories.

telescoped words Blending (1).

teletactor (tel-ə-tak′tėr) [G. *tele*, distant + L. *tactus*, touched] Instrument which amplifies sound waves and transmits them to the skin where they can be sensed as mechanical vibrations.

Temple University Short Syntax Inventory (TUSSI) *See Language Tests and Procedures* in appendices.

Templin-Darley Tests of Articulation See *Articulation Tests and Phonological Analysis Procedures* in appendices.

Templin Phoneme Discrimination Test See *Auditory Tests and Procedures* in appendices.

tempo (It. fr. L. *tempus*, time] See rate.

temporal bones See under skull.

temporal gyri See under gyrus.

temporal lobe See under cerebrum, under brain.

temporal sulci See under sulcus.

temporary threshold shift (TTS) See under threshold shift.

temporomandibular (tem′pôr-ō-man-dib′-yu-lėr) Relating to the temporal bone and the mandible; denoting the articulation of the lower jaw.

temporomandibular joint (TMJ) Combined gliding and hinge-type structure in front of the tragus of the ear, which allows movement of the mandible; this movement can be sensed when the jaws are opening.

temporomandibular joint syndrome Dysfunction of the temporomandibular joint with impairment of mandibular movement and masticatory muscle function, as from arthritis, severe malocclusion, or trauma; accompanied by varying combinations of headache, earache, muscular discomfort, tinnitus, vertigo, clicking sensations in the joint, stuffy sensations in the ear and impaired hearing, and burning sensations in the throat, mouth, and tongue. Syn: Costen's syndrome.

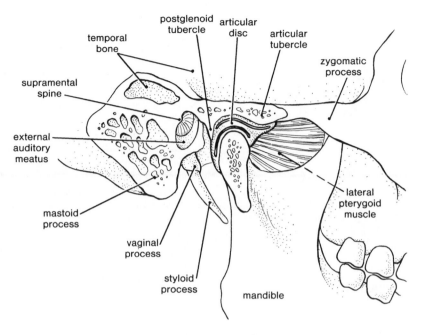

Temporomandibular Joint
Sagittal section with related structures.

tendon (ten'dən) [L. *tendo*, to extend,
stretch out] Fibrous connective tissue
by which muscles are attached to
bones and other structures.

tense (tens) [Fr. L. *tempus*, time] **1.** In traditional grammar, the time an action
takes place as determined by various
verb forms. There are six basic tenses,
plus a progressive construction, all
formed by combining one of the principal parts of the verb (**infinitive:** *to go,
walk;* **past:** *went, walked;* and **past
participle:** *have gone, walked).* Tenses are either **perfect,** time periods
constructed from the past participle
form of the verb, plus a form of *have*
used as an auxiliary verb to denote action that has been or will be completed
at some time in relation to some other
time, or **simple,** time periods which tell
time now, in the future, or in the past,
and which do not have to be expressed
in terms of another time period. **2.** See
under distinctive features.

future perfect t. Tense which represents an action that will be completed at some definite time in the
future; *e.g.,* he *will have gone* by that
time; he *will have walked* the route
by supper time.

past perfect t. Tense representing action completed at some definite time
in the past; *e.g.,* he *had gone* long before he was missed; I *had walked* at
noon, but now I walk earlier.

present perfect t. Tense representing an action as having been completed at some indefinite time up to
the present or extending into the
present; *e.g.,* he *has gone* to the store;
I *have walked* for hours.

progressive t. Tense denoting continuing action during a given time
(tense) period which may occur in
any of the perfect or simple tenses;
constructed with a form of the verb
to be used as an auxiliary verb and
an /-ing/ form of the main verb (infini-

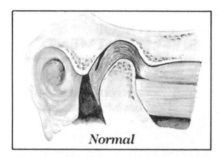

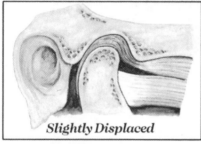

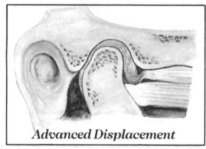

TMJ Syndrome
© American Association of Oral and Maxillo-facial Surgeons.

tive base or past participle base); commonly referred to as the "is-ing" form of verbs. The various progressive tenses are (a) **future perfect progressive:** he *will have been going/walking;* (b) **past perfect progressive:** he *had been going/walking;* (c) **present perfect progressive:** he *has been going/walking;* (d) **simple future progressive:** he *will be going/walking;* and (e) **simple present progressive:** he *is going/walking,* I *am going/walking.*
simple future t. Tense indicating an action still to occur; *e.g.,* he *will go;* he *will walk.*
simple past t. Tense indicating an action which may have occurred at any time in the past, but not as close to the present as in the present perfect tense; *e.g.,* he *went* home; he *walked* the dog.
simple present t. Tense indicating present action, action that occurs at all times, customary or habitual action, or action that is occurring at the time the sentence was formed; *e.g.,* I *go* there; he *goes* there; I *walk* all the time; he *walks* all the time.
tense pause In stuttering, a dysfluency judged to exist between words, part-words, or nonwords (interjections) when there are inaudible or barely audible manifestations of heavy breathing or muscular tightening.
tense phoneme See under phoneme.
tense vowel See under vowel.
tension (ten′shən) [L. *tensio* fr. *tensus,* stretched] **1.** Act of stretching; condition of being stretched or taut. **2.** Mental, emotional, or nervous strain; may result when needs are unsatisfied or goal-directed behavior is blocked. **3.** Strained relations or barely controlled hostility between persons or groups.
tensor veli palatini muscle See *Muscles of the Palate* table, under palate.
tenth cranial nerve See *Cranial Nerves* table, under cranial nerves.
TEOAE Transient evoked otoacoustic emissions. See under otoacoustic emissions.
TEP Tracheoesophageal puncture.
terminal [L. *terminus,* boundary, limit] See under neuron.
terminal behavior See under behavior.
terminal contour Terminal *juncture.*
terminal juncture See under juncture.
terminal lag See under lag.
terminal string See under *derivation* of a sentence.
terminal sulcus See under sulcus.
tertiary stress See under stress.
TES Therapeutic error signal.

test [L. *testum*, earthen vessel] **1.** Method of examination yielding a measure, usually considered to be an objective measure; may consist of a set of standardized questions administered for the purpose of measuring abilities in a given field. **2.** Direct structured observation of behavior, usually under specific conditions; considered to be a subjective measure. **3.** Operation designed to assess the significance of statistics. **4.** In logic, any operation applied to reasoning to assess its validity. For various tests, see specific terms and the appendices.

   criterion-referenced t. A test that compares an individual's performance to specific criteria, thus determining the skills the individual possesses. (The individual is not measured against norms set by the performance of other individuals.)

   norm-referenced t. A standardized test that compares an individual's test score to the average score of a group of individuals who are representative of the tested individual.

   standardized t. A test that has set standards on which an individual is evaluated, in addition to set administration and scoring procedures. Yields a score that may be used to compare the individual's performance with those of others in his age group.

Test for Auditory Comprehension of Language—Third Edition (TACL-3). See *Language Tests and Procedures* in appendices.

Test for Examining Expressive Morphology (TEEM) See *Language Tests and Procedures* in appendices.

Testing-Teaching Module of Auditory Discrimination (TTMAD) See *Auditory Tests and Procedures* in appendices.

Test of Adolescent Language See *Language Tests and Procedures* in appendices.

Test of Articulation in Context See *Articulation Tests and Phonological Analysis Procedures* in appendices.

Test of Articulation Performance-Diagnostic (TAP-D) See *Articulation Tests and Phonological Analysis Procedures* in appendices.

Test of Articulation Performance-Screen (TAP-S) See *Articulation Tests and Phonological Analysis Procedures* in appendices.

Test of Auditory-Perceptual Skills See *Auditory Tests and Procedures* in appendices.

Test of Auditory-Perceptual Skills—Upper Level See *Auditory Tests and Procedures* in appendices.

Test of Auditory Reasoning and Processing Skills See *Auditory Tests and Procedures* in appendices.

Test of Children's Language See *Language Tests and Procedures* in appendices.

Test of Early Language Development—Third Edition (TELD-3) See *Language Tests and Procedures* in appendices.

Test of Language Competence (TLC) See *Language Tests and Procedures* in appendices.

Test of Language Development—Intermediate—Third Edition See *Language Tests and Procedures* in appendices.

Test of Language Development—Primary—Third Edition See *Language Tests and Procedures* in appendices.

Test of Minimal Articulation Competence See *Articulation Tests and Phonological Analysis Procedures* in appendices.

Test of Nonverbal Auditory Discrimination (TENVAD) See *Auditory Tests and Procedures* in appendices.

Test of Nonverbal Intelligence (TONI) See *Psychological Measures and Tests* in appendices.

Test of Phonological Awareness See *Articulation Tests and Phonological Analysis Procedures* in appendices.

Test of Pragmatic Skills See *Language Tests and Procedures* in appendices.

Test of Word Finding—Second Edition

(TWF-2) See *Language Tests and Procedures* in appendices.

test-retest reliability coefficient See under reliability coefficient.

tetism (te′tiz-əm) In articulation, a condition in which a majority of consonants are replaced by the /t/ sound.

text (tekst) In pragmatics, any passage, spoken or written, of any length that forms a unified whole; may be anything from a single sentence to a novel or all-day committee meeting. A text is best regarded as a semantic unit, a unit not of form but of meaning.

   mathetic t. Text used to construct reality and solve problems; to narrate, explain, hypothesize, or predict.

   nonobtrusive t. Text that waits for the recipient to come to it; *e.g.*, lecture, essay, novel.

   obtrusive t. Text that moves toward the recipient, as in everyday conversation, personal written notes, and letters.

   pragmatic t. Text used as a means of satisfying needs; *e.g.*, to request objects, actions, and information, to seek interactions, to share feelings and information.

textlinguistics (tekst-liŋ-guis′tiks) Methods of defining, analyzing and interpreting texts.

text telephone (TT) See telecommunication device for the deaf.

textual operant See under operant, verbal.

The Aphasia Screening Test See *Language Tests and Procedures* in appendices.

The Help Test See *Language Tests and Procedures* in appendices.

the oral-nasal acoustic ratio See TONAR.

theoretical linguistics General *linguistics.*

theory (thē′ə-rē) [G. *theōria*, a speculation] **1.** General reasoned principle formulated to explain a group of related phenomena. **2.** Hypothesis or opinion not founded on actual knowledge. **3.** Doctrine underlying a skill, as differentiated from the actual practice

of that skill. For various theories, see specific terms.

therapeutic (thār-ə-pyu′tik) [G. *therapeutikos*] Relating to the treatment of a condition.

therapeutic error signal (TES) Method for determining an individual's best learning modality. Acoustic, visual, and proprioceptive sensory stimuli are used to increase discrimination ability; negative and positive sensory feedback are used for recognition of errors and to establish goals; teaching is then directed toward the sensory modality through which the most progress has been demonstrated. Syn: trial lesson.

therapy (thār′ə-pē) [G. *therapeia*, medical treatment] Treatment of any significant condition to prevent, alleviate, or cure it. For types of therapy, see specific terms.

thermal noise White *noise.*

theta waves or **rhythm** See under electroencephalogram.

THI Traumatic head injury.

thinking Any mental process or activity not predominantly perceptual by which an individual can comprehend some aspect of an object or situation; involves judging, abstracting, reasoning, and conceptualization.

third cranial nerve See *Cranial Nerves* table, under cranial nerves.

third-octave filter See under filter.

thoracic (thôr-as′ik) Relating to the thorax.

thoracic respiration See under respiration.

thorax, pl. **thoraces** (thôr′aks, -ə-sēz) [L. fr. G. *thōrax*, breastplate, the chest] The chest; the upper part of the body between the neck and the abdomen (from which it is separated by the diaphragm) which is encased by 12 pairs of ribs and contains the chief organs of the circulatory and respiratory systems.

three-day measles (mē′zəlz) Rubella.

threshold [A.S. *therxold*] Point at which sensation first appears; the lowest intensity necessary to produce an awareness of stimulation.

absolute t. In audiology: **1.** Faintest sound of a given frequency that a person can detect in 50% of a number of trials. **2.** Intensity at which a sound is just distinguishable from silence. Syn: audibility, detectability, or detection threshold; hearing threshold level; threshold hearing level.

acoustic reflex t. Lowest intensity level of a stimulus (in dB) that produces reliable changes in acoustic immittance as measured close to the plane of the tympanic membrane.

audibility t. Absolute *threshold.*

detectability t., detection t. Absolute *threshold.*

difference limen (DL) In audiology: **1.** Discriminable differences between two sensation levels; the magnitude of the difference thresholds for pitch and loudness varies with frequency, intensity, and duration. **2.** Smallest difference in pitch that can be detected in 50% of a series of trials. Syn: differential threshold; just noticeable difference.

differential t. Difference limen (see above).

equivalent speech reception t. Average of two of three speech frequencies (500, 1000, and 2000 Hz) that shows the lesser amount of hearing loss; usually used with potential candidates for surgery to help predict the degree of success of the operative procedure.

false t. In audiology, an inaccurate estimate of the true sensitivity of hearing.

intelligibility t. Speech reception *threshold.*

just noticeable difference (JND) Difference limen (see above).

most comfortable loudness (MCL) In audiology, the hearing level at which speech is most comfortable for the individual. See also *Audiometric Tests and Procedures* in appendices.

most comfortable loudness range (MCLR) In audiology, the range in intensities at which continuous speech

is heard and understood with ease; may vary in intensity as much as 10 to 20 dB for those with normal hearing.

noise detection t. (NDT) In audiology, the lowest intensity at which one can detect the presence of a masking noise during audiometric testing.

pain t. *Threshold* of discomfort.

pure-tone air-conduction t. Level of intensity at which a pure tone emitted from earphones is just recognizable in 50% of the number of presentations. See also *Audiometric Tests and Procedures* in appendices.

pure-tone bone-conduction t. Level of intensity at which a pure tone emitted from an oscillator (placed on the mastoid process immediately posterior to the auricle or on the center of the forehead) is just distinguishable in 50% of the number of presentations. See also *Audiometric Tests and Procedures* in appendices.

speech awareness t. (SAT) Speech detection *threshold.*

speech detection or **detectability t. (SDT)** Level at which speech is heard 50% of the time; indicates when sounds can be recognized to be speech even though the words may not be recognized. Syn: speech awareness threshold. See also *Audiometric Tests and Procedures* in appendices.

speech reception in noise Measure of the ability to hear in a background of competing noise; materials utilized are the same as those for determining a speech threshold; the spondees are presented at a level 20 dB above the listener's speech reception threshold, and the listener is required to repeat 50% of the words correctly; may be used in special tests for malingering.

speech reception t. (SRT) Faintest intensity at which an individual identifies 50% of the simple spoken words presented and repeats them correctly; secured by using spondees or connected discourse. Syn: intelligibility threshold. See also *Audiometric Tests and Procedures* in appendices.

t. of discomfort (TD) In audiology: **1.** Intensity level at which continuous speech delivered to the sound field of the listener is judged to be uncomfortably loud; subjects with normal hearing can usually tolerate up to 120 dB. **2.** Minimum level of intensity at which sound pressure will produce the sensation of unpleasantness, tickle, or pain. Syn: pain or tickle threshold; tolerance level or range; tolerance threshold for speech; uncomfortable loudness level.

t. of feeling In audiology, the minimum intensity level at which sound pressure produces a sensation of hearing, *i.e.*, feeling the vibration, not sensing it, as in bone conduction. Syn: vibrotactile threshold. See also *threshold* of discomfort.

tickle t. *Threshold* of discomfort.

tolerance level or **range** *Threshold* of discomfort.

tolerance t. for speech *Threshold* of discomfort.

uncomfortable loudness level (UCL) *Threshold* of discomfort.

vibrotactile t. *Threshold* of feeling.

threshold hearing level Absolute *threshold*.

threshold shift Change in hearing sensitivity; may be caused by exposure to noise.

permanent t. s. (PTS) Irreversible loss of hearing sensitivity, usually the result of exposure to noise.

temporary t. s. (TTS) Transient hearing loss occurring for a relatively brief period of time following exposure to noise. Syn: auditory fatigue.

threshold shift method Hood technique. See under masking techniques.

throat (thrōt) [A.S. *throtu*] **1.** Passage from the mouth through the fauces and pharynx. **2.** Anterior aspect of the neck between the chin and clavicles.

thrombosis 1. Coagulation of the blood

within a blood vessel in any part of the circulatory system. **2.** A blood clot.

thyration indicator (thī-rā′shən) Instrument constructed to aid the hearing-impaired individual in modulating his voice more effectively.

thyroarytenoid muscle See *Muscles of the Larynx* table, under larynx.

thyroepiglottic muscle See *Muscles of the Larynx* table, under larynx.

thyrohyoid muscle See *Muscles of the Larynx* table, under larynx.

thyroid cartilage See under cartilage.

TIA Transient ischemic attack.

tic [Fr.] **1.** A spasmodic or sudden twitch. **2.** More or less involuntary repeated contraction of a certain group of associated muscles; may be a continuation in stereotyped form of a movement or muscle set which was at one time voluntary and purposeful. **3.** Patterned movements which occur repeatedly in the same location, usually of the head, facial structures, or shoulders; may be psychogenic or organic in origin.

tickle threshold *Threshold* of discomfort.

tidal air Tidal volume. See under respiratory volume.

tidal volume See under respiratory volume.

timbre (tim′bėr) [Fr. sound (of bell)] **1.** Quality of a sound. **2.** Aspect of a complex tone resulting from the overtones of the fundamental frequency; the manner by which tones of a given pitch in different instruments are distinguished. **3.** Vocal color; the means by which voices are differentiated on the basis of the distribution of patterns of pitch and loudness. **4.** Sensation a listener receives from vocal patterns or sounds.

time See under deixis.

Time Compressed Speech Test See *Audiometric Tests and Procedures* in appendices.

time-out (TO) In conditioning: **1.** Period during which the subject does not respond to a stimulus, usually created by removing the individual from the response-evoking situation; may serve as a punishing stimulus. **2.** Period free from any reinforcement; an interval during which responses previously reinforced are no longer reinforced.

time pressure In stuttering, a compulsive feeling of urgency to speak; a feeling that does not allow deliberate relaxed speech.

TIN Tone in Noise.

tin ear Colloquialism for tone *deafness.*

tinnitus (ti-nī′təs, tin′i-) [L. jingling, clinking] Sensation of sound in the head which may be localized in one or both ears or perceived in the cranial region; perceived as a throbbing, hissing, whistling, booming, clicking, buzzing, roaring, or high-pitched tone or noise; may result from any auditory impairment in any location within the auditory pathway or have a vascular or muscular origin; often associated with Ménière's disease and otosclerosis.

tip-of-the-tongue phenomenon Condition in which an individual has difficulty recalling a specific word or name that is "on the tip of the tongue" but cannot be verbalized. Syn: feeling-of-knowing.

tissue (tish′u) [Fr. *tissu,* woven] Collection of similar cells, and the intercellular substance surrounding them, which are united in the performance of a particular function. There are four basic types of tissue: (a) **connective tissue,** which includes blood and lymph, bone, cartilage, fat, membrane, and tendon; (b) **epithelium,** the avascular cellular outer layer of the skin and mucous membrane; (c) **muscle tissue,** which contracts on stimulation and is classified as skeletal, smooth (internal organs), or cardiac (heart); and (d) **nerve tissue,** highly differentiated tissue composed of neurons in nerve fibers capable of receiving, transmitting, and processing impulses of stimuli.

TLC Total lung capacity.

TMH Trainable mentally handicapped.

TMJ Temporomandibular joint.

TO Time-out.

token reward Item of little intrinsic value which serves as a reinforcer; *e.g.,* a chip, ticket, or an indicator on a chart given to an individual for a specific accomplishment.

Token Test for Children See *Language Tests and Procedures* in appendices.

Token Test for Receptive Disturbances in Aphasia See *Language Tests and Procedures* in appendices.

tolerance [L. *tolero,* to endure] **1.** Ability to resist or endure strain or other procedures without undue psychological or physiologic harm. **2.** Level of an individual's ability to withstand frustration without developing inadequate modes of response or behavior. **3.** In acoustics, the maximum sound pressure level that can be experienced. **4.** In instrumentation, the margin for error in the fit of mechanical parts.

tolerance level or **range** *Threshold* of discomfort.

tolerance threshold for speech *Threshold* of discomfort.

tomography (tə-mog′rə-fē) [G. *tomos,* a cutting (section) + *graphē,* a writing] Radiographic technique to obtain an x-ray of a body tissue at a specific plane, with exclusion of adjacent tissues; useful in speech for studying laryngeal structures, anomalies, and pathologic conditions. Syn: laminography; planigraphy; polytomography. *Cf.* cineradiography; fluoroscopy; radiography. See also x-ray.

> **computed t. (CT)** Gathering of anatomical information from a cross-sectional plane of the body, presented as an image generated by computer synthesis of x-ray transmission data obtained in a number of different directions through a given plane.

> **computerized axial t. (CAT)** Former name for computed tomography.

tonal spectrum Picture of a complex tone which shows its component frequencies and intensities; interpreted on an oscilloscope.

TONAR (the oral-nasal acoustic ratio) 1. System for separating nasal from oral resonance, based on differences in resonance characteristics between the oral and nasal cavities; separation is achieved by the use of a mask consisting of two compartments, one above the other, made of lead encased in fiberglass and fitted into a single unit which is held firmly against the face. **2.** Array of instruments which analyzes vocal output in terms of relative nasal and oral sound pressures.

tone (tōn) [G. *tonos*] **1.** Tension present in resting muscles. **2.** Firmness or healthy state of tissue, part, or organ. **3.** In voice, the character of voice in expressing an emotion or in expressing distinguishing characteristics of various morphemes in certain languages. **4.** In acoustics, sound sensations having a pitch, loudness, and timbre. For types of tone not listed below, see specific term.

   complex t. In acoustics, a sound wave characterized by combined pure tones; it has more than one pitch and contains simple sinusoidal components of different frequencies.

   difference t. Distinctive sound or pitch heard by the ear which represents the sound or pitch between the frequencies of two generating tones; *e.g.*, if frequencies of 1500 dB and 2000 dB are presented, the ear will hear these two tones as well as a tone of 500 dB (difference tone).

   glottal t. Original tone produced by the activity of the vocal folds. See also fundamental *frequency* (3).

   modal t. Habitual *pitch.*

   partial t. 1. A fundamental frequency and its overtones; *e.g.*, in a fundamental frequency of 100 Hz and an overtone of 200 Hz, the fundamental frequency is the first partial and 200 Hz is the second partial (or first

overtone). **2.** Any component of a complex tone.

   pure t. In acoustics, a sound wave which has only one frequency with no overtones or harmonics; a simple sinusoidal sound wave. Syn: simple tone.

   simple t. Pure *tone.*

   warble t. Sound resulting from rapid changes of frequency within fixed limits around a basic pure-tone frequency.

tone control Modulator permitting the increase or decrease of the relative amplification of the high, middle, and low frequencies; allows selective amplification of specific frequency bandwidths.

tone deafness See under deafness.

tone decay Decrease in the threshold sensitivity during the hearing of a barely audible sound, the sound seeming to disappear; rapid tone decay may be a symptom of a retrocochlear lesion. See also temporary *threshold shift.*

Tone Decay Test See *Audiometric Tests and Procedures* in appendices.

tone focus Emphasis of resonance along the vocal tract or pharyngeal pathway; may be in the laryngopharynx, oropharynx, or nasopharynx.

Tone in Noise (TIN) See *Audiometric Tests and Procedures* in appendices.

tongue (təŋ) [A.S. *tunge*] **1.** Highly mobile mass of muscular tissue covered with mucous membrane which is located on the floor of the mouth; it serves as an organ of taste and assists in mastication, swallowing, and articulation. **2.** Primary organ of articulation, usually functioning in conjunction with the mandible to assist in the production of many different speech sounds; as a resonator, it modifies the shape of the oral cavity and alters the position of the soft palate, hyoid bone, mandible, and pharynx.

   Apex, the tip, is the anterior edge

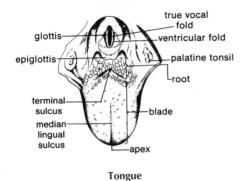

Tongue

of the tongue nearest to the upper incisor teeth.

Blade or **body** is the flattened anterior two thirds of the tongue beneath the hard palate, including the apex, which is capable of extension, retraction, and lateralization.

Dorsum is the upper surface of the tongue, containing many projections (papillae), some of which have taste buds and tactile end organs; it is divided into the blade and root portions.

Root is the posterior one third of the tongue beneath the soft palate. It is directly attached to surrounding structures and is connected with the hyoid bone, epiglottis, soft palate, and pharynx.

Muscles of the tongue are of two types: (a) **extrinsic,** muscles with origins outside the tongue and insertions in the tongue, serving to depress, elevate, and protrude the tongue; and (b) **intrinsic,** muscles with origins and insertions in the tongue, serving to alter the shape of the tongue. See *Muscles of the Tongue* table.

bifid or **forked t.** Diglossia.

tongue height Distance that the tongue is moved from the floor of the mouth toward the roof of the mouth in the production of vowels.

tongue press See injection method,

under speech, methods of esophageal speech.

tongue thrust 1. When, in a resting position, the anterior or lateral portions of the tongue contact more than half the surface area of either the upper or lower incisors, cuspids, or bicuspids or protrude between them, or when, during the swallow of any two of three media (liquids, solids, saliva), there is a visible increase by the tongue of (a) force against the teeth, (b) degree of protrusion between the teeth, or (c) contact of surface area of the teeth. **2.** Abnormal lingual pressure applied to the front teeth, accompanied by lip closure of a sucking nature, which occurs during swallowing as perseveration of what is considered a normal swallowing pattern in an infant; excessive tongue thrust may result in protrusion of the anterior teeth, with possible distortions of speech sounds. Syn: deviant, infantile, reverse, or visceral swallowing; orofacial muscle imbalance.

tongue thrust classifications Classifications based on the type of malocclusion resulting from tongue thrust.

   Barrett's Classification

     Type I: *Incisor Thrust* (Angle's Class I) Maxillary overjet, with slight retrusion of the lower incisors; the tongue pushes against the incisors, wedging apart the uppers and lowers.

     Type II: *Full Thrust* (Angle's Class II, Division I) Marked overjet, with retroclination of the lower incisors; the tongue thrusts from first molar to first molar.

     Type III: *Mandibular Thrust* Occurs with Class III occlusions, with the upper first molar posterior (distal) to its normal position.

     Type IV: *Bimaxillary Protrusion* Labioversion of the upper and lower incisors, with the lowers often spaced apart; the tongue

MUSCLES OF THE TONGUE

Muscle	Origin	Insertion	Innervation	Function
EXTRINSIC (origin outside the tongue and insertion within the tongue)				
Genioglossus	Superior genial tubercle of the mandible.	Hyoid and lateral portion of tongue	Hypoglossal nerve	Protrudes and depresses tongue
Hyoglossus	Body and greater cornu of hyoid	Side of tongue	Hypoglossal nerve	Depresses tongue
Palatoglossus	Inferior surface of the soft palate	Side of tongue	Accessory nerve	Elevates tongue and constricts anterior fauces
Styloglossus	Styloid process	Side of tongue	Hypoglossal nerve	Elevates tongue
INTRINSIC (origin and insertion entirely within the tongue)				
Longitudinalis inferior	Base of tongue	Tip of tongue	Hypoglossal nerve	Alters shape of tongue
Longitudinalis superior	Base of tongue	Tip of tongue	Hypoglossal nerve	Alters shape of tongue
Transversus linguae	Median raphe of tongue	Dorsum and sides of tongue	Hypoglossal nerve	Alters shape of tongue
Verticalis linguae	Dorsal aspect of tongue	Sides and base of tongue	Hypoglossal nerve	Alters shape of tongue

pushes against the lingual margins of the teeth.

Type V: *Open Bite* Edges of the upper incisors are parallel to the edges of the lower incisors ; the teeth are apart during swallows.

Type VI: *Closed Bite* (Angle's Class I) May be a slight overjet; teeth are apart during swallows, and there is tongue protrusion.

Type VII: *Unilateral Thrust* (Angle's Class I) May be a crossbite opposite the side of the tongue thrust; lateral incisors, cuspids, and first bicuspids on one side are undererupted, creating a unilateral open bite.

Type VIII: *Bilateral Thrust* Class III occlusion in older patients but may be Class I occlusion in younger patients; there is a bilateral open bite in the molar region; the tongue tip usually contacts the lower incisors while the sides of the tongue push against the molars and, sometimes, against the bicuspids and cuspids.

Garliner's Classification

Bilateral Swallowing Problem Bilateral depression in the molar area in response to bilateral tongue thrust.

Bimaxillary Protrusion Anterior teeth in both dental arches are inclined labially.

Class III Occlusal Problem Two types: skeletal Class III, in which tongue pressure moves the lower teeth forward, and functional Class III, in which the existent anterior position of the mandible causes the tongue thrust.

Closed Bite Occlusal Problem While swallowing, the bite opens and the tongue hits against the upper incisors.

Complete Swallowing Problem
Thrusting area extends from molar to molar.

Open Bite Problem Two types are included: dental open bite and skeletal open bite.

Simple Anterior Swallow Tongue pushes against the upper incisors.

Unilateral Swallowing Problem Tongue pushes against the bicuspids and molars on one side of the mouth, and may exert pressure against all of the dentition in the upper dental arch.

tongue thrust therapy Myofunctional therapy.

tongue-tied Colloquialism for ankyloglossia.

tonic [G. *tonikos*] In a state of contraction sufficient to keep a muscle taut but not sufficient to produce movement.

tonic block See under block.

tonometer (tə-nom′ə-tėr) [G. *tonos*, tone + *metron*, measure] **1.** Any instrument used to measure the pitch of tones or for producing tones of known pitch; may be used to isolate various partials of a complex tone. **2.** Instrument used to determine pressure or tension.

tonsil [L. *tonsilla*, stake] Mass composed of lymphoid tissue and covered with a mucous membrane; abnormal swelling results in an alteration of resonance.

palatine t. Paired soft submucosal lymphoid masses located in the lateral walls of the oropharynx between the anterior and posterior pillars of the fauces; when overly enlarged, they tend to muffle oral resonance so that it sounds "swallowed."

pharyngeal t. Unpaired lymphatic mass located on the posterior wall of the nasopharynx which is prominent in children but usually atrophies in adults; when overly large, it interferes with resonance, giving speech a hyponasal quality. Syn: adenoid.

tonsillectomy (ton-sə-lek′tə-mē) [tonsil + G. *ektomē*, excision] Surgical removal of the palatine tonsils.

tonsillectomy and adenoidectomy (T & A) Combined surgical removal of the palatine and pharyngeal tonsils.

tooth See teeth.

topic shift Any change from the current topic of discussion.

abrupt t. s. Any topic shift that was made quickly and had no immediate referent.

gradual t. s. Any topic shift that had one or more transitional utterances that connected the immediate topic and the one which followed.

topography (tə-pog′rə-fē) [G. *topos*, place + *graphē*, a writing] In anatomy the description of any part of the body, especially in relation to a defined surface area.

TORCH An acronym used to identify the major infections that may be contracted by a fetus in utero. **T** stands for *toxoplasmosis;* **O** is for *other,* which may include ophthalmologic disease; **R** is for *rubella;* **C** is for *cytomegalovirus;* and **H** is for *herpes simples.* Some authorities have used **(S)TORCH** to include *syphilis.* Any disease of the **(S)TORCH** complex is considered a high risk factor for hearing loss.

Toronto Tests of Receptive Vocabulary, English/Spanish See *Language Tests and Procedures* in appendices.

torque (tôrk) [L. *torqueo*, to twist] A rotational stress; a twisting; force involved in producing the rotation of a body about an axis; *e.g.,* rotation of the cartilages of the ribs requires contraction of the muscles of inhalation and results in a torque of these muscles; when the muscles relax, the natural tendency of the cartilages is to untorque.

torsional wave See under wave.

torsiversion See under teeth malpositions.

total cleft palate Complete *cleft palate.*

total communication (TC) See under aural rehabilitation.

total laryngectomy See under laryngectomy.

total lung capacity (TLC) See under respiratory capacity.

Tourette syndrome Giles de la Tourette syndrome.

toxic (tok'sik) [G. *toxikon*, an arrow poison] Poisonous; caused by a poison.

toxic deafness See under deafness.

toxoplasmosis A parasitic infection transmitted by pregnant women to their unborn children; may cause sensorineural hearing loss in some newborns.

trachea, pl. **tracheae** (trā'kē-ə, -kē-ē) [G. *tracheia artēria*, rough artery] Cartilaginous and membranous tubular part of the respiratory passageway which extends from the cricoid cartilage through the thorax and divides into the bronchi; colloquially referred to as windpipe.

tracheobronchial tree (trā-kē-o-broŋ'-kē-əl) Trachea and bronchi considered collectively.

tracheoesophageal puncture (TEP) A procedure where a fistula is formed between the trachea and esophagus through which air is directed by means of a prosthetic device to generate esophageal speech.

tracheostoma Stoma.

tracheotomy (trā-kē-ot'ə-mē) [trachea + G. *tomē*, incision] Surgical procedure by which an opening is made in the wall of the trachea and into which a tube is inserted to facilitate breathing.

tract [L. *tractus*, a drawing out, an extension] Series or system of anatomically and physiologically related parts or organs. For various tracts, see specific terms.

traditional analysis Phonetic analysis. See under phonological analysis.

traditional grammar See under grammar.

tragus, pl. **tragi** (trā'gəs, -gī) [G. *tragos*, goat (allusion to appearance of growth of hairs on the part)] Anatomical landmark of the auricle of the ear. See auricle, under external *ear*.

trans- [L. *trans*, across, through] Prefix meaning across, through, beyond.

transcortical motor aphasia See under aphasia.

transcortical sensory aphasia See under aphasia.

transcription (tran-skrip'shən) [L. *transcriptio*] **1.** Recording of a speech sound as it is heard rather than as it is spelled according to the alphabet. **2.** Recording of a speech unit into the characters of the International Phonetic Alphabet; may be a phonemic or phonetic representation.

　broad t. Phonemic *transcription.*

　close t. Phonetic *transcription.*

　narrow t. Phonetic *transcription.*

　phonemic t. Conversion of a speech unit into phonemic symbols, written with virgules (slash marks) and indicating the phoneme to which each sound belongs; it can only be interpreted by someone familiar with the phonology of the language transcribed; *e.g.,* /kot/ for *coat.* Syn: broad transcription.

　phonetic t. 1. As accurate as possible recording of the exact pronunciation of an utterance, written with square brackets and including the allophonic features or variations of a phoneme; may be interpreted by an individual ignorant of the language so transcribed if he knows the principles of the transcription; *e.g.,* in *coat* [$k^h o^w t$], the aspiration of [k] is indicated by the superior *h,* and the rounding of [o] is indicated by the superior *w.* **2.** Conversion of a speech sound into the International Phonetic Alphabet characters. Syn: close or narrow transcription.

transducer (tranz-du'sẻr) Device that receives energy in one form and changes or transforms it into another form; *e.g.,* a microphone, which converts sound energy into electrical energy, or a loudspeaker, which converts acoustic energy into electrical energy.

transducing (tranz-du′siŋ) [trans- + L. *duco*, to lead] Cross-modality *perception*.

transference tranz-fèr-ens) [L. *transfero*, to bear across] **1.** Term used to indicate a modification of the laryngeal signal imposed by the configuration of the supraglottal structures; *e.g.*, teaching the placement of /s/ and having it generalize with voicing for the production of /z/. **2.** A generalization of learning; the use of newly established target behavior in various situations outside of a clinical setting. See also carryover.

transferred meaning See metaphor, under figure of speech.

transformation (tranz-fôr-mā′shən) [L. *transformatus*, transformed] **1.** Operation that changes one configuration or expression into another, in accordance with a rule. **2.** In linguistics, a grammatical operation which affects the deep grammatical structures to produce surface structures; it involves changes which add or delete symbols, make substitutions, or effect order changes, but which do not alter the meaning of the sentence. **3.** Explanation, in part, of how a reader or listener can understand a sentence in which the grammatical relations have been obscured in the surface structure. **4.** In cognition, a child's inability to focus on changes, *i.e.*, an inability to integrate series of events in terms of beginning-end relationships.

transformational or **transformational generative grammar** Generative transformational *grammar*.

transformer Electronic device capable of varying the voltage of an electronic current between stages of a circuit.

transient 1. Lasting only a short time. **2.** A not periodic signal of short duration.

transient distortion See under distortion.

transient evoked otoacoustic emissions (TOAE) See under otoacoustic emissions.

transient ischemic attack (TIA) 1. Episode of cerebrovascular insufficiency, usually due to partial occlusion of an artery; symptoms vary with the site and the degree of occlusion, but may include disturbance of normal vision, dysphasia, numbness, or unconsciousness. **2.** A mini-stroke which may last for minutes or hours.

transient vibration See under vibration.

transillumination (tranz′i-lu-mə-nā′-shən) Photoglottography.

transistor (tran-zis′tèr) Electronic device that amplifies an electric current; allows electrical transmission in one direction only.

transition (tran-zi′shən) [L. *transitio*, to go across] Frequency shift found in spectrograms of speech at the junction of a consonant and vowel; reflects the changes in the oral cavity that occur as the articulators move from the position of a consonant to that of a vowel. **normal t.** Closed *juncture.*

transitional stuttering See under stuttering stages.

transmitter [L. *transmitto*, to send across] Any instrument for sending a message in the form of a signal to a receiver, usually by radio waves or through a wire.

transmutation (trans-myu-tā′shən) [L. *transmutatus*, changed] Use of a word in various syntactic functions; the same word used as different parts of speech; *e.g.*, What *drink* do you want? I'll *drink* it.

transposition (tranz-pə-si′shən) Metathesis. See under phonological processes.

transsexual voice See under voice.

transverse (tranz-vèrs′) [L. *transversus*] Across and at an angle to the long axis of the body or a part.

transverse plane See under plane.

transverse temporal gyri See under gyrus.

transverse wave See under wave.

transversion See under teeth malpositions.

transversus abdominis muscle See *Mus-*

cles of Respiration table, under respiration.

transversus linguae muscle See *Muscles of the Tongue* table, under tongue.

transversus thoracis muscle See *Muscles of Respiration* table, under respiration.

trauma (trä′mə) [G. wound] **1.** Injury, wound, or severe emotional stress caused by an external force. **2.** In acoustics, damage to hearing from a sudden high-intensity sound, such as an explosion.

traumatic brain injury (TBI) An acquired injury to the brain caused by an external force resulting in total or partial functional disability or psychosocial impairment or both, which adversely affects an individual's performance. It applies to open or closed head injuries resulting in impairments in one or more areas, such as cognition; language; speech; memory; attention; reasoning; abstract thinking; judgment; problem-solving; sensory, perceptual and motor abilities; psychosocial behavior; physical functions; and information processing. It does not apply to brain injuries that are congenital or degenerative, or brain injuries induced by birth traumas.

traumatic head injury Traumatic brain injury.

traveling wave theory See under hearing theories.

Treacher Collins syndrome [E. Treacher Collins, Eng. ophthalmologist, 1862–1919] Incomplete form of mandibulofacial dysostosis, *q.v.*

Tree/Bee Test of Auditory Discrimination See *Auditory Tests and Procedures* in appendices.

tree diagram See branching tree diagram.

tremolo (trem′ə-lō) Tremor of the voice; an irregular or pulsating vocal quality; an exaggerated vibrato.

tremor (trem′ər) [L. a shaking] **1.** Trembling or shaking of a muscle group. **2.** Involuntary rhythmic movements, intermittent or constant, involving an entire muscle or only a circumscribed group of muscle bundles. See under cerebral palsy symptomatology.

   intentional t. Tremor not present during rest, but which appears with voluntary or "intended" movements.

tremulous speech See under voice disorders of phonation.

trial lesson Therapeutic error signal.

triangular wave See under wave.

Tri-County Contextual Articulation Test See *Articulation Tests and Phonological Analysis Procedures* in appendices.

trigeminal nerve See *Cranial Nerves* table, under cranial nerves.

trigger set Preparatory set (2).

trill See under consonant, manner of formation.

triphthong See under vowel.

triplegia (trī-plē′jē-ə) [G. *tri-*, three + *plege*, a stroke] Paralysis involving three extremities, usually two legs and one arm. *Cf.* diplegia; hemiplegia; monoplegia; paraplegia; quadriplegia.

trite [L. *tritus*] Denoting an expression lacking in originality, freshness, or meaning because of excessive usage; hackneyed; *e.g.*, blushing bride.

TROCA Tangible reinforcement of operant conditioned audiometry.

trochaic stress See under stress.

trochlear nerve See *Cranial Nerves* table, under cranial nerves.

-trophy [G. *trophē*, nourishment] Suffix denoting nutrition, nourishment.

trough curve Saddle curve. See under audiogram configurations.

true language See under language.

true vocal folds See under vocal folds.

TT Text telephone.

TTS Temporary threshold shift.

tumor (tu′mėr) [L. a swelling] Common term for neoplasm.

   eighth nerve t. Acoustic *neurilemoma.*

tuning fork Two-pronged metal fork, usually made of steel, which when struck vibrates to produce a pure tone at a fixed frequency.

Tuning Fork Test See *Audiometric Tests and Procedures* in appendices.

TYMPANOGRAM CLASSIFICATION
(Feldman model)

Classification	*Pathology*
Pressure peak	
Negative	Blocked eustachian tube Serous otitis media
Normal	Ossicular fixation Ossicular discontinuity Eardrum abnormality
Positive	Early acute otitis media
Absence of pressure peak	Middle ear drainage Tympanic perforation
Amplitude	
Stiff (high impedance)	Ossicular fixation Otitis media
Flaccid (low impedance)	Ossicular discontinuity Eardrum abnormality
Shape	
Flattened or decreased slope	Serous otitis media Ossicular fixation Tumors of the middle ear
Increased slope	Eardrum abnormality Ossicular discontinuity
Smoothness	Eardrum abnormality Ossicular fixation Vascular tumors Open eustachian tube

turbinates or **turbinated bones** Nasal conchae. See under skull.

turbulence (tėr′byǝ-lǝns) [L. *turbulentia*] Sound generated at points of constriction in the vocal tract.

   nasal t. Noise of air passing over resistance in the nasal passages.

TV Tidal volume.

twelfth cranial nerve See *Cranial Nerves* table, under cranial nerves.

twin language See idioglossia (3).

two-factor model of stuttering Conditioned disintegration theory. See under learning theory, under stuttering theories.

two-toned voice See diplophonia, under voice disorders of phonation.

tympan-, tympani-, tympano- [G. *tympanon*, drum] Combining forms denoting the tympanic cavity or middle ear.

tympanic cavity Middle *ear.*

tympanic membrane See under external *ear.*

tympanitis (tim-pǝ-nī′tis) [tympan- + G. -*itis*, inflammation] Myringitis.

tympanogram (tim′pǝ-nō-gram) [tympano- + G. *gramma*, a writing] **1.** Graph depicting eardrum and middle ear compliance as a function of air pressure changes within the external auditory canal. **2.** Chart of the results of acoustic impedance audiometry. See also acoustic impedance.

tympanogram classification (Feldman model) Interpretation of tympanometry by descriptive analysis utilizing (a) pressure peak, the point of maximum compliance (normal, negative, positive); (b) amplitude, the degree of compliance at the eardrum (normal,

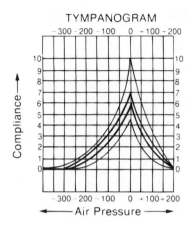

TYMPANOGRAM

Tympanogram
Peak immittance at or near 0 indicates a normal air-filled middle ear.

stiff, flaccid); and (c) shape, the modification of slope and shape of the tympanogram.

tympanogram classification (Jerger model) Coding system that types various patterns of tympanograms, characterized by a large inverted V. See acoustic impedance. See also acoustic immittance measurement.

    Type A: Indicative of a normally functioning middle ear, the point of maximum compliance occurring when ear canal and middle ear pressure are equal (0 mm H_2O).

    Type A_D: Type A in which the curve is very deep and may not meet in a point on the chart; may be associated with flaccidity of the tympanic membrane or separation of the ossicles.

    Type A_S: Type A in which the curve is much shallower than usual; suggestive of middle ear pathology.

    Type B: Depicted by little or no change in the compliance of the tympanic membrane as the air pressure in the ear canal is changed; may be associated with ears having extremely stiffened middle ear systems, as seen when the middle ear space (a) is filled with fluid (serous

or adhesive otitis media), (b) is filled with earwax or other debris, or (c) has a congenital malformation; may also be seen in tympanic membrane perforation.

    Type C: Point of greatest compliance occurs on the negative side of 0 mm H_2O, indicating below normal pressure within the middle ear (negative to normal atmospheric pressure); may be associated with poor eustachian tube function.

    Type D: Depicted by a deep curve with a small notch at the peak; may be found with scarred eardrums.

    Type E: Depicted by a broad, deep, often multiple, notching; may be found with ossicular discontinuity.

tympanometry (tim-pə-nom′ə-trē) [tympano- + G. *metron*, measure] **1.** Procedure used in acoustic immittance measurement to determine the point (pressure peak), magnitude (amplitude), and shape of the greatest compliance of the tympanic membrane; measured in arbitrary units. It is performed by loading the eardrum with air pressure equal to 200 mm (equivalent water pressure), measuring its compliance, and then making successive measurements of compliance as the pressure in the canal is decreased; when pressure reaches 0 mm, negative pressure is created by the pump, and additional compliance measurements are made. **2.** Measurement of the resistance to the flow of acoustical energy at the tympanic membrane during various pressure changes; one of three measurements utilized in acoustic immittance measurement. See also acoustic immittance measurement, acoustic impedance.

tympanoplasty (tim′pə-nō-plas-tē) [tympano- + G. *plassō*, to form] Myringoplasty.

tympanotomy (tim-pə-not′ə-mē) [tympano- + G. *tomē*, incision] Myringotomy.

tympanotomy tube Grommet.

ubiquitous glottal stop Glottal stop (1).

UCL Uncomfortable level or uncomfortable loudness level.

ulcer (əl′sėr) [L. *ulcus*] Lesion on the surface of the skin or a mucous membrane caused by superficial loss of tissue, usually with inflammation. For types of ulcer, see specific terms.

ultrasonic (əl-trə-son′ik) [L. *ultra*, beyond + *sonus*, sound] Denoting those sounds with frequencies above the range of human detection, generally considered to be above 20,000 Hz.

ultrasonic frequency See under frequency.

ultrasonography An instrumental procedure utilizing a transducer that produces sound waves to image the movement of structures used for swallowing; also used to determine the activity of blood flow in the carotid arteries to determine any stenosis or occlusion that could result in a cerebral vascular accident.

ultrasound Sound pressure waves whose frequency is above the audible range. Ultrasound is often used for diagnostic or therapeutic purposes.

umbo [L. boss of a shield] See tympanic membrane, under external *ear.*

un- [L.] Prefix denoting negation, separation, reversal of action.

unaided augmentative communication See under augmentative communication.

uncomfortable level or **uncomfortable loudness level (UCL)** Threshold of discomfort. See *Audiometric Tests and Procedures* in appendices.

unconditioned reinforcer Primary *reinforcer.*

unconditioned response See under response.

unconditioned stimulus See under stimulus.

underbite See under teeth malpositions.

underextension (ən′dėr-ek-sten′shən) In language, restricted use of a word; *e.g.*, use of *car* to refer only to moving cars on the street and not to parked cars or to pictures of cars. Syn: overrestriction.

underlying structure Deep *structure.*

undermasking See under masking.

understanding Process of comprehending or grasping a meaning.

understatement See under figure of speech.

uni- [L. *unus*, one] Prefix denoting one, single, not paired; equivalent to Greek *mono-*.

unilateral (yu-nə-lat′ėr-əl) [uni- + L. *latus*, side] Pertaining to or restricted to one side of the body.

unilateral abductor paralysis See abductor paralysis, under laryngeal motor *paralysis.*

unilateral adductor paralysis See adductor paralysis, under laryngeal motor *paralysis.*

unilateral cleft lip See under cleft lip.

unilateral cleft palate See under cleft palate.

unilateral paralysis See under paralysis.

unimodal (yu-ni-mō′dəl) [uni- + L. *modus*, a measure, quantity] **1.** Pertaining to discrimination and perception of an object or event which involves independent functioning of each receptor system. **2.** Denoting a method of teaching by concentrating on only one sensory modality (auditory, visual). Syn: unisensory.

unintelligible speech See under speech.

unisensory (yu-ni-sen′sôr-ē) Unimodal.

unit [L. *unus*, one] **1.** Any standard of measure by multiplications or fractions of which a scale or system is formed. **2.** A single thing or person, or any group of things or persons considered as a whole because of mutual or interrelated functions or activities.

United States of America Standards Institute (USASI) Former name of American National Standards Institute.

universal grammar See under grammar.

universality See natural phonological processes.

universals See linguistic universals and subentries.

unmitigated echolalia See under echolalia.

unrounded vowel See under vowel.

unstressed See weak *stress.*

unstressed syllable deletion Syllable reduction. See under syllable structure, under phonological processes.

unstressed vowel Neutral *vowel.*

upper bound Longest utterance in a transcription of a language sample.

upper partial One of the overtones of the fundamental frequency. See also harmonic; overtone.

upper respiratory infection (URI) Invasion of the upper respiratory tract by pathologic microorganisms; may affect hearing and speech.

upward masking See under masking.

urano- [G. *ouranos*, vault of the sky, *ouraniskos*, roof of the mouth] Combining form relating to the palate, usually the hard palate. See also palato-.

uranoplasty (yu′rə-nō-plas-tē) [*urano-* + G. *plasso*, to form] Plastic or reconstructive surgery of the palate.

uranoschisis (yu-rə-nos′kə-sis) [*urano-* + G. *schisis*, fissure] Cleft palate.

URI Upper respiratory infection.

usage doctrine Belief that the usage of the majority of the speakers of a language determines the standard of the language; there is therefore no justification for describing linguistic forms as correct or incorrect.

USASI United States of America Standards Institute.

"U"-shaped curve Saddle curve. See under audiogram configurations.

Usher's syndrome [C. H. Usher, 20th-century Eng. ophthalmologist] Hereditary-associated deaf-mutism and retinitis pigmentosa, characterized by deafness at birth or by early childhood, lack of speech development, and degenerating vision with blindness by the second decade.

Utah Test of Language Development—Third Edition See *Language Tests and Procedures* in appendices.

utricle (yu′tri-kəl) [L. *utriculus*, dim. of *uter*, leather bag] Larger of the two vestibular sacs. See vestibule, under inner *ear.*

utterance 1. Unit of vocal expression preceded and followed by silence; may be made up of words, phrases, clauses, or sentences. **2.** Any vocal expression. For types of utterance, see specific term.

uvula (yu′vyu-lə) [L. dim. *uva*, grape] Small cone-shaped process hanging from the lower border of the soft palate (velum) at midline. Syn: velar tail.

uvular (yu′vyu-lèr) Relating to or associated with the uvula.

uvular muscle See *Muscles of the Palate* table, under palate.

V$_T$ Tidal volume.

vagus nerve See *Cranial Nerves* table, under cranial nerves.

validity [L. *validus*, strong] Extent to which a test measures that which it is intended to measure; it is always specific to the purposes for which a test is used.

> **concurrent v.** See criterion-related *validity*.

> **construct v.** Extent to which a test measures some relatively abstract trait or construct based on an analysis of the nature of the trait and its manifestations.

> **content v.** Extent to which the content of a test represents a balanced and adequate sampling of that which it is intended to measure; sometimes referred to as face validity.

> **criterion-related v.** Extent to which scores on the test are in agreement with (concurrent validity) or predict (predictive validity) some given criterion measure.

> **face v.** See content *validity*.

> **predictive v.** See criterion-related *validity*.

vallecula A shallow groove or depression.

> **epiglottic v.** A depression between the lateral and median glossoepiglottic folds on each side.

variable-interval reinforcement schedule See under reinforcement schedule.

variable-ratio reinforcement See under reinforcement schedule.

vascular (vas'kyu-lėr) [L. *vasculum*, small vessel] Consisting of, pertaining to, or provided with blood vessels.

VC Vital capacity.

V-C Vowel-consonant.

vela (vē'lə) Plural of velum.

velar (vē'lėr) Pertaining to the velum.

velar area See under consonant, place of articulation.

velar assimilation See under assimilatory *phonological processes*.

velar insufficiency Velopharyngeal insufficiency.

velarized consonant Dark lateral. See lateral, under consonant, manner of formation.

velar tail Uvula.

velocity (və-los'i-tē) [L. *velositas*] Rate of motion; the distance traveled in unit time in a given direction.

> **particle v.** In sound, the speed of movement of a portion of the medium through which a sound wave is passing.

velopharyngeal (vē-lō-fə-rin'jəl, vel-ō-fə-rin'jē-əl) Pertaining to the velum (soft palate) and the posterior nasopharyngeal wall. Syn: palatopharyngeal.

velopharyngeal closure Closing, by the velum and pharynx, of the nasal cavity from the oral cavity, thus directing air through the mouth rather than through the nose.

velopharyngeal competence Ability to separate the nasal cavity from the oral cavity by action of the velum and the pharynx.

velopharyngeal incompetence Inability to achieve adequate separation of the nasal cavity from the oral cavity by velar and pharyngeal action, although the structures appear normal; tends to result in excessive nasal resonance.

velopharyngeal insufficiency Condition in which the velum is cleft, too short, or lacks adequate neural innervation to reach the posterior pharyngeal wall, and thus impairs velopharyngeal competence. Syn: palatal or velar insufficiency.

velopharyngeal port 1. Port or gateway formed by action of the pharynx and velum to control the flow of air and sound through the mouth and nasal passages. **2.** The opening between the oropharynx and the nasopharynx.

velopharyngeal valve Valve which closes and opens the velopharyngeal port between the nasopharynx and the oropharynx; formed by the velum which is aided by the posterior pharyngeal wall musculature.

velum, pl. **vela** (vē′ləm, -lə) [L. veil, sail] The soft palate, composed of the uvula and palatoglossal and palatopharyngeal arches.

vent Hole drilled through an earmold of a hearing aid which allows the passage of air and the modification of sound to reach the eardrum. See also bore.

vented earmold See under earmold.

ventilation tube Grommet.

ventral [L. *ventralis*] Away from the backbone; toward the front of the body; opposite of dorsal.

ventricle One of three divisions of the larynx, *q.v.*

ventricular dysphonia See under voice disorders of phonation.

ventricular folds See under vocal folds.

ventricular phonation See under voice disorders of phonation.

ventriculus laryngis One of the three divisions of the larynx, *q.v.*

verb See under parts of speech. For types of verb, see specific terms.

verbal 1. Pertaining to words, especially spoken words; oral expression. **2.** See under parts of speech.

verbal aphasia See under aphasia.

verbal apraxia See under apraxia, verbal.

verbal fluency See under fluency.

verbal mediation 1. Ability to retrieve auditory images; the capability of experiencing or recreating auditory experiences by thinking about them. In some children, this ability is impaired or lacking. **2.** Process of internally reconstructing or rehearsing heard digits, words, phrases, or sentences. Syn: reauditorization.

Verbal Motor Production Assessment for

Children (VMPAC) See *Language Tests and Procedures* in appendices.

verbal operant See operant, verbal.

verbal paraphrasia See under paraphrasia.

verbal play Vocal play.

verbigeration (vėr-bi-jėr-ā′shən) [L. *verbum*, word + *gero*, to carry about] Catalogia.

verbotonal method (vėr-bō-tō′nəl) System of teaching the hearing impaired which is primarily auditory in nature. Auditory stimuli are filtered through various octave bandwidths to find the most sensitive region of response for the individual; when the optimal field of hearing has been identified, training is initiated under the frequency and intensity conditions that allow maximum understanding [P. Guberina, 1964].

vermillion border (vėr-mil′yeən) Red external portion of the lips.

vernacular (vėr-nak′yu-lėr) [L. *vernaculus*, native, homeborn] **1.** Language or dialect native to a region or a country; may be standard or nonstandard. **2.** Mode of expression when applied to a particular profession.

Vernet′s syndrome [M. Vernet, Fr. neurologist, 1887–1974] Paralysis of the superior constriction of the pharynx, soft palate, fauces, vocal folds, and sternocleidomastoideus and trapezius muscles with anesthesia of the soft palate, fauces, pharynx, larynx, and posterior third of the tongue; due to lesion of the glossopharyngeal, vagus, and spinal accessory nerves (cranial nerves IX, X, and XI) where they pass between the temporal and occipital bones at the base of the skull, often as a result of trauma.

vertical hemilaryngectomy Hemilaryngectomy.

verticalis linguae muscle See *Muscles of the Tongue* table, under tongue.

vertigo (vėr′tə-gō) [L. dizziness] Whirling sensation or dizziness often associated with diseases of the ear.

vestibular (ves-tib′yu-lėr) Relating to a vestibule, especially that of the ear.

vestibular canal Scala vestibuli. See cochlea, under inner *ear*.

vestibular folds Ventricular folds. See under vocal folds.

vestibular hydrops Ménière's disease.

vestibular membrane See under membrane.

vestibular window Oval window. See under middle *ear*.

vestibule (ves′ti-byul) [L. *vestibulum*, ante-chamber] **1.** Bony cavity in the inner ear connecting the semicircular canals with the cochlea, and also communicating with the tympanum through the oval window. See under inner *ear*. **2.** One of the three divisions of the larynx, *q.v.*

vestibulocochlear nerve See *Cranial Nerves* table, under cranial nerves.

vibrant consonant See trill, under consonant, manner of formation.

vibration (vī-brā′shən) [L. *vibratus*, quivered, shook] Continuing or periodic motion; action that regularly repeats itself and travels in a straight line; may be simple harmonic motion like that of a pendulum. See also oscillation; wave. For types of vibration not listed below, see specific terms.

    forced v. Vibration imposed and controlled by a force external to the vibrator.

    free v. Vibration started and then left to oscillate without any outside influence to control its movement.

    sympathetic v. Vibration when one of two bodies close to each other and with the capacity for free vibration is put into vibration; the other body will go into vibration or resonate with the first.

    transient v. 1. Relatively brief vibration that occurs in electrical circuits, resonators, and other such structures, as a result of a sudden change in conditions. **2.** A harmonic, usually an upper harmonic, which fades out after a brief interval of time.

vibration meter Instrument, corresponding to a sound level meter, which measures the displacement, velocity, acceleration, or jerk of a vibration. Syn: vibrometer.

vibrato (və-brä′tō, vī-) Rise and fall in pitch and volume of the voice, usually in singing; the change in pitch is usually only a small fraction of a musical step. See also tremulous speech, under voice disorders of phonation.

vibratory cycle Cycle of vocal fold vibration from the time the glottis begins to open to the next time the glottis begins to open. Syn: glottal cycle.

vibrometer (vī-brom′ə-tėr) Vibration meter.

vibrotactile (vī-brō-tak′tĭl) Denoting use of the sense of touch to receive or interpret sound vibrations.

vibrotactile hearing aid See under hearing aid.

vibrotactile response See under response.

vibrotactile threshold *Threshold* of feeling.

videofluoroscopic swallow study (VSS) See modified barium swallow, under barium swallow.

videofluoroscopy Videotape recording of physiological or pathological speech activity observed by fluoroscopy. Particularly useful in the study of swallowing, respiratory, and vocal fold movements and in determining the adequacy of velopharyngeal closure. See also fluoroscopy, cinefluoroscopy, radiography, tomography, x-ray.

virgules (vėr′gyulz) [F. commas, little rods] Slanted lines that enclose phonemic symbols and indicate that broad differences are being transcribed. See phonemic *transcription*.

viscera, sing. **viscus** (vis′ėr-ə, -kəs) [L. internal organs, soft parts] Organs of the thoracic and abdominal cavities, *i.e.*, of the respiratory, cardiovascular, digestive, urogenital, and endocrine systems.

visceral (vis′ėr-əl) Relating to the viscera.

visceral nervous system Autonomic *nervous system*.

visceral swallowing Tongue thrust.

visible speech See under speech.

visual acuity See under acuity.

visual agnosia See under agnosia.

visual alexia See under alexia.

visual area See occipital lobe, under cerebrum, under brain.

Visual Aural Digit Span Test (VADS) See *Auditory Tests and Procedures* in appendices.

visual closure See under closure.

visual cue Visible gesture, posture, or facial expression used to aid communication.

visual discrimination See under discrimination.

visual figure-ground See under figure-ground.

visual figure-ground discrimination See under discrimination.

visual hearing or **listening** Comprehension of spoken thought through the interpretation of visual stimuli. See also aural rehabilitation.

visual memory See memory.

visual memory span See memory span.

visual method See aural rehabilitation.

visual-motor coordination or **function** Ability to synchronize vision with the movements of the body or body parts; *e.g.*, copying from a printed page.

visual perception See under perception.

Visual Reinforcement Audiometry See *Audiometric Tests and Procedures* in appendices.

visual-tactile system of phonetic symbolization Method used to teach speech to the hearing impaired, which uses two categories of symbols: (a) static symbols, representing articulatory positions and including the hard palate, tongue, teeth, and lips; and (b) dynamic symbols, indicating the movement of the articulators [A. Zaliouk]. See also grammatic method, under aural rehabilitation.

visual training Learning to perceive the position of objects in space, to discriminate one object from another, to direct visual tracking from left to right, to recognize a whole object from a partial stimulus, to increase the rate of perception, to sequence materials, and to differentiate figure-ground stimuli. See also speech reading, under aural rehabilitation.

visual-verbal agnosia See under agnosia.

vital capacity (VC) See under respiratory capacity.

VMPAC Verbal Motor Production Assessment for Children.

vocabulary (vō-kab′yu-lār-ē) [L. *vocabularius*, of words] All of the words of a particular language, group, or field of knowledge. See *Vocabulary Development* in appendices. See also lexicon.

    core v. Basic set of words that have high utility for a particular person in his regular activities.

vocal (vō′kəl) [L. vocalis] Pertaining to the voice, speech, or to the organs of speech.

vocal abuse Mistreatment, usually by overuse, of the laryngeal and pharyngeal musculature; *e.g.*, by screaming or yelling.

vocal attack Manner by which phonation is initiated in relation to the timing of the closure of the glottis; usually refers to the manner in which vowels are initiated.

vocal bands Vocal folds.

vocal constriction Subjective feeling of openness of the throat regulated along a continuum from maximal constriction (swallowing) to minimal constriction (yawning).

vocal cords Vocal folds.

vocal efficiency Fullest voice with the least vocal effort.

vocal effort Behavior by which respiratory force is scaled from low to high subglottal pressure; the power supply for phonation.

vocal fatigue See under voice disorders of phonation.

vocal focus Sensation associated with

the placement of the tone in the head; the feeling of the location of the focal point of the tone.

vocal fold approximation See adduction.

vocal fold paralysis See under paralysis.

vocal folds Thyroarytenoid ligaments of the larynx, the superior pair being called the ventricular (false) folds and the inferior pair the true vocal folds. Syn: vocal bands or cords.

> **bowed v. f.** Malformation of the vocal folds due to chronic vocal strain over a long period of time; the posterior part of the glottis will no longer close, resulting in a weak, breathy voice.

> **false v. f.** Ventricular folds (see below).

> **true v. f.** Paired vocal folds covered with mucous membrane which lie inferior to the ventricular folds and contain the vocal ligament and fibers of the vocalis and thyroarytenoid muscles; each fold branches out from a fixed anterior point on the lateral walls of the larynx and extends from the posterior surface of the angle of the thyroid cartilage to the vocal processes of the arytenoid cartilages. Sound is produced when these folds are set into vibration.

ventricular folds Thick paired folds of mucous membrane which lie superior to the true vocal folds and enclose a narrow band of fibrous tissue and a few fibers of vocalis muscle; each fold is attached anteriorly to the interior of the thyroid cartilage and posteriorly to the arytenoid cartilages. Except under pathologic conditions, these folds do not contract or shorten during phonation. Syn: false vocal folds; vestibular folds.

> **vestibular folds** Ventricular folds (see above).

vocal fry Glottal fry. See under voice disorders of phonation.

vocalic (vō-kal′ik) Speech sound functioning as a vowel; includes some consonants which may at times serve as vowel sounds. See under distinctive features. See also consonant.

vocalic glide Diphthong. See under vowel.

vocalis muscle See *Muscles of the Larynx* table, under larynx.

vocalization (vō′kə-li-zā′shən) **1.** Any sound produced using the organs of speech. **2.** See under substitution, under phonological processes.

vocalized pause Filler.

vocal misuse Incorrect use of pitch, tone focus, quality, volume, breath support,

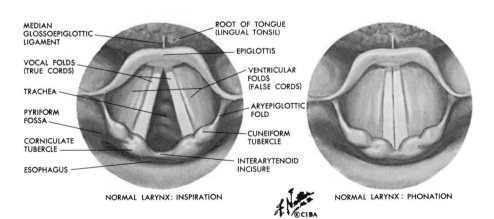

MEDIAN GLOSSOEPIGLOTTIC LIGAMENT
ROOT OF TONGUE (LINGUAL TONSIL)
EPIGLOTTIS
VOCAL FOLDS (TRUE CORDS)
VENTRICULAR FOLDS (FALSE CORDS)
TRACHEA
PYRIFORM FOSSA
ARYEPIGLOTTIC FOLD
CORNICULATE TUBERCLE
CUNEIFORM TUBERCLE
ESOPHAGUS
INTERARYTENOID INCISURE

NORMAL LARYNX: INSPIRATION   NORMAL LARYNX: PHONATION

Vocal Folds

or rate which may occur singly or in combinations.

vocal mode Classes of vocalization which describe vocal behavior; may range from falsetto to glottal fry (highest to lowest pitch). Syn: vocal range or register. See also pitch.

vocal muscle See vocalis in *Muscles of the Larynx* table, under larynx.

vocal nodules See under laryngeal anomaly.

vocal organs Those parts of the body most closely associated with speech production, *i.e.*, the lungs, trachea, larynx, nasal cavities, and oral cavity. *Cf.* articulators.

vocal phonics Auditory synthesis.

vocal play In the development of speech, the stage during which the child experiments with sounds and syllables. Syn: verbal play.

vocal range or **register** Vocal mode.

vocal rehabilitation Treatment of voice problems, such as disturbances of pitch, tone focus, quality, intensity, breath support, or rate.

vocal resonance See under resonance.

vocal tract That part of the speech mechanism above the level of the vocal folds and capable of modifying speech sounds generated by the vocal folds; includes the pharyngeal, oral, and nasal cavities.

vocal tremor Rapid fluctuations of pitch, and sometimes loudness, without relation to the meaning being expressed.

voice [L. *vox*] **1.** In speech, sound produced by the vibration of the vocal folds and modified by the resonators. **2.** In grammar, distinction in the form of a verb to indicate whether the subject acts **(active voice)** or is acted on **(passive voice)**; *e.g.*, the car hit the train (active voice); the train was hit by the car (passive voice).

    active v. See voice (2).

    adolescent v. Change in the character and quality of voice as a result of the changes due to puberty. Syn: mutation voice; puberphonia.

    chest v. Voice lacking nasal resonance; a heavy voice.

    esophageal v. Esophageal speech. See under alaryngeal *speech.*

    eunuchoid v. See under voice disorders of phonation.

    gravel v. Glottal fry. See under voice disorders of phonation.

    guttural v. Throaty low-pitched voice.

    inspiratory v. Speech on inhalation.

    light v. Falsetto. See under voice disorders of phonation.

    muffled v. Throaty or retracted voice which frequently suggests a dialectal base; can be attributed to enlarged lingual tonsils filling the space between the tongue and epiglottis, or a habitually retracted tongue.

    mutation v. Adolescent *voice.*

    passive v. See voice (2).

    pulsated v. Glottal fry. See under voice disorders of phonation.

    transsexual v. Transitory voice problem encountered in the transsexual patient desiring development of a voice consistent with the new sex role; involves a change in both pitch and quality.

    two-tones v. See diplophonia, under voice disorders of phonation.

voice clinician Speech and language pathologist.

voiced Denotes sounds produced with simultaneous vibration of the vocal folds; includes all vowels, semivowels, diphthongs, and voiced consonants. See also under distinctive features.

voiced consonant See under consonant.

voice disorder Any deviation in pitch, intensity, quality, or other basic vocal attribute which consistently interferes with communication, draws unfavorable attention, adversely affects the speaker or the listener, or is inappropriate to the age, sex, or perhaps the culture or class of the individual; may be organic or functional in nature and may be the result of laryngeal function or resonance disorders. See also laryngeal anomaly.

voice disorders of phonation Disorders of voice resulting primarily from the action of the vocal folds; vocal intensity or quality that is unsuitable for the individual in relation to age, sex, or environment.

aphonia Complete loss of voice as a result of hysteria (conversion), growths, paralysis, disease, or overuse of the vocal folds which may develop suddenly or over a period of time; in a less severe form, often referred to as dysphonia. Syn: involuntary whispering. See also subentries under aphonia.

breathiness Excessive amount of air loss accompanying vocal tone; an audible escape of air is usually observed as the approximating edges of the vocal folds fail to make optimum contact.

coup de glotte (ku-də-glät′) [Fr. stroke of the glottis] Glottal catch (see below).

diplophonia (dip-lə-fō′nē-ə) [G. *diplos*, double + *phōnē*, voice] **1.** Vibration of the ventricular folds concurrently with the vocal folds to produce a "two-toned voice"; the ventricular folds usually produce the lower pitch and the vocal folds the higher pitch. **2.** Two distinct pitches are perceived simultaneously during phonation. Some authorities believe this occurs when the vocal folds are under differing degrees of tension or mass and each vibrates at a different frequency. Also spelled dyplophonia.

eunuchoid voice (yu′nə-koid) [G. *eunouchos*, eunuch + *eidos*, resemblance] Falsetto and high-pitched voices.

falsetto [It.] High-pitched voice produced by the vibration of the anterior one third of the vocal folds, the posterior cartilaginous portion being so tightly abducted that only minimal, if any, vibration is possible; falsetto

range overlaps much of the normal range. Syn: light voice.

glottal attack Glottal catch (see below).

glottal catch Extreme glottal closure prior to the initiation of the airflow, which disturbs the normal synchrony of timing and results in the vocal folds being blown widely apart. Syn: glottal attack, glottal seizure, click, stop, or stroke; coup de glotte.

glottal click Glottal catch (see above).

glottal fry Syncopated vocal fold vibration which generally occurs over the lower part of the pitch range; usually described as a bubbling, cracking type of low-pitched phonation. Syn: gravel or pulsated voice; vocal fry.

glottal stop or **stroke** Glottal catch (see above).

gravel voice Glottal fry (see above).

gutturophonia (gət-ėr-ō-fō′nē-ə) [L. *guttur*, throat + G. *phōnē*, voice] Form of dysphonia characterized by a throaty or low-pitched voice.

harshness 1. Usually perceived in a phonatory milieu of hard vocal attacks (sudden approximation of the vocal folds), pitch and intensity problems, and overadduction of the vocal folds. **2.** Resonance phenomenon characterized by tongue retraction and constriction of the pharyngeal constrictors which is sometimes accompanied by nasality; synonymous with excessive vocal effort.

hoarseness One of the more common dysphonias which can be produced by anything that interferes with optimum vocal fold adduction; pitch level is usually low and the range is restricted; pitch breaks or aphonic episodes may also be observed. Three types of hoarseness are (a) **dry hoarseness,** characterized by increased intensity and air loss; (b) **rough hoarseness,** a two-toned voice resulting from vocal fold vibration occurring in two different locations along the vocal folds; and (c) **wet hoarseness,** a voice consisting of air loss and lowering of pitch often accompanied by glottal fry. Syn: huskiness.

huskiness Hoarseness (see above).

hyperfunction (hī-pèr-fəŋk′shən) Excessive forcing and straining, usually at the level of the vocal folds, but which may occur at various points along the vocal tract.

hyperkinetic dysphonia Partial loss of phonation caused by overcontraction of laryngeal or respiratory muscles.

hypofunction (hī-pō-fəŋk′shən) Reduced vocal capacity resulting from prolonged overuse, muscle fatigue, tissue irritation, or general laryngeal or specific problems relating to the opening and closing of the glottis; characterized by air loss and sometimes hoarseness and pitch breaks.

hypophonia (hī-pō-fō′nē-ə) [hypo- + G. *phōnē*, voice] Form of dysphonia characterized by a whispered voice.

laryngeal stuttering Spastic dysphonia (see below).

light voice Falsetto (see above).

macrophonia (mak-rō-fō′nē-ə) [macro + G. *phōnē*, voice] Voice characterized by excessive intensity.

monotone Voice characterized by little or no variation of pitch or loudness; pitch range is usually restricted to one of four semitones. See also pitch.

paradoxic vocal cord dysfunction Closure of the vocal cords on inspiration which may masquerade as asthma or occur with asthma; may be treated with speech therapy.

phonasthenia Voice fatigue (see below).

pitch break Sudden abnormal shift of pitch during speech, usually related to an individual's speaking at an inappropriate pitch level; the typical pitch break is one octave higher (**ascending pitch break**) or one octave lower (**descending pitch break**) than the normal voice.

pulsated voice Glottal fry (see above).

spasmodic dysphonia Interruption of phonation. Voice may sound strained and speaking may become a struggle; may be the result of abductor or adductor disorders. Syn: spastic dysphonia.

    abductor s. d. Intermittent episodes of breathy dysphonia. Drops in pitch and vowel prolongations are typical.

    adductor s. d. Characteristics include vocal strain, intermittent dysphonia, tension, loudness, pitch variations, and pitch breaks.

strident (strī′dənt) Voice usually perceived as having high-frequency resonance; produced by elevation of the larynx and hypertonicity of the pharyngeal constrictors, resulting in a decrease of both length and width of the pharynx.

stridor (strī′dèr) Voice quality which accompanies respiration and is characterized by the presence of a tense, nonmusical laryngeal noise; typically appears in young children during sleep.

syllabic aphonia Brief absence of sound during the effort to produce speech; commonly known as "frog in the throat."

tremulous speech Quavering speech, consisting of an irregular vibrato with amplitudes and frequencies approaching the tremolo.

ventricular dysphonia or **phonation 1.** Voice produced by the vibration of the ventricular folds which may occur as a substitute form of vocalization or concurrently with normal phonation; hoarseness, weak intensity, and low pitch with little inflection are characteristic. **2.** Voice in which the ventricular folds are used as the primary source of phonation, while the vocal folds are in an open, retracted position.

vocal fry Glottal fry (see above).

voice fatigue Deterioration of vocal quality due to prolonged use; may be the result of vocal abuse or be indicative of a pathologic condition. Syn: phonasthenia.

voice disorders of resonance Acoustical effect of the voice, usually the result of a dysfunctioning in the coupling or uncoupling of the nasopharyngeal cavities. See also resonance.

assimilated nasality Hypernasality occurring only on those sounds which immediately precede or follow the nasal consonants /m/, /n/, /ŋ/. See also assimilation.

cul de sac (kəl'də-sak') [Fr. bottom of the sack] Voice quality resulting from an anterior nasal obstruction and a posterior aperture, or from carrying the tongue too far backward; usually described as hollow-sounding. Syn: pharyngeal resonance.

denasality Hyponasality (see below).

hypernasality Excessively undesirable amount of perceived nasal cavity resonance during phonation. Syn: hyperrhinolalia; hyperrhinophonia; rhinolalia aperta.

hyperrhinolalia Hypernasality (see above).

hyperrhinophonia Hypernasality (see above).

hyponasality (hī'pō-nā-zal'i-tē) Lack of nasal resonance for the three phonemes /m/, /n/, and /ŋ/ resulting from a partial or complete obstruction in the nasal tract. Syn: denasality; hyporhinolalia; hyporhinophonia; rhinolalia clausa.

hyporhinolalia Hyponasality (see above).

hyporhinophonia Hyponasality (see above).

mixed nasality Voice quality which exhibits characteristics of hypernasality and hyponasality.

rhinolalia aperta Hypernasality (see above).

rhinolalia clause Hyponasality (see above).

voice fatigue See under voice disorders of phonation.

voiceless Denotes sounds produced with no vibration of the vocal folds.

voiceless consonant See under consonant.

voice onset time (VOT) **1.** Time between the release of the stop consonant and the beginning of voicing in the vowel. **2.** Time required to initiate sound at the vocal folds. Syn: speech initiation time.

voice pathologist Speech and language pathologist.

voice quality The auditory aspects of the function of the vocal folds. Adequate closure, efficient timing of closure, and the amount of tonicity within the folds themselves will influence the type of voice produced. A normal vocal quality is described as nontense, lacking in extraneous noise, nonbreathy, and easily produced and sustained throughout phonation.

voice register Pitch range which may vary from chest voice to falsetto. See also pitch.

voice shift Change of pitch from the end of one phonation to the beginning of the next.

voice termination time (VTT) Time required to cease vocal fold activity.

voice therapist Speech and language pathologist.

voice tone focus Emphasis or placement of resonance in the laryngopharynx, oropharynx, or nasopharynx.

voicing (vois'iŋ) Refers to the action of the vocal folds during speech sound production. When the folds vibrate during speech sound production, the sound is voiced. When the folds are not vibrating during speech sound production, the sound is voiceless.

volition (vō-li'shən) [L. *volo*, to will] Act of making a choice or decision.

volitional oral movement Voluntary movement of the oral structures.

volley theory See under hearing theories.

volt [A. Volta, It. physicist, 1745–1827] Unit of electromotive force or electrical potential; the pressure which causes current of one ampere to flow through resistance of one ohm.

voltmeter An instrument for measuring electromotive force in volts.

volume (vôl′yum) [L. *volumen*, something rolled up, scroll] **1.** Loudness of a sound; dependent on intensity, frequency, and overtone structures. **2.** Space occupied by any form of matter. For types of volume, see specific terms.

volume control Adjustment device which makes it possible to control the overall gain of a hearing aid from little or no amplification to its maximum output; may be manual or automatic. Syn: acoustic gain control; gain control.

    automatic v. c. (AVC) Device to control to a predetermined degree the intensity of a signal leaving a receiver; volume is controlled by a resistor which helps compress amplification. Syn: automatic gain control.

    manual v. c. Device allowing manual regulation of the intensity of a signal leaving a receiver; in a hearing aid, it is designed to allow the wearer to adjust the amount by which the input signal is amplified.

volume unit meter (VU meter) Meter on an audiometer which enables the examiner to monitor input signals.

voluntary mutism Mutism (2).

vomer See under skull.

VOT Voice onset time.

vowel (vou′əl) **1.** Voiced speech sound resulting from the unrestricted passage of the air stream through the mouth or nasal cavity without audible friction or stoppage. It is described in terms of (a) relative position of the tongue in the mouth: front, central, back; (b) relative height of the tongue in the mouth: high, mid, low; and (c) relative shape of the lips: spread, rounded, unrounded. **2.** Most prominent sound in a syllable; in American English: /i/, /ɪ/, /e/, /ɛ/, /æ/, /ʊ/, /u/, /o/, /ɔ/, /ɑ/, /ɝ/, /ʌ/, /ɚ/, /ə/. Syn: syllabic speech sound; simple syllabic. See also International Phonetic Alphabet.

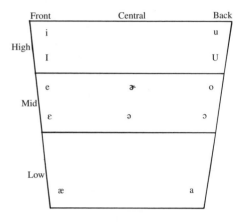

Vowel Diagram

VOWELS

Vowel	Description
i	high, front, tense*
ɪ	high, front, lax*
e	(upper-) mid, front, tense*
ɛ	(lower-) mid, front, lax*
æ	low, front
u	high, back, tense* (rounded)
U	high, back, lax* (neutral or slightly rounded)
o	(upper-) mid, back, tense* (rounded)
ʌ	(lower-) mid, back (unrounded)
ɔ	(lower-) mid, back (rounded)
ɑ	low, back
ə	mid-central (unstressed)
ɚ	central, rhotacized (unstressed)
ɝ	central, rhotacized (stressed)

*A majority of authorities agree that these vowels belong in the tense/lax classifications.

    back v. Vowel sound produced by the arching or adjustment of the tongue in the back part of the mouth, with the lips more or less rounded, except for /ɑ/; in American English:

/u/ high, /ʊ/ lower high, /o/ mid, /ɔ/ higher low, /ɑ/ low.

cardinal v.'s Set of eight vowels (four front and four back) whose perceptual quality is defined independently of any language and which are presumed to have approximately equal acoustic intervals between them, with characteristic tongue and lip positions and well-defined acoustic qualities; considered the descriptive physiologic limits of tongue positions for vowel sounds and form a standard against which the quality of other vowels can be measured: /i/, /ɛ/, /æ/, /ɑ/, /a/, /ɔ/, /o/, /u/.

central v. Vowel sound produced by the arching or adjustment of the tongue near the center of the mouth with the lips generally unrounded; in American English: /ɝ/, /ɛ/, /ʌ/, /ɚ/, /ə/.

close v. High *vowel*.

complex syllabics Diphthong (see below).

diphthong (difʹthông) [G. *diphthongos*, having two sounds] **1.** Sequence of two vocalic sounds, only one of which is syllabic. **2.** Speech sound which glides continuously from one vowel to another in the same syllable. **3.** Sound whose quality changes noticeably from its beginning to its end in a syllable. In American English: /aɪ/, /aʊ/, /ɔɪ/, /ju/, /eɪ/, /oʊ/. Syn: complex syllabics; vocalic glide; glide.

front v. Vowel sound produced by the arching or adjustment of the tongue in the front part of the mouth with the lips in the front part of the mouth more or less spread; in American English: /i/ high, /ɪ/ lower high, /e/ higher mid, /ɛ/ lower mid, /æ/ low.

high v. Vowel sound produced when the tongue is high, at the top of the mouth: /i/, /u/, /ɪ/, /ʊ/. Syn: close or narrow vowel.

indefinite v. Neutral *vowel*.

interconsonantal v. Vowel phoneme occurring between two consonants in the middle of a word.

lax v. Vowel sound produced without added muscle tension, which is short in duration; authorities differ as to which vowels belong in this class; *e.g.*, /ɪ/, /ɛ/, /ɝ/, /ʊ/; /ɪ/, /ɛ/, /æ/, /ʊ/, /ɝ/, /ɚ/, /ə/, /ʌ/.

light v. Neutral *vowel*.

low v. Vowel sound produced when the tongue is low, at the bottom of the mouth; *e.g.*, /ɑ/, /æ/. Syn: open vowel.

mid v. Vowel sound produced when the height of the tongue is at mid position: /e/, /ɛ/, /ɝ/, /ʌ/, /ɚ/, /ə/, /o/, /ɔ/.

narrow v. High *vowel*.

neutral v. **1.** Lax, mid-central vowel pronounced with the least energy of any of the vowels. **2.** A vocal murmur; the most common vowel sound in the English language: /ə/. Syn: indefinite, light, obscure, or unstressed vowel; schwa.

obscure v. Neutral *vowel*.

open v. Low *vowel*.

postconsonantal v. Vowel phoneme occurring after a consonant at the end of a word.

preconsonantal v. Vowel phoneme occurring before a consonant at the beginning of a word.

pure v. Vowel sound whose quality remains substantially unchanged throughout the syllables in which it is used: /i/, /ɪ/, /ɛ/, /æ/, /ə/, /ɑ/, /ɔ/, /ʊ/, /u/, /ʌ/, /ɝ/.

retroflex v. Vowel sound produced with an added curling of the tongue tip: /ɚ/, /ɝ/.

rhotacised v. Vowel having an /r/-like quality; *e.g.*, fɚ = fur, bɝd = bird.

rounded v. Vowel sound whose production is accompanied by lip rounding: /u/, /ʊ/, /o/, /ɔ/.

semivowel 1. Sound that is vocalic in composition, yet characteristically consonantal in distribution. **2.** Sound which can stand as either a vowel or consonant. In American English: /r/, /j/, /w/.

tense v. Vowel sound produced with added muscle tension, which is long in duration; authorities differ as to which vowels belong to this class; *e.g.*, /i/, /e/, /ə/, /ɚ/, /u/, /o/; /i/, /e/, /ɜ/, /u/, /o/, /ɔ/, /ɑ/.

triphthong (trif'thôŋ) [G. *triphthongos*, with three sounds] Group of three consecutive vowel sounds uttered with a single effort of articulation or breath impulse; *e.g., our, ire.*

unrounded v. Vowel sound whose production is not accompanied by lip rounding: /i/, /ɪ/, /e/, /æ/, /ɑ/.

unstressed v. Neutral *vowel.*

vocalic glide Diphthong (see above).

vowel-consonant (V-C) See under syllable.

vowelization See under substitution, under phonological processes.

vowel neutralization See under substitution, under phonological processes.

vowel quadrilateral Schematic representation of tongue positions for the eight cardinal vowels.

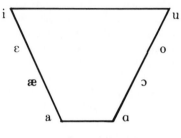

Vowel Quadrilateral

VSS Videofluoroscopic swallow study.
VTT Vocal termination time.
VU meter Volume unit meter.

W-1/W-2 Auditory Tests See *Auditory Tests and Procedures* in appendices.

W-22 Auditory Test See *Auditory Tests and Procedures* in appendices.

warble tone See under tone.

warm-wire anemometer (an-ə-mom′ə-tėr) [G. *anemos*, wind + *metron*, measure] Instrument used to measure the velocity of oral and nasal airflow; operates on the principle that the cooling effect of air flowing past an electrically heated wire varies systematically with changes in velocity of the air stream.

Washington Speech Sound Discrimination Test See *Auditory Tests and Procedures* in appendices.

waterfall curve Ski slope curve. See under audiogram configurations.

watt [J. Watt, Scot. engineer, 1736–1819] Unit of measurement of electric power; the rate of work represented by a current of one ampere under the pressure of one volt.

wave 1. Physical activity in a medium such that at any point in the medium the amplitude of the wave (and other associated quantities) varies with time, while at any instant of time the amplitude varies with position. **2.** Movement of a particle in any medium whereby an advancing series of alternate elevations and depressions or expansions and contractions is pro-

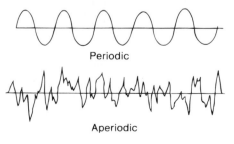

Periodic

Aperiodic

Wave

duced; a restoring force acts on the displaced particle. A wave may (a) be modified in its intended direction; (b) differ as to the manner of production; (c) differ as to the medium in which it travels; (d) differ as to the direction in which it travels; and (e) differ as to the number of frequencies covered.

alpha w.'s See under electroencephalogram.

aperiodic w. Wave which has components at all frequencies and which is not restricted to components at multiples of a fundamental frequency; the waveform does not regularly repeat itself in a given period of time. Syn: nonperiodic wave.

beta w.'s See under electroencephalogram.

complex w. Wave consisting of two or more frequencies but which can be broken down into a set of sine waves, each with a definite frequency and intensity; may be complex and periodic if the frequencies which make it up are harmonically related, otherwise it is complex and aperiodic.

cosine w. Sinusoidal wave that begins at 90′ or 270′ rather than at 0′.

damped w. Sound wave that progressively diminishes in amplitude during successive cycles.

delta w.'s See under electroencephalogram.

diffracted w. Any wave whose direction is changed because of striking a sharp edge, narrow opening, or new medium; usually refers to light waves entering a prism.

electromagnetic w. Wave formed by simultaneous periodic variations of electric and magnetic intensities; may vary in frequency; *e.g.*, radio, light, and heat waves; x-rays.

incident w. Any wave occurring in

341

one medium and traveling successfully or unsuccessfully to another medium. See also reflected *wave;* refracted *wave.*

Jewett w. Early fast-wave responses thought to originate in the brainstem within 10 msec after an auditory signal.

longitudinal w. Any wave particle oscillating in a line parallel to the direction in which the wave is moving; the particle of the medium vibrates back and forth in the same plane as the wave; *e.g.,* a sound wave.

negative spike-w.'s See under electroencephalogram.

nonperiodic w. Aperiodic *wave.*

notched w.'s See under encephalogram.

periodic w. Wave which repeats itself regularly as a function of time; opposite of aperiodic wave; *e.g.,* musical sound.

pure w. Sinusoidal *wave.*

reflected w. Any wave whose direction in the original medium is changed; as the wave tries to enter a second medium, it bounces from the medium's surface and is turned back into the original medium; *e.g.,* a vocal echo.

refracted w. Any wave whose direction is changed (distorted) as it travels from one medium into another; *e.g.,* change in vocal quality when utilizing a public address system.

simple w. Sinusoidal *wave.*

sine w. Sinusoidal *wave.*

sinusoidal w. (sī-nə-soi′dəl) [L. *sinus,* cavity, hollow + G. *eidos,* resemblance] **1.** Wave which is smooth and symmetrical both vertically and horizontally, with one peak (crest) and trough (valley) for each vibration. **2.** Wave with a single frequency, the simplest form of any wave; *e.g.,* a pure tone. Syn: simple, sine, or pure wave.

six-hertz positive spike-w.'s See under electroencephalogram.

slow w.'s See under electroencephalogram.

sound or **sound pressure w. 1.** Character of sound vibrations determined by the number and relative intensities of the various harmonic groups; waveforms may be simple or complex. **2.** One of a succession of compressions and rarefactions of air caused by a vibrating body.

standing w. 1. Wave produced when sound pressure waves of the same frequency and amplitude are traveling in opposite directions; if produced in a nonsoundproof room, the resulting amplitude may be zero at some points and double at others. **2.** Stationary pattern of waves formed by the interaction of rarefaction and condensation, as occurs at locations in an auditorium where sound from the stage cannot be heard.

theta w.'s See under electroencephalogram.

torsional w. Any wave particle oscillating in a curve whose plane is at right angles to the direction in which a wave is moving.

transverse w. Any wave particle oscillating at right angles to the direction in which a wave is moving.

triangular w. Complex wave rich in harmonic energies, with both even and odd harmonics present. See also complex *wave.*

wave filter See under filter.

waveform Graphic representation of a wave demonstrating its pattern of intensity, amplitude, or pressure at any moment. Syn: waveshape.

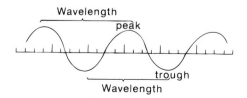

Waveform with Wavelength

waveform distortion See under distortion.

wavelength Distance a wave travels during each complete cycle (peak to peak or trough to trough); inversely related to frequency, the longer waves moving slower than the shorter waves. Wavelength may be determined by the formula: wavelength = velocity of sound (in a given medium) ′ frequency.

wave of excitation 1. Any electrochemical change that is carried through tissue; *e.g.*, the electrochemical reaction experience, but not necessarily overtly reacted to, when hearing a sound in a hearing test. **2.** Neural impulse, especially when conceived as being an electrochemical change.

waveshape Waveform.

wax See cerumen.

weak stress See under stress.

weak syllable deletion Syllable reduction. See under syllabic structure, under phonological processes.

webbing Congenital condition apparent when adjacent structures are joined by a broad band of tissue that is not normally present. See also laryngeal web, under laryngeal anomaly.

Weber Test See *Audiometric Tests and Procedures* in appendices.

Wechsler Adult Intelligence Scale (WAIS) See *Psychological Measures and Tests* in appendices.

Wechsler Intelligence Scale for Children—Revised (WISC-R) See *Psychological Measures and Tests* in appendices.

Wechsler Preschool and Primary Scale of Intelligence (WPPSI) See *Psychological Measures and Tests* in appendices.

weight (wāt) [A.S. *gewight*] Force with which a body is attracted toward the earth by gravity; heaviness.

Weiss Comprehensive Articulation Test See *Articulation Tests and Phonological Analysis Procedures* in appendices.

Weiss Intelligibility Test See *Articula-*

tion Tests and Phonological Analysis Procedures in appendices.

Wepman Auditory Discrimination Test See *Auditory Tests and Procedures* in appendices.

Wepman Auditory Memory Battery See *Auditory Tests and Procedures* in appendices.

Wernicke's aphasia See under aphasia.

Wernicke's area [K. Wernicke, Ger. neurologist, 1848–1905] Region in the superior convolution of the temporal lobe of the cerebrum which is identified as the center for understanding oral language; corresponds approximately to Brodmann's areas 22, 39, and 40.

Western Aphasia Battery (WAB) See *Language Tests and Procedures* in appendices.

wet hoarseness See hoarseness, under voice disorders of phonation.

Wever-Bray effect or **phenomenon** [E. G. Wever, U.S. psychologist, 1902–1991, and C. W. Bray, U.S. otologist, 1904–] Microphonic response of the cochlea (so called because of resemblance to the electrical phenomena produced by sound waves in microphones) consisting of electrical potentials caused by the stimulation of the cochlea by sound; the exact nature of the cochlear microphonics is not known.

whisper [A.S. *hwisprian*] Nonvocal sound with no carrying power produced by the arrangement of the glottis during exhalation (soft whisper); the vocal folds do not approximate and there is no tenseness or effort in production.

    buccal w. Sound produced by an accumulation of air in the mouth and pharynx instead of that ordinarily expelled from the lung passages; usually accompanied by rapid articulatory movements, and sometimes occurs as an unsatisfactory method for alaryngeal speech.

    forced w. Sound with a moderate degree of carrying power which creates extreme vocal fold tension and requires a great amount of physical effort in production; may be abusive to the vocal folds because of strong contact only at the anterior portion of the folds. Syn: stage whisper.

soft w. See whisper.

stage w. Forced *whisper.*

white noise See under noise.

Whorf's hypothesis [B. Whorf, 20th-century linguist] Assumption that differences in linguistic habits cause differences in nonlinguistic behavior. See also linguistic determinism; linguistic relativity.

wh- question See under question.

wide-band noise White *noise.*

wide range audiometer See under audiometer.

Wide Range Intelligence Test See *Psychological Measure and Test* in appendices.

Willis' paracusis *Paracusis* willisi.

windows See under middle *ear.*

windpipe Colloquialism for trachea.

Wing's symbol [G. Wing, U.S. educator of the deaf, 1883] Method used with the hearing impaired which is based on symbols (primarily numbers and letters) representing functions of different parts of speech in a sentence; these symbols are placed over the word, phrase, or clause to demonstrate the form, function, and position of the parts of the sentence, rather than just to illustrate parts of speech; *e.g.,* 1 = noun, 2 = possessive, 0 = object.

WINL Within normal limits.

wisdom teeth See molar *teeth* (2).

word 1. Free form consisting of a sequence of one or more phonemes and one or more syllables which have meaning without being divisible into smaller units capable of independent use; *e.g.,* I, go, mother, baby. **2.** Minimum free form which can be simple, complex, or compound. See also morpheme.

    ambiguous w. Linguistic unit which may have many meanings; *e.g.,* bat

(flying mammal, baseball bat, to hit or strike at). Syn: homograph.

antonym (an'tə-nim) [G. *antōnym,* having opposite name] Linguistic unit opposite in meaning to another linguistic unit; *e.g.,* hot/cold, wet/dry.

base w. Simple form of a linguistic unit to which affixes may be added or of which grammatically different forms may be utilized; *e.g., hold* is the base for both *uphold* and *held.* Syn: root or simple word; semanteme.

class w. Content *word.*

clipped w. Shortened free form which is considered a whole form rather than an abbreviation; *e.g.,* auto (automobile), exam (examination), plane (airplane).

complex w. Linguistic unit consisting of one free form and one or more bound forms; *e.g., guessed = guess* (free form), *ed* (bound form); unquestionable = *un* (bound form), *question* (free form), *able* (bound form).

compound w. Linguistic unit consisting of at least two free forms; *e.g.,* baseball, doorknob, highchair.

content or **contentive w.** Linguistic form within a sentence which carries the most meaning and provides the substance of a sentence; *e.g.,* nouns, verbs, adjectives, adverbs, and pronouns. Syn: class, form, or lexical word.

form w. Content *word.*

function w. Functor (see below).

functor Word whose grammatical function is more obvious than its semantic content and which serves primarily to give order to a sentence; *e.g.,* articles, prepositions, modal and auxiliary verbs, and conjunctions. Syn: function, interstitial, or structure word.

heterogeneous w. Syntagmatic *word.*

homogeneous w. Paradigmatic *word.*

homograph (hom'ə-graf) [G. *homos,*

same + *graphē*, a writing] Ambiguous *word*.

homonym (hom'ə-nim) [G. *homōnymon*, having the same name] Free form which is pronounced like another free form but differs from it in origin, meaning, and often in spelling; *e.g.*, by/buy, plain/plane, knew/new. Syn: homophone.

homophene (hom'ə-fēn) [G. *homos*, same + phēnē, voice] In speechreading, a word which has the appearance of being identical to another word in its production; *e.g.*, tug/tongue, dug/tuck.

homophone (hom'ə-fōn) [G. *homos*, same + phonē, voice sound] Homonym (see above).

interstitial w. Functor (see above).

lexical w. Content *word*.

monosyllabic w. Word of one syllable.

nonsense w. Nonsense syllables combined into a word form that does not carry a meaning for the individual; it is only through contextual cues that the nonsense word acquires a temporary meaning.

open w. Any of a rather large number of words infrequently used by children at the two-word stage of language development; *e.g.*, mommy *go*, mommy *eat*, mommy *play*. *Cf.* pivot *word*. See also pivot *grammar*; open, under parts of speech.

paradigmatic w. Word that is the grammatical equivalent of another word; *e.g.*, go/went/gone. Syn: homogeneous word. See also paradigmatic *response*.

pivot w. Any of a small number of words, frequently used by children at the two-word stage of language development; *e.g.*, *mommy* go, *mommy* eat, *mommy* play. *Cf.* open *word*. See also pivot *grammar*; open, under parts of speech.

polysyllabic w. Word of more than one syllable.

portmanteau w. Telescoped *word*.

protowords Well-defined meaningful sound patterns produced by young children which are not apparently modeled on any adult words.

relational w.'s Adjectives, adverbs, verbs, and prepositions which occur in syntactic relation to nouns and pronouns in a sentence; *e.g.*, in "The girl read the book," "read" determines the meaning relation between "girl" and "book"; in "The book is on the table," "on" determines the order of words and how the object "book" is located in relation to the object "table." See also functor (above).

root w. Base *word*.

semanteme (sə-man'tēm) [Fr. *semantème*] Base *word*.

sign w. See under sign English.

simple w. Base *word*.

split w. Word in which the initial sound is separated from the rest of the word; used in articulation and stuttering therapy, and in speech audiometry; *e.g.*, s- -un.

spondee w. (spon'dē) [G. *spondeios*, ceremonial] Word of two syllables which when pronounced has equal stress on both syllables; often used in audiometric testing; *e.g.*, cowboy, doorway, sunset.

standard w. Linguistic unit which is of correct phonetic structure, as determined by dictionary phonetic listing.

structure w. Functor (see above).

synonym (sin'ə-nim) [G. *synōnym*, having equivalent meaning (name)] One of two or more words or expressions of the same language that have the same or similar meaning; *e.g.*, cab/taxi, annoy/irritate, compel/oblige.

syntagmatic w. One of two words, each belonging to different grammatical classes, which form a meaningful relationship with each other; used to express one idea; *e.g.*, last year. Syn: heterogeneous word. See also syntagmatic *response*.

telescoped w.'s Two words from different sources or languages combined into a single word; they may be combined by additions or by combining one part of one word with one part of another word; *e.g.,* motor + hotel = motel, smoke + fog = smog. Syn: portmanteau word.

word approximation Phonetic pattern in which one or more of the phonetic elements of the standard word are present.

word association Substitution of a word, usually in the same general category or similar in meaning, for a word one is unable to recall; *e.g., spoon* for *fork, dog* for *cat.* See also word-finding problem; anomic *aphasia.*

word blindness Alexia.

word calling In reading, the pronunciation of individual words without evidence that the meaning has been grasped.

word classes Set of words similar to those belonging to parts of speech, but which is based on position in sentence patterns or on formal criteria; forms are not defined according to function. *Cf.* parts of speech.

word configuration Pattern of a free form; *i.e.,* its overall features, length, typography, etc.

word count Study of the frequency with which certain words occur in spoken or written language.

word deafness See auditory *aphasia.*

word discrimination score See speech discrimination, under speech *audiometry.*

word-finding problem Word-retrieval problem.

Word Intelligibility by Picture Identification (WIPI) See *Auditory Tests and Procedures* in appendices.

word-retrieval problem Inability to evoke words corresponding to specific concepts. Syn: word-finding problem. See also anomic *aphasia.*

word sequence Correct order of words in a sentence; demonstrates the acquisition of some of the important rules of grammar.

Word Test See *Language Tests and Procedures* in appendices.

work 1. Exertion of strength; effort directed toward an end. **2.** Physically, the action of a force acting against a resistance. **3.** Force applied multiplied by the distance through which it must act.

written language See under language.

XYZ

x-ray (eks′rā) [named in 1895 by its discoverer, W. K. Roentgen, Ger. physicist, 1845–1923] **1.** That portion of the electromagnetic spectrum consisting of radiation of extremely short wavelength which is emitted from a target anode substance bombarded by a stream of electrons moving at a sufficiently high velocity. It is capable of (a) penetrating various thicknesses of solids; (b) producing secondary radiations by impinging on material bodies; (c) acting on photographic films and plates to produce images (radiographs); and (d) causing fluorescent screens to emit light. Its capabilities make it useful in demonstrating structural relationships during a speech or nonspeech activity. Syn: roentgen ray. **2.** Radiograph. See also cineradiography; fluoroscopy; radiography; tomography.

yawn-sigh approach Techniques used in stuttering and voice therapies to aid in eliminating hard glottal contacts and to encourage greater airflow. The client is instructed to yawn to obtain a longer inspiration, exhale with a light phonation (sigh), and then exhale phonating words that begin with an /h/; use of the initial /h/ helps to eliminate the hard glottal attacks.

Y-cord hearing aid See under hearing aid.

yes-no question See under question.

zero amplitude See under amplitude.

zero cerebral Term used to refer to a flaccid muscle that does not have the power to contract voluntarily.

zero hearing level Sound pressure level required to make any frequency barely audible to the normal ear.

zero morpheme (Ø) See under morpheme.

zygomatic bones See under skull.

Appendices

Developmental Sequences of Language Behavior: Overview

[Nicolosi and Collins]

RECEPTIVE	EXPRESSIVE

0–6 MONTHS

RECEPTIVE	EXPRESSIVE
Startle response to loud sound	Birth cry—undifferentiated
Reflex smiling to tactile and kinesthetic stimulation	Vocal grunt at 8 days
Responds to voice and sound	Small throaty noises
Often quieted by familiar friendly voice	Different kinds of crying for pain, hunger, and discomfort
Attends readily to speaking voice	Babbles and coos in vocal play
Responds to own voice	Babbles to self, others, and objects
Social smile	Laughs out loud
Responds to angry vocal tones by crying	Says two syllables
Responds to pleasant tones by cooing	Repeats monosyllables
Increased awareness of environment	Babbling used for getting attention and expressing demand
Briefly holds and inspects two objects	Gives vocal expression of eagerness
Responds to noise and voice by turning toward source of sound	Vocalizes displeasure
Beginning to sense inflection and intensity meanings	
Responds to pleasant speech by smiling and laughing	

6–12 MONTHS

RECEPTIVE	EXPRESSIVE
Increased awareness and response to environment	Begins using inflectional patterns
Listens with increased intentness to new words	Many speech and nonspeech sounds used in random vocalizations
Responds to own name with head turn, eye contact, or smile	Sings tones (7 months)
Understands "no"	Lalling continues (to 9 months)
Responds to specific person (8 months)	Tries to repeat sounds produced by others
Responds to bye-bye (9 months)	Uses intonation pattern with jargon speech
Shakes head yes and no to some questions (10 months)	Directs sounds and gestures to objects and persons
Follows simple instructions (11 or 12 months)	Echolalia begins (9–12 months); e.g., child enjoys imitating sound sequences
	First word appears (10–12 months)

Developmental Sequences of Language Behavior: Overview—*Continued*

RECEPTIVE	EXPRESSIVE
	Five- to six-word vocabulary (12 months)
	Word type is noun—concrete lexical meanings
	Vocalizes during play
	Intentional language begins

1–2 YEARS

RECEPTIVE	EXPRESSIVE
Understands simple commands and prohibitions (13–18 months)	Average sentence length: 1.5 words
Recognizes familiar objects, persons, pets (14–18 months)	50% of the words are nouns at 18 months, 39% at 24 months
Responds to a variety of semantic categories: action, agent, possession, recurrence	Two- or three-word combinations at 18 months; examples, noun modifiers: the, a, my, more, big; my truck, the car
Identifies one body part (18 months)	Possessive forms: Daddy chair, baby book
Follows directions involving spatial concepts; "in-on"	Adjective-noun combinations: big boy, broken doll
Responds to simple "wh-" questions	10- to 20-word vocabulary at 18 months, 200 words at 24 months
Identifies three body parts (20 months)	Jargon peak at 18 months, gone at 24 months
Identifies two or more objects or pictures from a group	Uses telegraphic speech (omission of articles, helping verbs, etc.)
Perceives others' emotion	Conducts expressive, inflected conversation by means of fluent jargon
Understands the distinction between pronouns such as: "Give it to me," "Give it to her"	Adjectives and adverbs appear in speech: good, bad, nice, hot, cold
Identifies five body parts (22 months)	Simple verb forms appear: see, want, go
Comprehends approximately 300 words	First phrase
	First sentence
	First pronoun (with partial discrimination): I, me, you
	Imitates many words (word echolalia)
	Uses stereotyped phrases: don't cry, be careful

2–2½ YEARS

RECEPTIVE	EXPRESSIVE
Demonstrates an understanding of several action words by selecting appropriate pictures (24–27 months)	Names familiar objects of environment (24 months)
Recognizes and identifies general family name categories (24–27 months) such as baby, grandma, mother	Jargon substantially decreased
	200–300 word vocabulary: nouns, 38.6%; verbs, 21%; adverbs, 7.1%; pronouns, 14.6%

Developmental Sequences of Language Behavior: Overview—*Continued*

RECEPTIVE	EXPRESSIVE
Distinguishes prepositions *in* and *under*	Asks simple questions (ego centered): where ball
Distinguishes between *on* and *many*	Says full name
Listens to simple stories	Improvises own syntax: look me no
Identifies object by use	Repeats two digits from memory
Understands *come-go, run-stop, give-take*	Articles used correctly (a, the)
Understands semantic difference of subject-object by position of noun: show us the *car* pushing the *truck,* the *truck* pushing the *car*	Uses *and:* mommy *and* daddy
Comprehends all sentence structures	
Understands size differences (27–30 months)	

2½–3 YEARS

RECEPTIVE	EXPRESSIVE
Rapid increase in comprehension vocabulary (400 words at 30 months, 800 words at 36 months)	Begins to use verb contractions (30 months)
Responds to commands using *on, under, up, down, over here,* and *jump*	Imitates two-word combinations (30 months)
Responds to commands using two related actions; run fast	Dysfluencies are common (30 months)
Understands taking turns	Rapid vocabulary expansion (900 words)
Can execute simple two-step commands	Uses short simple sentences (3.1-word average)
Identifies seven body parts	90% of speech readily understood
Shows an interest in explanations of *why* and *how*	Relates simple imaginative tales
Demonstrates an understanding of most common adjectives	Carries on purposeful conversation
	Talks when playing alone
	Talks about immediate experiences
	Describes action in a book
	Beginning to ask questions
	Identifies objects by name and use
	Uses personal pronouns (most use first- and second-person pronouns correctly)
	Beginning to use verb inflections (simple past tense, *-ing* for present progressive verb form)
	Beginning to use noun inflections (simple plurals, possessives)
	Continued increase in use of adjectives
	Uses prepositions (prepositions of location are first)
	Verbalizes toilet needs
	Asks for *another*
	Can name three objects in a picture

Developmental Sequences of Language Behavior: Overview—*Continued*

RECEPTIVE	EXPRESSIVE
	Knows a few rhymes
	Repeats three digits

The period from 2–3 years is predominantly one of transition, when jargon is discarded and when objects and pictures are heeded. A child can now combine three words to build a sentence; the three-word sentence is typical of 2 years.

3–4 YEARS

RECEPTIVE	EXPRESSIVE
Improving in listening skills and beginning to learn from listening	Expressive vocabulary 900–1500 words
Understands up to 1500 words by age 4	Mean sentence length 4.3 words
Recognizes plurals, sex differences, pronouns, adjectives	Speech usually 90–100% intelligible in context; still slight trouble with sentence structure
Comprehends complex and compound sentences	Can carry on long conversations
Learns to appreciate social meaning of oral communication	Bosses and criticizes others
	Articulation skills improving; still has difficulty with fricatives, sibilants, /r/, and /l/
	Uses more compound and complex sentences which are more grammatically complete
	More consistent and correct use of plurals and possessives
	Consistent use of imperative and emphatic sentences
	Consistent use of verb contractions
	Question-asking *why* stage
	Uses *what, where,* and *how*
	Uses pronoun *we*
	Can complete opposite analogies: brother is a boy, sister is a _____

4–5 YEARS

RECEPTIVE	EXPRESSIVE
Comprehends 1500–2000 words	Vocabulary of approximately 2000 words
Carries out more complex commands, with two to three actions	Mean sentence length 4.3 words
Understands dependent clause: *if, because, when,* and *why*	Articulation (consonants, vowels, diphthongs) is 80% correct
	Can define words in terms of use
	Language is fairly complete in structure and form
	Uses conjunctions and understands prepositions
	Uses longer, more complex sentences
	Will reply to simple questions: What is a house made of?

Developmental Sequences of Language Behavior: Overview—*Continued*

RECEPTIVE	EXPRESSIVE
	Will tell a story about himself or environment with slight stimulation
	Continues to make grammatical errors (though less frequently)

5–6 YEARS

RECEPTIVE	EXPRESSIVE
Understands vocabulary of 2500–2800 words	Expressive vocabulary 2500 words
Responds correctly to more complicated sentences, but is still confused at times by involved sentences	Mean sentence length 5 to 6 words
	Articulation is intelligible
	Uses almost all phrase structure and transformational rules of adult English, although incorrect forms still occur periodically
	All pronouns used consistently and correctly
	Comparative adjectives are used: big-bigger, loud-louder
	Can answer telephone and carry on conversation
	Relates fanciful tales
	Exchanges information, asks questions, and relates stories
	Correct use of irregular verbs: be, go, do, get, can, have, will
	Articles *an, a* and *the* correct
	Uses prepositions: to, of, in, up, on
	Can tell a familiar story

Vocabulary Development

12 months	Two to six words other than "mama" and "dada"
18 months	10–20 definite words in vocabulary
24 months	200–300 words in speaking vocabulary
30 months	Vocabulary of 450 words
36 months	Vocabulary nears 900–1000 words
42 months	Vocabulary of 1200 words
48 months	Vocabulary of 1500–2000 words
54 months	Vocabulary of 1900 words
60 months	2200–2500 words in speaking vocabulary

Mean Length of Utterance

[Brown]

LANGUAGE DEVELOPMENT FROM 1.0 MORPHEMES TO 4.5 MORPHEMES

The ages at which these particular aspects of language development occur varies. The order of development and the changes that occur at each "stage," which is determined by MLU, is quite invariant—not only across children but even across languages.

Stage I Semantic Roles and Grammatical Relations

Covers an MLU interval from 1.0 to 2.0 morphemes

One-, two-, and three-word utterances

Semantic relations: agent-action, action-object, action-locative, entity-locative, entity-attribute, demonstrative-entity

Yes-no questions signaled by rising intonation; *e.g.,* "See kitty?"

Limited set of *wh-* questions

Stage II Grammatical Morphemes and the Modulation of Meaning

Covers an MLU interval between 2.0 and 2.5 morphemes

Addition of grammatical morphemes, tense markers, plurals, articles, possessive markers, auxiliaries, the copula, third-person regular, and the prepositions *in* and *on;* usually not used 100% of the time until the child is past Stage V

Stage III Modalities of the Simple Sentence

Covers an MLU between 2.5 and 3.0 morphemes

Length increases are mainly the result of the addition of the auxiliary, which enables the child to make interrogative and negative sentences more closely resemble the adult form

Increase in the number of *wh-* questions

Interrogative reversals

Polite phrases; *e.g.,* "please," "thank you"

Stage IV Embedding

Covers an MLU between 3.0 and 3.5 morphemes

Major linguistic change which increases length at this stage is the embedding of one sentence into a semantic role of another sentence; *e.g.,* (1) object-noun-phrase complements, such as "We know, we just do it to ya;" (2) indirect or embedded *wh-*questions, such as "I don't know what I drawed;" (3) relative clauses, such as "Here ones that don't below here."

LANGUAGE DEVELOPMENT FROM 1.0 MORPHEMES TO 4.5 MORPHEMES

Stage V Coordination of Simple Sentences and Propositional Relations

Covers an MLU interval between 3.5 and 4.5 morphemes

Coordination of two simple sentences; *e.g.,* "He hit me right here and it hurt."

Coordination of two sentences with deletion; *e.g.,* "My mommy and daddy don't eat candy."

Locatives; *e.g.,* up, down

Main conjunction is *and*

STAGE	APPROXIMATE AGE (in Months)
I	12–26
II	27–30
III	31–34
IV	35–40
V	41–46

General Outline of
From Birth

APPROXIMATE AGE	COGNITIVE DEVELOPMENT	
	Piaget's Stage	Concepts
	I. Sensorimotor Period	
0–1 mo	A. Reflexive	Total absence of control over movement
2–3 mo	B. Primary Circular Reactions	Reflexes change as a result of experience
3–8 mo	C. Secondary Circular Reactions	*First habits:* if by accident a movement has an interesting result, that's fun—so do it again
8–12 mo	D. Coordination of Early Schemas	*Intention beings:* two or more schemas become intercoordinated: one serves as the *instrument* (e.g., first word), the other as *goal* (e.g., result like attention from adult)
12–18 mo	E. Tertiary Circular Reactions	Repetition with variation *Active experimentation* with objects Existence Nonexistence Recurrence
18–24 mo	F. Invent New Means to the End	Invent new means through *mental* combination (*i.e.,* two semantic concepts) Cause-effect
	II. Preoperational Period	
2–4 yr	A. Preconceptual Stage	Concerned almost exclusively with language learning

Language Development to 11 Years [*Burns*]

LANGUAGE DEVELOPMENT			
Semantics	Syntax		Pragmatics
	Birth cry	0–9 mo	Periocutionary Acts
			Gazing, crying
	Cooing		Touching, smil-
			ing, laughing,
			vocalizing
	Babbling		Grasping and
			sucking
	First word: *mamma, dada,* etc.	9–18 mo	Illocutionary Acts
			Labeling
			Answering
			Requesting
			Calling
			Greeting
			Protesting
	Names of objects and actions		Repeating
	no, allgone, etc.		Practicing
	more, etc.		
	Use of two-word phrases—Semantic Relations	18–24 mo	Locutionary Acts
Agent-action			Dialogue
Action-object			Adoption of roles
Location-object	Some word order only		Addressee
Location-action			Speaker
Attribute-object			Respondent
Introducer-object			Questioner
Possessor-possessed			Persuader
2–3 yr A. Further develop-		2–4 yr	Use of contingent
ment of semantic			queries
relations: dative			Topic maintenance
+ experiencer,			Use of monologue
experiencer +			Stylistic variation
object			Indirectives
			Feedback
			Role playing
B. Case relations	Case grammar		
Agentive case	Meaning dictates the		
Dative case	kinds of noun cases that		
Objective case	must or may be used		
Locative case	with the verb		
	First sentence usage—always a verb		

General Outline of Language Development

APPROXIMATE AGE	COGNITIVE DEVELOPMENT Piaget's Stage	Concepts
		Space Time Quantity
		Time Possession Specificity Time
		Person: *me, he,* etc.
		Time
4–7 yr	B. Intuitive Stage	Time
		Classification
		Seriation Conservation Coordination
		Ego separation
		Further concepts of time

From Birth to 11 Years—*Continued*

	LANGUAGE DEVELOPMENT		
	Semantics	Syntax	Pragmatics
3–4 yr		Transformational grammar	
	Location	*in-on* (affix)	
	Ongoing action	*-ing* (affix)	
	More than one	*-a* (affix)	
		more	
		some	
		two	
	Past tense	Irregular past, regular past	
	Possessive	*-a* (affix)	
	Specificity	*a, the* (affix)	
	Uncontractible copula	*is* (affix to VP)	
	Regular past	*-ed* (affix)	
	Third person regular	*-s*	
	Third person irregular		
	Uncontractible auxiliary	*is . . . ing*	
	Contractible copula & auxiliary	*'s*	
4 yr		Major transformations	
	who, what, where	Question: *wh-, yes-no*	
	not, can't, don't	Negative	
	Future	*wanna, gonna, gotta*	
4+ yr			
	Semantic classification	Conjoining	
		Embedding	
		Passives	
	Syntagmatic/ paradigmatic shift		
	Superordination		
	Comparatives/ superlatives		
	Same-different		
	Temporal conjunctions:	$\times$ (first event), *then* $\times$ (second event)	
	Causal conjunctions	Because—personal justification only	
	Verbs	Use of action dative with *to*	
		Experiencer verbs followed by NP or S	
	Command/request	Ask/tell with NP and *wh-* word	
	Passive-voice	Noncompressed Agent (animate) Object (inanimate)	
	Use of conditional verb tenses like modals *can, will, may,* etc.		
	Use of perfect tense		
	Use of gerunds and participles		

General Outline of Language Development

APPROXIMATE AGE	COGNITIVE DEVELOPMENT Piaget's Stage	Concepts
7–11 yr	III. Concrete Operational Period	Logical reason begins Coordination
		Embedding Passives

From Birth to 11 Years—*Continued*

LANGUAGE DEVELOPMENT		
Semantics	Syntax	Pragmatics

Causal conjunctions *because*—logical justification		
Temporal	Time reversed	
Logical sequence	Subordinate clause first If . . . , then . . . Therefore, . . .	
Discordance	*But* *Even though* *Although*	
Command/request	Without NP specified	
Compressed and unconstrained	Two NP are both animate or both inanimate; *no* is modified	

Speech Sound Development

[Templin]

Earliest age at which 75% of all subjects produced each test sound element correctly.

CHRON-OLOGIC AGE	SPEECH SOUND			
3.0	Vowels	ē, ĭ, ĕ, ă, ŏ, ŭ, o͞o, o͞o, ō, ô, ȧ, ûr		
	Dipththongs	u̅, ā, ī, ou, oi		
		INITIAL	MEDIAL	FINAL
	Consonants	m	m	m
		n	n	n
			ng	ng
		p	p	p
		t		t
		k	k	
		b	b	
		d	d	
		g	g	
		f	f	f
		h	h	
		w	w	
	Double consonant blends			ngk
3.5	Consonants		s	
			z	
				r
		y	y	
	Double consonant blends			rk
				ks
				mp
				pt
				rm
				mr
				nr
				pr
				kr
				br
				dr
				gr
				sm

Speech Sound Development—*Continued*

CHRON-OLOGIC AGE	SPEECH SOUND	INITIAL	MEDIAL	FINAL
4.0	Consonants			k
				b
				d
				g
		s		
		sh		sh
			v	
		j		
		r	r	
		l	l	
	Double consonant blends	pl		
		pr		
		tr		
		tw		
		kl		
		kr		
		kw		
		bl		
		br		
		dr		
		gl		
		sk		
		sm		
		sn		
		sp		
		st		
				lp
				rt
				ft
				lt
				fr
	Triple consonant blends			mpt
				mps
4.5	Consonants			s
			sh	
		ch	ch	ch
	Double consonant blends	gr		
		fr		
				lf

Speech Sound Development—*Continued*

CHRON-OLOGIC AGE	SPEECH SOUND	INITIAL	MEDIAL	FINAL
5.0	Consonants		j	
	Double consonant blends	fl		rp
				lb
				rd
				rf
				rn
	Triple consonant blends			shr
		str		
				mbr
6.0	Consonants		t	
		th	th	th
		v		v
		t̶h̶		
				l
	Double consonant blends			lk
				rb
				rg
				rth
				nt
				nd
				t̶h̶r̶
				pl
				kl
				bl
				gl
				fl
				sl
				skw
	Triple consonant blends			str
				rst
				ngkl
				nggl
				rj
				ntth
				rch
7.0	Consonants		t̶h̶	t̶h̶
		z		z
			zh	zh
				j

Speech Sound Development—*Continued*

CHRON-OLOGIC AGE	SPEECH SOUND	INITIAL	MEDIAL	FINAL
	Double consonant blends	thr		
		shr		
		sl		
		sw		
				lz
				zm
				lth
				sk
				st
	Triple consonant blends	skr		
		spl		
		spr		
				skr
				kst
				jd
8.0	Double consonant blends			kt
				tr
				sp

NOTE: Initial and medial *hw,* final *ifth*, and final *tl* are not produced correctly by 75% of the subjects by 8 years of age.

Developmental Sequences of Motor Behavior

GROSS MOTOR	FINE MOTOR
1 MONTH	
tonic-neck reflex	hand clenches on contact; reflex grasp
head droops	visual localization
lifts head and shoulders	
2 MONTHS	
legs thrust in play	gains control of 12 oculomotor muscles
head erect in vertical position	eyes follow pencil or moving person
waves arms when lying on back	
3 MONTHS	
neurological maturation sufficient to control vocal mechanism	watches play with hands
reaches for objects	pulls at clothing
holds head steady	puts objects to mouth
lifts head and chest when on stomach	
4 MONTHS	
when prone, elevates self by arms	plays with hands and fingers
sits with support	closure reflex begins to disappear
holds self erect when pulled to sitting position	contact generally unilateral
	eyes help with reaching action
5 MONTHS	
begins to shift to bilateral movements	uses hands for support
turns from side to side	
sits with slight support	
6 MONTHS	
sits leaning forward	can grasp and hold two objects
gains control of trunk	gains control of hands
tries to creep or roll toward objects	can transfer and manipulate objects
7 MONTHS	
moves self by creeping	bilateral reaching, but with some spatial error

Developmental Sequences of Motor Behavior—*Continued*

GROSS MOTOR	FINE MOTOR

8 MONTHS

maintains standing position briefly	reaches unilaterally and persistently for toys
can roll from back to stomach	
sits easily without support	grasps with palm of hand

9 MONTHS

creeps and crawls	begins to use index finger more
pushes from stomach to sitting position easily	rotates wrist and tries to throw objects

10 MONTHS

moves from sitting to prone position	attempts to build block tower
creeps and pulls self to feet at rail	attempts to scribble imitatively
takes stepping movements	
takes side steps while holding on	

11 MONTHS

takes first independent step	holds crayon adaptively
stands near rail	extends toys, but will not release them
	begins to drink from cup

12 MONTHS

walks when one hand is held	grasps with fingers

1 YEAR

begins walking alone	learns to feed self
can open a closed door	picks up small objects with precision
removes socks and shoes	reaching movements smooth
seats self in chair (18 months)	uses push-pull toys (18 months)
walks well with feet slightly apart (18 months)	throws a ball overhand (20 months)
walks upstairs unassisted (18 months)	builds tower of three to five blocks
crawls downstairs backwards (18 months)	removes wrappers from candy
walks downstairs with hand held (18 months)	scribbles, but marks go off page
starts and stops walking safely (18 months)	turns pages of book two or three at a time
jumps in place (23 months)	begins to show hand preference
pedals tricycle (23 months)	imitates vertically drawn line

Developmental Sequences of Motor Behavior—*Continued*

GROSS MOTOR	FINE MOTOR

2–2½ YEARS

GROSS MOTOR	FINE MOTOR
runs on whole foot	bilateral use of nondominant hand
starts and stops running with ease	strings beads
climbs on furniture	makes circular scribbles
walks up and down stairs alone, but does not alternate steps	takes things apart and puts them back together
alternates quickly from standing and sitting, etc.	enjoys rhythmical equipment (swings, rocking chair, etc.)
walks on tiptoes	begins to match like objects
	holds crayons with fingers
	turns book pages one at a time
	builds tower of seven blocks
	imitates folding paper
	cuts with scissors

2½–3 YEARS

GROSS MOTOR	FINE MOTOR
jumps from chair	good hand and finger coordination
jumps off floor with both feet	makes vertical strokes with crayon
runs well straight forward	uses blunt-end scissors easily
can stand on tiptoe if shown	enjoys finger-painting for manipulation with little feeling for form
tries to stand on one foot	makes pies and cakes with sand and mud
walks downstairs, alternating forward foot if holding rail	lines blocks to make train
walks upstairs alternating feet	draws two or more strikes for cross
hops on one foot, for two or more hops	folds paper
walks on tiptoes if shown (30 months)	copies circle
	closes fist and moves thumb
	picks longer line, if choice given (three of three trials)
	draws undifferentiated but names form (3 years)

3–4 YEARS

GROSS MOTOR	FINE MOTOR
walks on line	draws head of man and usually one other part
turns wide corners on tricycle	paints picture with large brush or easel
swings in swings	drives nails and pegs
climbs nursery apparatus with agility	builds tower of 10–16 blocks
kicks large ball with facility	uses spoon well
squats to play on floor	puts on shoes
walks on tiptoe	imitates demonstrated vertical and horizontal strokes
walks downstairs alternating feet	
walks heel-to-toe	

Developmental Sequences of Motor Behavior—*Continued*

GROSS MOTOR	FINE MOTOR
catches bounced ball	touches thumb to two of four fingers on
sits with feet crossed at ankles	same hand
learns to gallop	prints a few capital letters—large,
runs easily and smoothly	simple letters anywhere on a page
	copies cross
	copies square

4–5 YEARS

climbs ladder and trees	imitates spreading of hand and bringing
runs on tiptoes	thumb into opposition with each
skips on one foot	finger
jumps from height of about one foot	holds paper with other hand in writing
walks backward, heel-to-toe	folds paper three times
dresses, but cannot tie	prints simple words
	copies star
	draws very simple house
	draws man with two to three parts

5–6 YEARS

runs lightly on toes	grips strongly with either hand
runs with few falls while playing games	frequently reverses letters
at the same time	counts fingers on one hand with index
balances on tiptoes	finger of other
dances to music	draws recognizable man with head,
stands on one foot 8–10 seconds	trunk, legs, arms and features (adds
hops two to three yards forward	about seven parts)
is able to sit longer	draws simple house with door,
uses overhead ladder	windows, roof, and chimney
can roller-skate	writes a few letters spontaneously
skips using alternating feet	prints first name in large and irregular
	letters, getting larger at middle or
	end of the name
	prints numbers 1 through 5 unevenly
	cuts with scissors more easily
	ties simple bow after model is given
	laces shoes
	copies rectangle
	copies star (three of three trials)
	draws triangle
	traces around diamond on paper

Developmental Sequences of Social Behavior

1 MONTH

Moro reflex present (5–7 days)
follows moving light with eyes
pupils dilate and constrict
eyes turn toward direction of part of body touched
body reacts to loud sounds
limbs flex and extend
lifts chin from prone position

2 MONTHS

smiles when talked to (facial-social response)
regards faces and voices
more visually attentive
grips objects placed in palm

3 MONTHS

Moro reflex begins to disappear
perceives objects in three dimensions
loses interest in repetitious stimuli
plays with hands and clothing

4 MONTHS

responds by turning head to voice
gives spontaneous social smile

5 MONTHS

responds to angry tone by crying
responds to pleasant speech by smiling and laughing

6 MONTHS

distinguishes between friendly and angry talking
plays with feet and toys
vocalizes to own image in mirror and to toys
anticipates feeding

7 MONTHS

smiles at onlookers

9 MONTHS

plays pat-a-cake and other such games
feeds self crackers, cookies, etc.
differentiates between family and strangers

12 MONTHS

adjusts to simple commands
cooperates in dressing
finger feeds self

1–2 YEARS

indicates wants and responses by gestures and vocalizing (15 months)
uses push-pull toys

2–2½ YEARS

toilet—dry during the day
copies domestic activities in simultaneous play
puts on and takes off shoes, hats, mittens, etc.

2½–3 YEARS

likes stories about self
recognizes self in mirror
dramatizes mother and baby using dolls (plays make believe)

Developmental Sequences of Social Behavior—*Continued*

1–2 YEARS	2–2½ YEARS	2½–3 YEARS
indicates wet pants	initiates own play activities	avoids simple hazards
resistant to change in routine	engages in simple make-believe activities	looks for missing toys
repeats actions that are laughed at	constantly demands mother's attention	dresses with supervision and some help (33 months)
toilet is regulated but not trained (15 months)	has tantrums when frustrated, but attention is easily distracted	feeds self for most of meal
pretends to read (15 months)	has no concept of sharing	insists on being independent
seats self at table (18 months)	defends own possessions with determination	helps put things away
explores environment energetically (18 months)	is active, restless, and rebellious	throws tantrums when unable to express immediate needs, and is less easily distracted
imitates simple actions		little notion of sharing
develops special attachment to various toys		watches other children at play with interest and occasionally joins in for a few minutes
engages in parallel play (21 months)		has interest in acquiring possessions of others, but seldom plays with them
engages in soliloquies on experiences		has more disputes with others than at any other age
shifts attention easily		

3–4 YEARS	4–5 YEARS	5–6 YEARS
can take turns and play cooperatively	distinguishes front from back of clothes	asks meanings of words
washes and dries hands	goes about neighborhood unattended	plays table games and complicated floor games
eats with fork and spoon with little spilling	enjoys outside play	plans and builds constructively
able to button and unbutton accessible buttons (41 months)	enjoys puzzles and looking at books	likes to complete projects started
dresses and undresses self without supervision	expresses verbal impertinence when desires are crossed	can make purchases
brushes teeth	cooperates with other children and takes turns	is dependable and obedient in house
separates from mother easily	plays competitive exercise games	behaves in a more sensible, controlled, and independent manner

Developmental Sequences of Social Behavior—*Continued*

3–4 YEARS	4–5 YEARS	5–6 YEARS
likes to help with adult activities in house and garden	builds with blocks	protects younger playmates
realizes play vividly—includes invented people and objects	enjoys playing dress up in adult's clothes	plays with two to five others in a group
enjoys floor play with bricks, boxes, toy trains, and cars—either alone or with siblings	needs other children to play with, and is alternately cooperative and aggressive with them as with adults	chooses own friends
understands sharing playthings	shows concern for younger siblings and sympathy for playmates in distress	plays with imaginary playmates
shows affection with younger siblings	shows off dramatically	is socially comfortable
plays interactive games such as tag, housekeeping, etc. (replaces parallel play)	calls attention to own performance	puts toys away in orderly manner
will sacrifice immediate satisfaction on a promise of later privilege		brushes and combs hair successfully
usually obedient, with only brief occasional outbursts		crosses street safely
some nail biting		uses bathroom by self
bosses and criticizes		understands rules of fair play
		appreciates meaning of clock time in relation to daily program
		explores neighborhood
		does simple errands
		conforms to adult ideas
		asks adult help as needed

Normal Development of Feeding

BOTTLE

2 months	Brings hands to mouth in supine and prone positions
3 months	Brings hand to mouth while holding an object
3½ months	Visually recognizes nipple or bottle
4 months	Pats bottle with one or both hands
4½ months	Holds bottle with both hands
5½ months	Holds bottle independently with one or both hands
18–24 months	Gives up bottle

FINGERS

1–4 months	Sucks fingers when near mouth
3 months	Brings hand to mouth while holding an object
3½ months	Visually recognizes food and the bottle
5–6 months	Mouths and gums solid foods
6½–7 months	Feeds self crackers (munching)
9 months	Holds soft cookies in mouth (doesn't bite through)
12 months	Bites through soft cookie
24 months	Bites through a variety of food thicknesses

SPOON/FORK

4–7 months	Opens mouth when a spoon is presented
9 months	Reaches for spoon when presented/bangs spoon
9½ months	Stirs with a spoon in imitation
12–14 months	Brings filled spoon to mouth, turning the spoon over en route
15–18 months	Scoops food and brings the spoon to the mouth spilling some
24 months	Brings spoon/fork to mouth palm up, self-feeding, little spillage

CUP

6 months	Drinks from cup held by adult—some loss of liquid
12 months	Holds cup—some loss of liquid
12–24 months	Drinks from a straw
18–24 months	Drinks from a cup—little spillage
20–22 months	Holds small cup in one hand—little spillage
30 months	Pours from a small cup

Language Tests and Procedures

NAME	AGE RANGE	DESCRIPTION
Adolescent Language Screening Test [Morgan & Guilford]	11–17 yr	Language use, content, and form are screened in seven subtests: pragmatics, receptive vocabulary, concepts, expressive vocabulary, sentence formulation, morphology, and phonology
Aphasia Clinical Battery I[Eggert]	Aphasia patient with significant involvement	Single words through four-element utterances; focuses on disturbances of word retrieval, verbal apraxia, auditory processing, paraphrasia, alexia, agraphia, agrammatism, and paragrammatism
Aphasia Diagnostic Profiles (ADP) [Helm-Estabrooks]	Adults	Assesses language and communication impairment associated with aphasia. Nine subtests create composite scores, and profiles address critical areas of performance
Aphasia Language Performance Scales (ALPS) [Keenan & Brassell]	Adults	Measures language performance of aphasic patients regardless of type of aphasia or severity of language deficit; consists of four scales: listening, talking, reading, and writing
Aphasia Screening Test, The (AST) [Whurr]	Adults	Provides a comprehensive, sensitive, and reliable screening test for language deficits in adults with brain damage. It is aimed at the severely to moderately impaired client
Appraisal of Language Disturbances (ALD) [Emerick]	Adults	Designed to permit the clinician to make a systematic inventory of a patient's communicative abilities both in the modalities of input and output and the central integration processes
Assessing Semantic Skills Through Everyday Themes (ASSET) [Barrett, Zachman, & Huisingh]	3–9 yr	Assesses receptive and expressive vocabulary skills using familiar themes. Consists of five receptive and five expressive subtests
Assessment of Children's Language Comprehension (ACLC) [Foster, Giddan, & Stark]	3.6–5 yr	Assesses the child's ability to comprehend from one to four critical elements in correct order in single words, phrases, and sentences

Language Tests and Procedures—*Continued*

NAME	AGE RANGE	DESCRIPTION
Bankson Language Test—Second Edition (BLT-2)	3–7 yr	Provides a measure of children's psycholinguistic skills. Organized into three general categories: (1) semantic knowledge; (2) morphological rules; (3) pragmatics
Bedside Evaluation Screening Test—Second Edition (BEST-2) [West, Sands, & Ross-Swain]	Adults	Assesses language competence in three communicative modalities: auditory comprehension, speaking, and reading
Bilingual Syntax Measure (BSM) [Burt, Dulay, & Hernández]	4–9 yr	Designed to measure children's oral production in English and/or Spanish grammatical structures by using natural speech as a basis for making judgments; available in Spanish and English; may be used as an indicator of language dominance with respect to basic syntactic structures when both forms are administered
Boehm Test of Basic Concepts—Third Edition	Kindergarten through grade 2	Designed to measure children's mastery of basic concepts needed in school
Boehm Test of Basic Concepts-Preschool—Third Edition	3–5.11 yr	Downward extension of the Boehm—Third Edition; measures understanding of 26 relational concepts considered necessary for achievement in the beginning years of school
Boston Assessment of Severe Aphasia (BASA) [Estabrooks, Ramsberger, Morgan, & Nicholas]	Adults	Provides a measure of severe aphasia for early poststroke administration at bedside. Designed to probe low functioning performance immediately following a stroke
Boston Diagnostic Aphasia Examination [Goodglass & Kaplan]	Adults	Aphasia; type and severity measured through assessment of conversational and expository speech, auditory comprehension, oral expression, understanding written language, and writing
Brief Test of Head Injury [Helm-Estabrooks & Holz]		Assesses the cognitive, linguistic, and communicative abilities of individuals with severe head trauma. Standard scores and percentiles are reported

Language Tests and Procedures—*Continued*

NAME	AGE RANGE	DESCRIPTION
Carrow Elicited Language Inventory (CELI)	3–7.11 yr	Evaluates expressive syntax in a sentence repetition task
Children's Language Battery, The [Eggert]	Children	Assesses vocabulary development, auditory comprehension, phonological processing, syntactic-grammatical development, and reading-writing skills
Clinical Evaluation of Language Fundamentals-Preschool (CELF-PRESCHOOL) [Wiig, Secord, & Semel]	3–6 yr	A downward extension of CELF-R; consists of six subtests: (1) basic concepts, (2) formulating labels, (3) linguistic concepts, (4) sentence structure, (5) recalling sentences in context, (6) word structure
Clinical Evaluation of Language Fundamentals (CELF-3) [Semel, Wiig, & Secord]	6–21 yr	Measures language skills in areas of semantics, syntax, phonology, and memory. CELF-3 includes expanded age ranges, new norms, and standard scores.
Communicative Abilities in Daily Living (CADL) [Holland]	Adult aphasics	Measures nonverbal behaviors as well as specific language forms; communicative functions in everyday encounters
Comprehensive Assessment of Spoken Language (CASL) [E. Carrow-Woolfolk]	3–21 yr	Individually and orally administered. Fifteen tests measure language-processing skills—comprehension, expression, and retrieval in four language structure categories: lexical/semantic, syntactic, supralinguistic, and pragmatic
Comprehensive Receptive and Expressive Vocabulary Test (CREVT)	4–17 yr	Assesses receptive and expressive vocabulary strengths and weaknesses
Comprehensive Receptive-Expressive Vocabulary Test-Adult (CREVT-A) [Wallace & Hammill]	18.0–89.11 yr	This instrument consists of two subtests which take less than 30 minutes to administer. Normed on 700 individuals from 10 states
Compton Speech and Language Screening Evaluation	3–6 yr	Screening test with divisions to evaluate articulation and vocabulary, color naming, shape recognition, auditory-visual memory span, and language

Language Tests and Procedures—*Continued*

NAME	AGE RANGE	DESCRIPTION
Del Rio Language Screening Test, English/Spanish	3.6–11 yr	Identifies children with deviant language performance; has separate norms for three groups of children: Anglo-English speaking, Mexican-American English speaking, and Mexican-American Spanish speaking; administered in English or Spanish
Dos Amigos Verbal Language Scales [Critchlow]	5–12 yr	Measure of bilingual (English-Spanish) language development which requires the child to provide the opposite word to the one read by the administrator; helps to determine the dominant language
Early Language Milestone Scale—Second Edition (ELM-2) [Coplan]	0–36 mo	Evaluates the development of auditory expressive, auditory receptive, and visual skills, using parental report and observation
Environmental Language Inventory (ELI) [McDonald]	Preschool	Assesses expression of early semantic-grammatic relations in elicited and spontaneous samples of language
Environmental Prelanguage Battery [Horstmefer & McDonald]	Children	Diagnostic and training instrument designed for use with nonverbal or minimally verbal individuals functioning below or at single word level
Evaluating Acquired Skills in Communication (EASIC) [Riley]	Severely handicapped children	Assesses abilities in the areas of semantics, syntax, morphology, and pragmatics
Evaluating Communicative Competence [Simon]	9–17 yr	An appraisal of communication skills through a series of 20 informal evaluation tasks; these tasks serve as probes of auditory and expressive language skills
Examining for Aphasia-3 (EFA-3) [Eisenson]	Adolescents and adults	A revised version of the original test; 33 subtests help determine areas of strength and weakness for receptive and expressive functions
Expressive Language Test [Huisingh, Bowers, LoGiudice, & Orman]	5–11 yr	Assesses expressive language functioning including grammar, concepts, metalinguistics, and categorizing and describing

Language Tests and Procedures—*Continued*

NAME	AGE RANGE	DESCRIPTION
Expressive One-Word Picture Vocabulary Test—2000 [R. Brownell, ed.]	2.0–18.11 yr	Pictures of objects, actions, and concepts are presented to the examinee who is asked to name each picture. Standard scores, percentiles, and age equivalents are reported
Expressive Vocabulary Test (EVT) [Williams]	2.6–90+ yr	Measures expressive vocabulary and word retrieval for standard American English
Fluharty Speech and Language Screening Test-R [Fluharty]	Preschool	Assesses vocabulary, articulation, and language (expressive and receptive)
Fullerton Language Test for Adolescents [Thorum]	11–18 yr	Consists of eight subtests: auditory synthesis, morphology, competency, oral commands, convergent production, divergent production, syllabication, grammatic competency, and idioms
Functional Communication Profile [Kleiman]	Adults	A method of evaluating communicative effectiveness by assessing and rating performance on nine major communication skill categories. A section on nonoral communication evaluates the effectiveness of sign language and other communication systems
Help Test, The [Lazzari]	6–11 yr	Assesses general language functioning including vocabulary, semantics, and grammar
Illinois Test of Psycholinguistic Abilities— Third Edition (ITPA-3) [Hammill, Mather, & Roberts]	5.0–12.11 yr	Six subtests measure spoken language (spoken analogies, spoken vocabulary, morphologic closure, sound deletion, syntactic sentences, and rhyming sequences.) Six subtests measure written language
International Test for Aphasia [Benton, Spreen, DeRenzi, & Vignolo]	Adults	Test battery for aphasia that may be adaptable to languages throughout the world
Interpersonal Language Skills and Assessment (ILSA) [Blagden & McConnell]	8–14 yr	Standardized test of pragmatics

Language Tests and Procedures—*Continued*

NAME	AGE RANGE	DESCRIPTION
James Language Dominance Test	Kindergarten and grade 1	Assesses language dominance in Mexican-American children
Joliet Speech and Language Screen—Revised Edition [Kinzler & Johnson]	Kindergarten, grades 2 and 5	Identifies children at high risk of having speech and language disorders; focuses on the areas of receptive vocabulary and expressive syntax
Kindergarten Language Screening Test—Second Edition (KLST) [Gauthier & Madison]	Kindergarten	Samples expressive and receptive language competence with identification of name, age, colors, body parts, number concepts, commands, sentence repetition, and a spontaneous speech sample
Language Modalities Test for Aphasia [Wepman]	Adults	Aphasia; receptive and expressive communication abilities are evaluated
Language Processing Test-Revised (LPT-R) [Richard & Hanner]	5–11 yr	Identifies processing breakdowns that contribute to poor memory and word finding problems through the following subtests: association, categorization, similarities, differences, multiple meanings, attributes
Language Proficiency Test (LPT) [Gerard & Weinstock]	Grade 9 through adult	Consists of three major sections that measure aural/oral, reading, and writing skills; the entire test covers nine areas of language functioning
Mean Length of Utterance (MLU)	Children	Number of morphemes per utterance are determined by an analysis of the child's spontaneous speech; the number of morphemes in each utterance are counted and divided by the total number of utterances
Merrill Language Screening Test [Mumm, Second, & Dykstra]	Young school-age children	Screening instrument to detect potential language problems
Minnesota Test for Differential Diagnosis of Aphasia [Schuell]	Adults	Aphasia; assessment of receptive and expressive communication abilities

Language Tests and Procedures—*Continued*

NAME	AGE RANGE	DESCRIPTION
Muma Assessment Program (MAP) [Muma & Muma]	Preschool and early school-age children	Descriptive assessment procedures are used to measure the cognitive, linguistic, and communicative systems of young children
Non-Speech Test, The [Huer]	0–48 mo	A standardized test of receptive and expressive language abilities for children who are nonverbal
Oral and Written Language Scales (OWLS) [Carrow-Woolfolk]	3–21 yr	The language test consists of two components: *Listening Comprehensive (LCS)* and *Oral Expression (OES)*. LCS assesses receptive language in response to verbal stimuli, by pointing or speaking. OES measures expressive language. The child answers questions or completes or generates sentences to spoken stimuli. No reading is required.
Orzeck Aphasia Evaluation [Orzeck]	Aphasic patients	Screening instrument for evaluating and exploring signs of aphasia in organic brain damaged patients; measures apraxia, agnosia, and sensory suppression
Patterned Elicitation Syntax Screening Test (PESST) [Young & Parachio]	3–7.6 yr	Assesses 44 syntactic structures, utilizing a delayed imitation format
Peabody Picture Vocabulary Test (PPVT-R) [Dunn]	2.6–40 yr	Measures vocabulary comprehension by a picture pointing task
Performance Assessment of Syntax Elicited and Spontaneous (PASES) [Coughran]	3–11 yr	Criterion-referenced assessment instrument that allows the clinician to measure spontaneous and elicited syntactic skills
Porch Index of Communicative Abilities (PICA)	Adults	Aphasia; evaluates communicative ability
Porch Index of Communicative Abilities in Children (PICAC)	Preschool and school age	Assesses verbal, gestural, and graphic abilities

Language Tests and Procedures—*Continued*

NAME	AGE RANGE	DESCRIPTION
Preschool Language Assessment Instrument (PLAI) [Blank, Rose, & Berlin]	3–6 yr	Arranged in a developmental sequence; measures four levels of thinking and reasoning
Preschool Language Scale—Fourth Edition (PLS-4) [Zimmerman, Steiner, & Pond]	Birth–6.11 yr	Measures total language; auditory comprehension; expressive communication. Standard scores, percentile ranks, and age equivalents are provided
Preschool Language Screening Test [Hannah-Gardner]	3–5.11 yr	Screening of selected language and nonlanguage tasks
Preschool Speech and Language Screening Test [Fluharty]	3–5 yr	Phonology, syntax, and semantics; based on the transformation-generative model and on developmental studies of speech and language
Receptive-Expressive Emergent Language Test—Second Edition (REEL-2) [Bzoch & League]	Birth–3 yr	Interview scale designed to determine general level of functioning for receptive and expressive language skills
Receptive-Expressive Observation Scale (REO) [Smith]	5–12 yr	Evaluates the major learning channels of visual and auditory input and verbal and written expression
Receptive One-Word Picture Vocabulary Test (2000) [R. Brownell, ed.]	2.0–18.11 yr	The test is administered by presenting a series of test plates that include four pictures. The examiner presents a stimulus word and the examinee is asked to point to the correct picture. Raw scores can be converted to standard scores, percentile ranks, and age equivalents
Revised Token Test [McNeil & Prescott]	Adults	Quantitative as well as descriptive test for auditory disorders associated with aphasia and brain damage
Reynell Developmental Language Scales	12 mo–7 yr	Assesses verbal comprehension and expressive language. Consists of three scales: (1) verbal comprehension A, (2) verbal comprehension B, and (3) expressive language

Language Tests and Procedures—*Continued*

NAME	AGE RANGE	DESCRIPTION
Rosetti Infant-Toddler Language Scale [Rosetti]	Birth–3 yr	Assesses six domains: interaction-attachment, pragmatics, play, gesture, language comprehension, and language expression
Ross Information Processing Assessment-Geriatric (RIPA-G) [D. Ross-Swain]	65–98 yr	Measures cognitive-linguistic deficits in geriatric residents. Ten communication and cognitive areas are profiled
Ross Information Processing Assessment-Primary (RIPA-P) [D. Ross-Swain]	5–12 yr	Tool used to identify and quantify information processing impairments in 5- to 12-year-olds. Used with children who have experienced traumatic brain injury, other neuropathologies such as seizure disorders, anoxia, or learning disorders
Ross Information Processing Assessment—Second Edition (RIPA-2) [D. Ross-Swain]	Adolescents and adults	Quantifies cognitive-linguistic deficits of brain-injured patients. It determines severity levels for each skill area
Scales of Cognitive Ability for Traumatic Brain Injury (SCATBI) [Adamovich & Henderson]	Adolescents and adults	Assesses cognitive and linguistic abilities of patients with head injuries. Consists of five subtests: perception, discrimination, orientation, organization, and recall and reasoning
Screening Kit of Language Development (SKOLD) [Bliss & Allen]	2–5 yr	Assesses preschool language development in six areas: vocabulary, comprehension, story completion, individual and paired sentence repetition with pictures, individual sentence repetition without pictures, and comprehension of commands
Screening Test for Auditory Comprehension of Language [Carrow]	3–6 yr	Screening for receptive language disorders (vocabulary, syntax, morphology)

Language Tests and Procedures—*Continued*

NAME	AGE RANGE	DESCRIPTION
Screening Test of Adolescent Language [Prather, Breecher, Stafford, & Wallace]	Junior and senior high-school age	Assesses vocabulary, auditory memory span, language processing, and proverb explanation
Sequenced Inventory of Communication Development—Revised Edition (SICD-R) [Hedrick, Prather, & Tobin]	4 mo–4 yr	Diagnostic test designed to evaluate the communication abilities of normal and retarded children; has two major sections: receptive and expressive
Sklar Aphasia Scale	Adults	Short screening device with eight to ten items to test each of the four modalities; covers a range from the phoneme level to paragraphs
Smith-Johnson Nonverbal Performance Scale [Smith & Johnson]	2–4 yr	Measures developmental level of handicapped children across a broad range of skills, indicating their strengths and weaknesses; useful with hearing impaired, delayed language, and culturally deprived children
Stephens Oral Language Screening Test	4–7 yr	Screening device for potential problems in syntax or articulation
Structured Photographic Expressive Language Test-P (SPELT-P) [Werner-Kresheck]	3–5.11 yr	Twenty-five items using 37 photographs are used to assess the young child's ability to generate early developing morphological and syntactic forms
Structured Photographic Expressive Language Test II (SPELT II) [Dawson-Stephens]	4–9.5	Fifty color photographs are used to examine expressive use of morphology and syntax
Temple University Short Syntax Inventory (TUSSI) [Gerber & Goehl]	3–5 yr	Designed to descriptively assess acquisition of early patterns of syntax and morphology; generates a descriptive analysis of basic sentence elements and morphemes for both initiated and elicited responses

Language Tests and Procedures—*Continued*

NAME	AGE RANGE	DESCRIPTION
Test for Auditory Comprehension of Language—Third Edition (TACL-3) [Carrow-Woolfolk]	3–9.11 yr	Individually administered measure of receptive spoken vocabulary, grammar, and syntax
Test for Examining Expressive Morphology (TEEM) [Shipley, Stone, & Sue]	3–8 yr	Fifty-four test items examine the allomorphic variations of six major morphemes: present progressives, plurals, possessives, past tenses, third-person singulars, and derived adjectives
Test of Adolescent and Adult Language (TOAL-3) [Hammill, Brown, Larsen, & Wiederholt]	12–24 yr	A revision assesses listening, speaking, reading, writing, spoken language, written language, vocabulary, grammar, receptive and expressive language, and overall language ability
Test of Adolescent/Adult Word Finding (TAWF) [D. German]	12–80 yr	Standardized test for identifying word finding in adolescents and adults. Includes a brief test that provides a quick assessment of word finding abilities
Test of Children's Language [Barenbaum & Newcomer]	5–8.11 yr	Assesses all aspects of a child's language using a storybook format
Test of Early Language Development-3 (TELD-3) [Hiresko, Reid, & Hammill]	2–7.11 yr	Yields an overall spoken language score; also includes scores for receptive language and expressive language subtest
Test of Language Competence (TLC) [Wiig & Secord]	9–19 yr	Measures specific language abilities through four subtests: understanding ambiguous sentences, re-creating sentences, making inferences, understanding metaphoric sentences
Test of Language Competence Expanded (TLC-E) [Wiig & Secord]	4–9 yr	Features the same subtests as the TLC, but the content differs to accommodate the different age range

Language Tests and Procedures—*Continued*

NAME	AGE RANGE	DESCRIPTION
Test of Language Development-Intermediate-3 (TOLD-I:3) [Newcomer & Hammill]	8–12.11 yr	Five subtests measure different components of spoken language
Test of Language Development-Primary-3 (TOLD-P:3) [Newcomer & Hammill]	4–8.11 yr	Nine subtests measure different components of spoken language
Test of Pragmatic Language (TOPL) [Teraski-Gunn]	5–13.11 yr	A comprehensive assessment of a student's ability to use pragmatic language effectively
Test of Pragmatic Skills [Shulman]	3–8 yr	Assesses functional communication abilities in children; the child is expected to complete tasks designed to elicit conversational intentions during play-oriented communication interactions
Test of Word Finding—Second Edition (TWF-2) [German]	4.0–12.11 yr	Used to diagnose word-finding disorders using pictures naming (nouns), pictures naming (verbs), sentence completion naming, and picture naming
Test of Word Finding in Discourse [German]	6.6–12.11 yr	Analyzes word finding in story telling/narrative tasks
Test of Word Knowledge [Wiig & Secord]	5–17 yr	Evaluates understanding and use of vocabulary words. All stimuli presented through auditory and visual channels
Token Test for Children, The [Di'Simoni]	4–12 yr	Screening test to aid in detecting receptive language disorders
Token Test for Receptive Disturbances in Aphasia [DeRenzi & Vignolo]	Adults	Designed to be especially sensitive to the detection of receptive disturbances so slight that they may be overlooked during the course of a clinical evaluation
Toronto Tests of Receptive Vocabulary, English/Spanish	4–10 yr	Identifies English- and Spanish-speaking children whose performance in identifying orally presented vocabulary is significantly below that of their peers

Language Tests and Procedures—*Continued*

NAME	AGE RANGE	DESCRIPTION
Utah Test of Language Development 3 [Mecham]	3–10.11 yr	Designed to measure receptive and expressive language skills in normal and handicapped children. Percentiles and standard scores are provided
Western Aphasia Battery (WAB) [Kertesz]	Aphasic patients	Designed to test aphasic disability and to provide the data needed to establish the prognosis and aims of therapy
Word Test, The [Jorgensen, Barrett, Huisingh, & Zachman]	7–12 yr	Test of vocabulary and semantics; measures vocabulary through six subtests: association, synonyms, semantic absurdities, antonyms, definitions, and multiple definitions
Word Test-Adolescent, The [Zachman, Huisingh, Barrett, Orman, & Blagden]	12–17 yr	Assesses four semantic and vocabulary tasks: brand names, synonyms, signs of times, and definitions
Word Test-R Elementary, The	7–11 yr	Assesses word knowledge and flexibility in these areas: association, synonyms, semantic absurdities, antonyms, definitions, and multiple definitions

Articulation Tests and Phonological Analysis Procedures

Alpha Test of Phonology, The [Lowe]
:   An articulation and phonological processing test. Aids in sound errors and identifying phonological processes.

Apraxia Battery for Adults—Second Edition (ABA-2) [Dabul]
:   Measures the presence and severity of apraxia in adolescents and adults through several subtests.

Arizona Articulation Proficiency Scale: Revised [Fudala]
:   Assesses total articulation proficiency for individuals from age 3 to 12; requires responses to stimulus cards or to sentences.

Assessment Link Between Phonology and Articulation (ALPHA) [Lowe]
:   Assesses sound production and phonological processes in children from preschool through fourth grade.

Assessment of Intelligibility of Dysarthric Speech [Yorkston & Beukelman]
:   Tool for quantifying single word and sentence intelligibility along with the speaking rate of dysarthric adolescents and adults.

Assessment of Phonological Processes-R (APP-R) [Hodson]
:   The revised edition includes (1) simplification in administration, (2) more information on remediation, (3) a multisyllabic screening protocol. Can be administered in 15–20 minutes and scored in 30 minutes.

Austin Spanish Articulation Test
:   Identifies articulation problems in Spanish-speaking children between the ages of 3 and 12 years.

Bankson-Bernthal Test of Phonology (BBTOP)
:   The BBTOP was designed to describe consonant productions and error patterns in preschool and early elementary age children. There are 80 stimulus words elicited using a picture-naming format. The child's productions are transcribed onto the test protocol using whole-word transcription. The productions are later scored for errors in word—initial and final position—and for phonological processes.

Children's Articulation Test [Haspiel]
:   Measures articulation and phonology in 3- to 11-year-olds using words or connected speech.

Clinical Probes of Articulation Consistency (C-PAC) [Secord]
:   Provides an in-depth picture of articulatory performance on specific speech sounds in a wide range of contexts; administered individually as an imitative and storytelling task; may be used (a) to decide where to begin therapy and for mapping the direction of therapy, (b) for formulating measurement strategies, (c) for multiphonemic measurement, (d) for measuring the effectiveness of therapy aid, and (e) for posttesting.

Comprehensive Test of Phonological Processing (CTOPP) [Wagner, Torgesen, & Roshotte]
:   Used to assess the phonological awareness, phonological memory, and rapid naming skills of persons between 5.0 and 24.11 years of age.

Articulation Tests and Phonological Analysis Procedures—*Continued*

Compton-Hutton Phonological Assessment
Provides a structured step-by-step approach to the linguistic analysis of misarticulations in preschool to adult individuals.

Deep Test of Articulation [McDonald]
Measures ability to spontaneously articulate specific speech sounds in many different contexts, and attempts to find phonetic environments in which a sound may possibly be produced correctly; both a picture and sentence form are provided; usually administered after a preliminary articulation test has been administered.

Denver Articulation Screening Examination (DASE) [Drumwright]
Test designed to detect articulation disorders in children from 2 years 5 months to 6 years of age; technique of administration is primarily the imitative method: the child is instructed to say what the examiner says; for the difficult-to-test child, simple line drawings are provided to assist the examiner in eliciting responses.

Elicited Articulatory System Evaluation (EASE) [Steed & Haynes]
An imitative sentence articulation assessment tool. It is designed to (1) provide a traditional and phonological analysis, (2) assess consonant and vowels in multiple contexts in connected speech, (3) be used as an initial tool or assess therapy progress, and (4) provide a tool that may be administered in a short period of time.

Fisher-Logemann Test of Articulation Competence, The
Assesses an individual's phonological system in an orderly framework of both a word and sentence form; articulation errors may be analyzed and summarized according to certain distinctive features; provides a table on dialects to guide the clinician in separating genuine misarticulations from dialectal variations.

Goldman-Fristoe Test of Articulation-2
The test provides information about a child's articulation ability by sampling both spontaneous and imitative sound production. The age range has been expanded to include ages 2 through 21. Age-based standard scores include separate normative information for females and males.

Haws Screening Test for Functional Articulation Disorders
Designed to provide the examiner with a means of identifying children who have misarticulations which may persist without receiving speech remediation; consists of 66 pictures which are used to spontaneously elicit the production of various target phonemes in their initial, medial, and final positions; stimulability may be determined by having the individual imitate the examiner's production of the word in which the target phoneme was missed.

Kahn-Lewis Phonological Analysis—Second Edition
Uses the 44 words from the Goldman-Fristoe Test of Articulation—Sounds in Words Subtest as input for phonological processes analysis. The words are scored on a multipaged protocol which lists common sound changes associated with phonological processes.

Ohio Tests of Articulation and Perception of Sounds, The (OTAPS) [Irwin]
Constructed to evaluate 67 speech sound elements in varying linguistic units under both interpersonal and intrapersonal conditions; through the use of four subtests for articulation, phonetic accuracy of speech sounds may be determined as to type of error, stimulability, and consistency of production; evaluates spontaneous production, imitative production, consistency of sound production, and prognostic indications for the learning of sounds; a screening portion also is included. See also in *Auditory Tests* and *Procedures* appendix.

Articulation Tests and Phonological Analysis Procedures—*Continued*

Phonological Awareness Test [Robertson & Salter]
  Assesses phonological skills and phoneme-grapheme correspondence for children ages 5.0–9.11 years.

Phonological Process Analysis [Weiner]
  Determines phonological patterns in children by analyzing processes such as syllable structure, harmony, and feature contrast.

Photo Articulation Test—Third Edition [Lippke, Dickey, Selmar, & Soder]
  Seventy-two color photographs are used to test consonants, vowels, diphthongs, and conversational speech in children ranging in ages from 3.0 to 8.11 years.

Picture Articulation and Language Screening Test [Rodgers]
  Assesses articulation and language skills; pictures are used to spontaneously elicit 27 phonemes (in only the initial and final positions) and various language-formation abilities; can be administered in three sections to screen, to diagnose, and to aid in the selection of a case load.

Procedures for the Phonological Analysis of Children's Language [Ingram]
  A set of procedures that can be used to complete a comprehensive phonological analysis of stimuli obtained from a spontaneous language sample or phonological diary, or through elicitation and testing. It can analyze for a wide range of phonological processes.

Riley Articulation and Language Test-R
  Screening test consisting of three subtests—language proficiency and intelligibility, articulation function, and language function. Standardized on kindergarten, first- and second-grade children.

Screening Deep Test of Articulation [McDonald]
  Assesses ability to spontaneously produce nine commonly misarticulated consonants from paired pictures and provides a quick means of checking commonly misarticulated phonemes in a limited number of phonetic contexts to determine in what percentage of contexts the phoneme is correctly produced; a phonetic profile is given for kindergarten children which also guides the examiner as to whether a deep test of articulation should be administered.

Screening Test for Developmental Apraxia of Speech–Second Edition [Blakeley]
  Identifies children 4–12 years who have both atypical speech and language problems and associated oral performance problems.

Secord Contextual Articulation Test (S-CAT) [Secord & Shine]
  Examines production of all English phonemes in a variety of phonemic-phonological contexts.

Slosson Articulation, Language Test with Phonology (SALT-P) [Tade & Slosson]
  Incorporates the assessment of articulation, phonology, and language into a single score which indicates the communicative competence of children ages 3–5.11 years.

Smit-Hand Articulation and Phonology Evaluation (SHAPE) [Smit & Hand]
  Tests articulation and phonology of children 3–9 years old. Evaluates production of initial and final consonants and clusters using 80 stimulus cards.

Articulation Tests and Phonological Analysis Procedures—*Continued*

Structured Photographic Articulation and Phonological Test (SPAT-D) [Kresheck & Tattersall]
A systematic assessment of children's articulation skills. Forty-eight photographs are used to assess 59 consonant singletons and 21 consonant blends. Sounds in context are easily elicited.

Templin-Darley Tests of Articulation
Provides for both screening and diagnostic assessments of spontaneous articulation in words and sentences; a complete set of speech norms is available for children ages 3–8 years; overlays are provided for a separate assessment of single consonants or consonant clusters, vowels, and diphthongs, and includes the Iowa Pressure Test to aid in assessing the adequacy of velopharyngeal closure.

Test of Articulation in Context [Lanphere]
Assesses articulation in naturalistic contexts. Uses four illustrated test scenes interesting to children: park, birthday party, classroom, and zoo.

Test of Articulation Performance-Diagnostic (TAP-D) [Bryant & Bryant]
An analysis of the strengths and weaknesses of children who require special instruction in articulation; strengths and weaknesses are analyzed by six different procedures: isolated words, distinctive features, selective deep test, continuous speech, stimulability, verbal communication scales.

Test of Articulation Performance-Screen (TAP-S) [Bryant & Bryant]
Thirty-one items indicate those children who are in need of further diagnostic assessment.

Test of Minimal Articulation Competence (T-MAC) [Secord]
A quick test for measuring articulatory performance, using a picture identification task format to assess articulation of 24 consonant phonemes according to syllabic function in familiar words, frequently occurring /s/, /r/, and /l/ blends, and 12 vowels, four diphthongs, and variations of vocalic /r/.

Test of Phonological Awareness (TOPA) [Torgesen & Bryant]
The TOPA measures the awareness of the individual sounds in words in children grades K–2.

Tri-County Contextual Articulation Test
Designed to assess the production of 10 of the most defective speech sounds; the sounds are elicited from numerous story pictures which feature the target phoneme in its initial, medial, and final position; the individual is asked to make up a story for the sound in each picture; scoring is based on a percentage of correct productions rather than on a single production of the desired sound.

Verbal Motor Production Assessment for Children (VMPAC) [Hayden & Square]
Identifies children with motor issues with items arranged from basic to complex. Assesses global motor control, focal oromotor control, and sequencing along with connected speech and language control and speech characteristics. Provides percentiles; useful for children ages 3–12 years.

Weiss Comprehensive Articulation Test
Designed to determine whether an articulation disorder or delay is present, to identify misarticulation patterns that exist, and to identify other problems or features that may be present; the measurements of speech intelligibility and stimulability provide data for establishing an individual's present level of articulation.

Articulation Tests and Phonological Analysis Procedures—*Continued*

Weiss Intelligibility Test
  Tape recorded samples of isolated words and contextual speech are used to obtain
  an intelligibility score expressed as a percentage, giving an indication of the severity
  of the communication problem.

Audiometric Tests and Procedures

Alternate Binaural Loudness Balance (ABLB)

> Direct measure of recruitment in unilateral hearing loss; assessed by having the individual compare the increasing loudness of a pure tone in his normal ear with a pure tone in his impaired ear.

Alternate Monaural Loudness Balance Test (AMLB) See Monaural Loudness Balance Test (below).

Békésy Ascending-Descending Gap Evaluation (BADGE)

> Test for nonorganic hearing loss using the Békésy audiometer; the subject who exaggerates his pure-tone thresholds is confused by the fact that tracings are begun above and below threshold, pulsed, and continuous.

Békésy Audiometry

> Utilizes the Békésy audiometer to determine threshold and to distinguish between a retrocochlear and cochlear sensorineural hearing loss; results may be classified into one of five types based on the comparison of response to continuous and pulsed tones.

Békésy Comfortable Loudness Procedure

> Comparison of levels judged by the listener to be comfortably loud using three sweep-frequency Békésy tracings: forward-interrupted, forward-continuous, and backward-continuous; a positive finding (sharp increase in the level for either of the continuous tracings compared to the interrupted tracing) suggests an eighth nerve site of lesion.

Békésy Forward-Reverse Tracings

> Comparison of two continuous Békésy sweep-frequency threshold tracings; one going from low to high frequencies and the other going from high to low frequencies; positive findings (10-dB or greater separation between tracings) are found with an eighth nerve site of lesion or functional hearing loss.

Bing Test

> Tuning fork test used to try to distinguish between conductive and sensorineural loss; bone conduction thresholds for low frequency signals are obtained with the test ear open and then occluded; no difference in threshold results suggests a conductive impairment, but if the threshold improves under occluded conditions, the hearing loss is sensorineural.

Caloric Test

> Irrigation of the external auditory canal with warm or cold water to stimulate the vestibular labyrinth; in normal patients the result is nystagmus, with some sensation of vertigo.

Cold-Running Speech Test

> Less frequently used test for establishing speech-reception thresholds (SRT); the individual responds every few seconds for as long as he can understand the connected discourse; the point at which he understands the speech 50% of the time is his SRT.

Audiometric Tests and Procedures—*Continued*

Competing Sentence Test (CST)

Dichotic auditory test designed to evaluate central auditory function; composed of 25 pairs of simple natural sentences six to eight words long, constructed around common themes; a percentage score is derived.

Dichotic Consonant-Vowel Test

Test to help identify central auditory nervous system pathologies; materials are composed of voiced and voiceless stop consonants, and are paired with /a/.

Dichotic Digits

Test designed to help detect central auditory pathologies; involves simultaneous presentation to separate ear of two paired numbers (1–10, excluding 7) in groups of two or three.

Doerfler-Stewart Test

Test for functional hearing loss which compares the ability to understand spondaic words in quiet and in noise (sawtoothed masking).

Electronystagmography (ENG)

Technique pertinent to the recording of electronic observation of eye movement, but with natural application in vestibular examinations due to the significance of nystagmus (involuntary eye movement) as a vestibular reaction; reveals the horizontal and possibly the vertical components of nystagmus; used with caloric stimulation.

Galvanic Skin Response (GSR)

Special test of functional hearing loss which uses the skin response in hearing testing to condition the individual to respond to sound as an emotion-producing stimulus; often referred to as Electrodermal Response Test (EDR), Electrodermal Audiometry (EDA), or Psychogalvanic Skin Response (PGSR).

Glycerol Test

Diagnostic and prognostic tool used for identification of Méniérè's disease: 1.2 mL/kg of chilled glycerol is given orally with an equal volume of saline; 1–3 hr after ingestion there is often significant improvement in hearing threshold, speech discrimination, tinnitus, and the sensation of fullness. The effect is transient and thought to reflect acute dehydration of the inner ear as a result of the osmotic effect.

High Level SISI

Modification of the SISI procedure administered with increments from low to high to help determine cochlear and retrochlear lesions.

Immittance Tests

A test battery: (1) tympanometry techniques, show abnormalities in the mobility of the tympanic membrane due to stiffness, flaccidity, or the presence of fluid in the middle ear cavity; (2) static acoustic impedance, identifies perforations of the tympanic membrane or the patency of the ventilating tubes in the eardrum; (3) acoustic reflex pattern, the presence or absence of normal reflex thresholds produces a four-reflex pattern (ipsilateral and contralateral for each ear) that aids in identifying a site of lesion; and (4) acoustic reflex decay, abnormal decay of the reflex for a 10 second tone at 10 dB suggests an eighth cranial nerve site of lesion.

_____

Audiometric Tests and Procedures—*Continued*
_____

Lengthened-Off-Time (LOT)

Test for functional hearing loss; a modification of Békésy audiometry that requires the individual to track his thresholds for a continuous and interrupted signal (the interrupted signal has a lengthened off-time).

Lombard Test

Test for functional hearing loss in which masking sounds are introduced into the ears while the subject talks; the test is positive if the individual raises the intensity level of his voice in order to hear himself above the masking sound, and negative if his voice remains at a fixed level.

Metz Test for Loudness Recruitment

An acoustic impedance measurement; may indicate recruitment in an individual with a hearing impairment if a stapedius reflex is elicited by a stimulus smaller than 60–70 dB above threshold.

Minimum Auditory Capabilities Test (MAC)

Battery of tests designed to determine an individual's auditory and visual strengths and weaknesses [Owens et al].

Monaural Loudness Balance Test (MLB) or Alternate Monaural Loudness Balance Test (AMLB)

Test for recruitment in which loudness balances are made in the same ear but at different frequencies; the procedure involves the individual's ability to compare the increasing intensity of a tone of the impaired frequency with that of the frequency at which hearing sensitivity is normal.

Most Comfortable Loudness (MCL)

Simple but not very reliable method of determining the presence of recruitment, along with the Uncomfortable Loudness Level test (UCL), with pure tones; based on the range of intensity of sound which the individual finds most pleasing.

NU Auditory Test Lists 4 and 6 [Northwestern University, Evanston, IL]

Six lists of 50 words used to determine auditory word discrimination. The lists are composed solely of consonant, vowel nucleus, consonant words that are familiar. The lists are appropriate for all age groups.

PBK Word Lists

Four 50-item word lists are presented to the individual; test items are within the speaking vocabulary of young children; appropriate for children 4 to 5 years of age.

Pure Tone Air-Conduction Threshold

Used to assist in diagnosing pathologic conditions of the ear; the individual is stimulated with pure-tone stimuli emitted from an audiometer via ear phones.

Pure-Tone Bone-Conduction Threshold

Technique used when air-conduction testing indicates a hearing loss; helps determine whether the loss detected is due to conductive or sensorineural factors, or both.

Audiometric Tests and Procedures—*Continued*

Rapidly Alternating Speech Perception Test (RASP)

Test developed to assess central auditory function; a speech signal is presented to both ears in a quickly alternating fashion; useful in locating lower brain lesions.

Real-Ear Measurement

This technique uses a probe microphone that is inserted into the ear canal with the hearing aid in place. With this technique the audiologist is able to measure the response of the hearing aid in the ear canal.

Rinne Test

Tuning fork test that compares an individual's hearing by air conduction with his hearing by bone conduction. The vibrating fork is held close to his external ear; when he reports he can no longer hear the tone, the tuning fork is placed against the mastoid process; if he can again hear the tone, the test is said to be Rinne negative and indicates a conductive loss; if the individual hears the fork longer by bone conduction, the test is said to be Rinne positive and indicates either a bone conduction-loss or normal hearing.

Rotation Test

Test for labyrinthine function in which the individual is placed in a revolving chair and rotated a specific number of times (usually 10) within a period of 20 seconds; the chair is rotated to the right and ensuing nystagmus noted, then to the left, and the nystagmus noted again; if the labyrinths are functioning normally, nystagmus will be in the direction opposite to that of rotation; if nystagmus is not present, some labyrinthine malfunction is indicated.

Schwabach Test

Quantitative test of bone-conduction hearing in which the degree of loss is indicated by comparing the subject's ability to hear with that of an examiner with normal hearing; a vibrating tuning fork is placed on the subject's mastoid process, and when he no longer hears any sound, the fork is transferred to the mastoid process of the examiner, who then counts the number of seconds he can hear it; the score is reported as minus seconds for the subject.

Short Increment Sensitivity Index (SISI)

Differential sensitivity test which consists of the introduction of small increments of loudness during the testing period; the individual with a sensorineural hearing loss will be able to detect most of the slight changes in loudness, whereas the person with normal hearing or conductive loss may not hear any changes (or may hear only a few of them).

Speech Detection Threshold (SDT)

Measure of the minimum hearing level at which an individual can just detect the presence of a speech signal (ongoing speech or isolated words) and can identify it as speech; the individual must respond to 50% of the stimuli presented.

Speech Discrimination in Noise

Selected list of monosyllabic, phonetically balanced words is presented to the test subject's ear while a competing speech noise is simultaneously presented to the same ear; the signal-to-noise ratio may be varied. The test also may be administered in a sound field environment.

Audiometric Tests and Procedures—*Continued*

Speech Reception Threshold (SRT)

Measure of an individual's threshold hearing level for speech; the faintest intensity at which an individual repeats correctly 50% or more of the spondaic test words (words of two syllables having equal stress).

Speech with Alternating Masking Index (SWAMI)

Speech discrimination test involving a dichotic listening task; speech is switched alternately between ears as noise is presented at 20 dB greater intensity in the opposite ear; individuals with normal hearing are able to understand the speech.

Staggered Spondaic Word Test (SSW)

Test for central auditory disorders utilizing the dichotic listening task of two spondaic words presented so that the second syllable presented to one ear is heard simultaneously with the first syllable presented to the other ear.

Stenger Test

Test for unilateral functional hearing impairments; when both ears are stimulated by the same frequency, but at different intensities, only the louder intensity will be perceived; if the loss in the "poorer" ear is genuine, the individual will be unaware of any signal in his "poorer" ear.

Suprathreshold Adaptation Test (STAT)

Variation of tone-decay testing, with test frequencies of 500, 1000, and 2000 Hz. The individual is instructed to signal as long as he hears the sound in the test ear; the non-test ear is masked with white noise at 90 dB SL; the test tone is presented at 110 dB SL until 60 seconds have passed or until the patient signals that he no longer hears the tone.

Swinging Story Test

Test for unilateral nonorganic hearing loss, in which portions of a story are presented to the "better" ear, "poorer" ear, and both ears; if the individual repeats information presented below the admitted threshold of the "poorer" ear, it is reasonable to conclude the hearing loss in that ear is exaggerated.

Synthetic Sentence Identification Test

Method for determination of word discrimination by means of seven-word sentences that are grammatically correct but meaningless; sentences, 10 in number, are presented to the individual who responds by pushing a button corresponding to the sentence heard; a competing message of continuous speech is presented in the test ear (ipsilateral) or in the opposite ear (contralateral) at the same intensity as the synthetic sentences.

Time-Compressed Speech Test

Presentation of words or sentences that have been speeded up without altering their pitch; abnormally decreased recognition of the altered speech may indicate a central site of lesion.

Tone-Decay Test

Measures ability to hear sustained tones for a period of time; the individual is presented with a continuous pure tone and responds when he no longer hears it; abnormal tone decay is a symptom often associated with retrocochlear lesion.

Audiometric Tests and Procedures—*Continued*

Tone in Noise (TIN)

Type of masking test utilizing measurement of the ability to recognize a tone in the presence of noise.

Tuning Fork Test

Means of describing a hearing loss by noting the individual's responses to vibrating tuning forks at various frequencies; the most common tuning fork tests are the Rinne, Weber, Bing, and Schwabach tests.

Uncomfortable Loudness Level (UCL)

Simple and rather subjective means of determining the presence of recruitment, based on the intensity level at which a tone or sound becomes uncomfortably loud; often used with Most Comfortable Loudness Level test (MCL).

Visual Reinforcement Audiometry (VRA)

Assessment of hearing levels, usually in an infant or young child, based on any conditioned response to sound; the child's responses are reinforced by showing a lighted picture, figure, etc. A modification of the response and equipment originally used for conditioned orientation reflex audiometry.

Weber Test

Tuning fork test used to differentiate between conductive and sensorineural hearing impairments, used in cases of unilateral hearing losses. The vibrating tuning fork is placed in the middle of the skull: if the individual hears the tone in his poorer ear, a conductive impairment is indicated; if he hears the tone in his better ear, the impairment is sensorineural; if no sensitivity difference is present, the tone will be heard equally in both ears.

Auditory Tests and Procedures

DISCRIMINATION-PERCEPTION

NAME	AGE RANGE	DESCRIPTION
Auditory Analysis Test [Rosner & Simon]	Kindergarten– grade 6	Requires the repetition of a spoken word omitting specific phonemic elements
Auditory Discrimination Test [Wepman]	3–5 yr	Requires a same-different response to 40 pairs of words
Auditory Pointing Test, The [Fudala, Kunze, & Ross]	Kindergarten– grade 5	Cross-modal test in which an auditory stimulus is paired with a visual-motor response to assess short-term memory span and sequential memory
Boston University Speech Sound Discrimination Test [Pronovost & Dumbleton]	All ages	Requires a same-different response to phonetically similar monosyllabic words
California Consonant Test [Owens & Shubert]	Adults	Designed to identify discrimination problems in patients with a high-frequency hearing loss; emphasis is placed on unvoiced consonants
Carrell Discrimination Test	Children and adults	Paired sounds are presented via a recording and the subject is to give a same or different response
Carrow Auditory-Visual Abilities Test [Cavat]	4–10 yr	Measures auditory and visual perceptual, motor, and memory skills in children
Complex Speech Sound Discrimination Test [Hall]	Children and adults	Coined or artificial words are presented in a meaningful phrase; includes a study of discrimination in vowels, consonants, omissions, additions, and transpositions
Differentiation of Auditory Perception Skills (DAPS) [Reagon & Cunningham]	5–8 yr	Screening instrument designed to determine selected aspects of auditory perception; consists of five subtests: auditory cadence, auditory distinction, auditory imagery, syllable completion, and auditory reasoning
Flowers Auditory Screening Test (FAST) [Flowers]		General central auditory screening test designed to identify children with potential auditory deficits

Auditory Tests and Procedures—*Continued*

DISCRIMINATION-PERCEPTION

NAME	AGE RANGE	DESCRIPTION
Flowers-Costello Test of Central Auditory Abilities	Kindergarten–grade 6	Assesses auditory perceptual functions; tests response to low-pass-filtered speech and to competing messages
Flowers Test of Auditory Selective Attention (FTASA)	Grades 1–8	Test of auditory attention span, with emphasis on assessment of auditory vigilance
Goldman-Fristoe-Woodcock Auditory Skills Battery	3 yr–adult	Battery of tests designed for diagnostic assessment of auditory skills; includes auditory selective attention test, auditory discrimination test, auditory memory test, and sound symbol test
Goldman-Fristoe-Woodcock Test of Auditory Discrimination	3.8 yr–adult	Prerecorded test of auditory discrimination; includes quiet and competing messages subtests
Kindergarten Auditory Screening Test [Katz]	Kindergarten	Assesses listening for speech in background noise and word-pair sound discrimination
Language-Structured Auditory Retention Span Test (LARS) [Carlson]	3.7 yr–high school	Assesses and indicates level of auditory memory; two equivalent forms available
Lindamood Auditory Conceptualization Test	All ages (requires ability to judge sameness and difference, number concept to 4, and left–right progression)	Measures ability to discriminate one speech sound from another (sameness and difference) as well as the ability to perceive the number and order of sounds in sequences, both in nonsyllabic and syllabic patterns
Northwestern University Children's Perception of Speech Test (NU-CHIPS)	Children	Picture discrimination test designed to measure word-discrimination ability when the stimulus items are presented at a comfortable loudness level
Ohio Tests of Articulation and Perception of Sounds (OTAPS) [Irwin & Stevenson]	Children	Measures sound discrimination under both intrapersonal and interpersonal conditions
Pediatric Speech Intelligibility Test (PSI) [Jerger et al.]	3–6 yr	Competing message task which measures central auditory dysfunction with two formats: sentence and word

Auditory Tests and Procedures—*Continued*

DISCRIMINATION-PERCEPTION

NAME	AGE RANGE	DESCRIPTION
Phonetically Balanced Kindergarten Word Lists [Haskins]	Kindergarten	Provides a measure of auditory discrimination of phonemes under standardized conditions
Picture Sound Discrimination Test [Templin]	3–5 yr	Paired picture test which assesses speech sound discrimination
Picture Speech Discrimination Test [Mecham & Jex]	All ages	Picture-type speech sound discrimination test; pictures have been selected from the Thorndike list
Prognostic Value of Imitative and Auditory Discrimination Test [Farquhar]	Kindergarten–7 yr	Consists of two parts: subject repeats sounds, nonsense syllables, and words; subject listens to orally presented material and is required to respond "same" or "different"
Robbins Speech Sound Discrimination and Verbal Imagery Type Tests	4–8 yr	Consists of 3 parts; verbal imagery, sound discrimination, and speech sound discrimination
Schiefelbush-Lindsey Test of Sound Discrimination	Grades 1–2	Assesses three aspects of a child's speech discrimination abilities; as the child hears speech from others, as he hears himself, and as he listens silently to sounds
Screening Test for Auditory Perception [Klimmel & Wahl]	1–6 yr	Five short subtests determine the child's ability to discriminate among long vs. short vowels, single vs. blend consonants, rhyming vs. nonrhyming, and same vs. different words
Screening Test for Auditory Processing Disorders (SCAN) [Keith]	3–11 yr	A screening test for auditory processing disorders: may be used with children who seem to have poor listening skills, short auditory attention span, or difficulty understanding speech in the presence of noise
Short-Term Auditory Retrieval and Storage Test (STARS) [Flowers]	Grade 1–high school	Short-term auditory recall or memory test; uses concept of simultaneously spoken verbal material binaurally

Auditory Tests and Procedures—*Continued*

DISCRIMINATION-PERCEPTION

NAME	AGE RANGE	DESCRIPTION
Speech Sound Memory Test [Hall]	Children and adults	Provides a measure of auditory memory for speech sounds, rather than a test of discrimination
Templin Phoneme Discrimination Test	6–9 yr	Consists of oral presentation of nonsense syllables; "same" or "different" response is required
Test for Auditory Processing Disorders in Adolescents and Adults (SCAN-A) [Keith]	12–adult	Determines the presence of auditory processing disorders in adolescents and adults
Testing-Teaching Module of Auditory Discrimination (TTMAD) [Risko]	Kindergarten–grade 6	Divided into two portions: a test of auditory discrimination (TAD) and a series of 450 games and activities to increase proficiency in auditory discrimination skills
Test of Auditory-Perceptual Skills (TAPS) [Gardner]	4–12 yr	Identifies children who have auditory perceptual difficulties, imperceptions of auditory modality, and language/learning problems through various subtests: auditory discrimination, sequential memory, word memory, interpreting directions, and auditory processing
Test of Auditory Perceptual Skills—Upper Level (TAPS-UL) [Gardner]	12–18 yr	Assesses performance in a number of auditory skills
Test of Auditory Reasoning and Processing Skills (TARPS) [Gardner]	5–14 yr	Assesses the child's ability to draw conclusions, to make inferences, and to apply and use judgment based on auditory information
Test of Nonverbal Auditory Discrimination (TENVAD) [Buktenica]	6–8 yr	Identifies primary grade children who may have auditory discrimination problems; contains five subtests to assess discrimination of pitch, loudness, rhythm, duration, and timbre
Tree/Bee Test of Auditory Discrimination [Fudala]	3 yr–adult	Assesses auditory discrimination in words, phrases, pairs, comprehension, pointing to words, same-different, and letters

Auditory Tests and Procedures—*Continued*

DISCRIMINATION-PERCEPTION

NAME	AGE RANGE	DESCRIPTION
Visual Aural Digit Span Test (VADS) [Koppitz]	5.6–12 yr	Test of intersensory integration and short-term memory
W-1/W-2 Auditory Tests (Central Institute for the Deaf)	All ages	Disc recording of 36 spondaic words, randomly arranged into different versions; used for estimating a listener's threshold for speech
W-22 Auditory Test (Central Institute for the Deaf)	All ages	Disc recording of four lists of 50 monosyllabic words used for estimating a listener's auditory word discrimination; lists and words adhere to phonetic and linguistic criteria established for speech-discrimination test purposes
Washington Speech Sound Discrimination Test [Prather]	All ages	Assesses auditory discrimination
Wepman Auditory Discrimination Test	4–8 yr	Measures auditory discrimination in forty pairs of words
Wepman Auditory Memory Battery	5–8 yr	*Auditory Memory Test* measures word recall. *Auditory Sequential Memory Test* evaluates ability to repeat digits
Word Intelligibility by Picture Identification (WIPI) [Ross & Lerman]	Young children	Test utilizing pictures to obtain discrimination scores when working with young hearing-impaired children with limited vocabularies

Psychological Measures and Tests

NAME	AGE RANGE	DESCRIPTION
Arthur Adaptation of the Leiter International Performance Scale,The [Arthur]	3–7.11 yr (adult form available)	Nonverbal intelligence measure for young children; involves matching of colors, shapes, pictures, etc., and picture completion
Battelle Developmental Inventory (Svinicki)	Birth–8 yrs	Assesses developmental skills in children from birth to 8 years. Five domains are measured: (1) personal-social, (2) adaptive, (3) motor, (4) communication, (5) cognitive
Bayley Scales of Infant Development [Bayley]	2–30 mo	Designed to provide evaluation of a child's developmental status in the first $2\frac{1}{2}$ years; consists of a mental scale, motor scale, and infant behavior record
Cattell Scales [Cattell]	2–30 mo	Measures infants' and young children's abilities; designed to constitute a downward extension of Form L of the Stanford Binet Intelligence Scale
Coloured Progressive Matrices, The [Raven]	All ages	Described as a test of observation and clear thinking; consists of three sets of 12 problems arranged to assess cognitive processes; requires few verbal instructions; suggested use in conjunction with a vocabulary test
Columbia Mental Maturity Scale [Burgemeister, Blum, & Lorge]	3–12 yr	Measures general intelligence by requiring verbal responses with a minimum of motor responses required; subject selects from a series of drawings the one which is unrelated to the others
Comprehensive Test of Nonverbal Intelligence (CTONI) [Hammill, Pearson, & Wiederholt]	6.0–90.11 yr	Measures nonverbal reasoning abilities of individuals for whom most other mental ability tests are either inappropriate or biased
Culture Fair Intelligence Test [Cattell]	4 yr–adult	Set of measures of intelligence without influence of cultural background, or of scholastic or verbal training
Draw a Person [Naglieri]	5–17 yr	Measures intellectual ability based on human figure drawings

Psychological Measures and Tests—*Continued*

NAME	AGE RANGE	DESCRIPTION
Goodenough-Harris Drawing Test	5–13 yr	Study of intellectual factors as assessed from the subject's spontaneous drawing of a human figure; scale of 51 points is used to score the drawing
Hiskey-Nebraska Test of Learning Aptitude [Hiskey]	4–10 yr	Nonverbal measure of intelligence through a series of subtests involving manipulation of objects, picture completion, etc. Originally designed for deaf children, however, norms also are provided for children with hearing problems
Kaufman Assessment Battery for Children [Kaufman & Kaufman]	2.6–12.6 yr	Individually administered measure of intelligence for children; contains scales for measuring two types of mental-processing abilities: simultaneous and sequential
Kaufman Brief Intelligence Test (K-BIT)	4.0–90 yr	Measures two cognitive functions: vocabulary and matrices. The vocabulary subtest (verbal) contains expressive vocabulary and definitions. The matrices subtest (nonverbal) measures fluid thinking—the ability to solve new problems through perceiving relationships and completing analogies
McCarthy Scales of Children's Abilities [McCarthy]	2.5–8.5 yr	Assesses a variety of cognitive and motor behaviors; six scales are included: verbal, perceptual-performance, quantitative, general cognitive, memory, and motor
Minnesota Preschool Scale [Goodenough, Mauer, & Wagener]	1.6–6 yr	Assesses mental development of children; verbal, nonverbal and combined scores may be derived
Pictorial Test of Intelligence [French]	3–8 yr	Objectively scored testing instrument to be used in assessing general intellectual level of both normal and handicapped children; subjects indicate their responses to questions by pointing to pictorial symbols of their choice on large response cards

Psychological Measures and Tests—*Continued*

NAME	AGE RANGE	DESCRIPTION
Porteous Mazes	3–adult	A nonverbal test of mental ability
Slosson Intelligence Test for Children and Adults [Slosson]	1 mo–adult	Measures individual's ability to learn and to solve and understand problems; all questions, and most answers, are verbal
Stanford-Binet Intelligence Scale [revised by Terman & Merrill]	2 yr–adult	Measures general intelligence through various tasks; although some items are labeled as performance, there is heavy emphasis on verbal abilities
System of Multicultural Pluralistic Assessment (SOMPA) [Mercer]	5–11 yr	Measures cognitive, sensory, motor, and adaptive abilities; yields an estimate of the child's learning potential; provides schools and agencies with a basis for reaching educational decisions involving sociocultural differences
Test of Nonverbal Intelligence (TONI) [Brown, Sherbenou, & Dollar]	6–80 yr	Language-free measure of intelligence and reasoning
Wechsler Adult Intelligence Scale (WAIS) [Wechsler]	16–75 yr and over	Assesses general intelligence through various verbal and performance subtests; allows qualitative interpretation of results
Wechsler Intelligence Scale for Children—*Revised* (WISC-*R*) [Wechsler]	6–15 yr	Measures general intelligence through a series of five verbal and five performance subtests
Wechsler Preschool and Primary Scale of Intelligence (WPPSI) [Wechsler]	4–6 yr	Measures mental ability of young children; divided into five verbal and five performance subtests
Wide-Range Intelligence Test (WRIT) [Glutting, Adams, & Sheslow]	4.0–85.0 yr	Consists of four subtest: vocabulary, verbal analogies, matrices, and diamonds

Stuttering
Children's Referral Checklist

	NORMAL DISFLUENCIES 1.5–7 yr	MILD STUTTERING 1.5–7 yr	SEVERE STUTTERING 1.5–7 yr
Speech behavior you may see or hear:	Occasional (not more than once in every 10 sentences), brief, (typically one-half second or shorter) repetitions of sounds, syllbles or short words; e.g., li-li-like this.	Frequent (3% or more of speech), long ($\frac{1}{2}$ to 1 second) repetitions of sounds, syllables, or short words; e.g., li-li-like this. Occasional prolongations of sounds.	Very frequent (10% or more of speech), and often very long (1 second or longer) repetitions of sounds, syllables, or short words. Frequent sound prolongations and blockages.
Other behavior you may see or hear:	Occasional pauses, hesitations in speech or fillers such as "uh," "er," or "um;" changing of words or thoughts.	Repetitions and prolongations begin to be associated with eyelid closing and blinking, looking to the side, and some physical tension in and around the lips.	Similar to mild stutterers only more frequent and noticeable; some rise in pitch of voice during stuttering. Extra sounds or words used as "starters."

When problem most noticeable:	Tends to come and go when child is tired, excited, talking about complex/new topics, asking or answering questions, or talking to unresponsive listeners.	Tends to come and go in similar situations, but is more often present than absent.	Tends to be present in most speaking situations; far more consistent and non-fluctuating.
Child's reaction:	None apparent	Some show little concern, some will be frustrated and embarrassed.	Most are embarrassed and some are fearful of speaking.
Parent's reaction:	None to a great deal	Most are concerned, but concern may be minimal.	All have some degree of concern.
Referral decision:	Refer only if parents are moderately to overly concerned.	Refer if it continues for 6 to 8 weeks or if parental concern justifies it.	Refer as soon as possible.

Adapted from Stuttering Foundation of America, publication no. 24, p. 13

Diagnostic Differences

	APRAXIA	DYSARTHRIA	FUNCTIONAL ARTICULATION
Movements of tongue, lips, and palate	Normal movements, except for speech; if nonverbal apraxia is also present, only volitional oral movements will be affected; vegetative function remains normal	Movement of one or more muscle groups obviously affected; difficulty with vegetative functions as chewing and swallowing	Normal
Neurological signs	"Soft" neurological signs: difficulty with fine motor coordination, gait, and alternate movements of the extremities	Usually part of a more generalized neurological impairment, such as cerebral palsy or other neuromuscular difficulties	Normal
Speech development	Sometimes retarded, but usually within normal range	Usually some delay	Normal
Phonation	Normal	May be incoordination of phonation and articulation, or of both with respiration	Normal
Ability to imitate speech sounds	Auditory stimulus is usually insufficient; imitation should be assisted by visual stimulus and may be normal when the child is watching therapist's movements; seeing the word in print helps the older child	Normal on auditory stimulus within the limits of muscular movements	Normal

Diadochokinetic rates	Slower than normal; /p t k/ may not be accomplished in correct order	Usually slower than normal and accurate within limits of muscular movement; correct syllable order preserved	Normal
Articulation	Inconsistent errors; distortions, additions, and substitutions are variable; imitation and use of single sounds, syllables, or words is better than their use in long sequences; transpositions of sounds; vowels affected in more severe impairments	Consistent errors; consonants often omitted; substitutions determined by the group of muscles chiefly affected; vowels usually normal	Consonant substitutions usually consistent; omissions and additions are rare; vowels are normal
Error patterns	Difference in error pattern between performance in spontaneous speech and repeated speech tasks	Consistent from task to task	Consistent from task to task
Prosody	Intentional slow rate and even stress to compensate for difficulties	Rate is slow according to degree of incoordination	Normal
Groping "trial-and-error" behavior	Present in older children or in those who have received speech therapy	Absent	Absent